Recent Advances in Alzheimer Research

(*Volume 2*)

Cellular Mechanisms in Alzheimer's Disease

Edited by

Fernando A. Oliveira

*Center for Mathematics, Computing and Cognition, Federal University of ABC –
UFABC, São Bernardo do Campo, São Paulo, Brazil*

Department of Neuroscience, Carleton University, Ottawa, Canada

Recent Advances in Alzheimer Research

Volume # 2

Cellular Mechanisms in Alzheimer's Disease

Editor: Fernando A. Oliveira

ISSN (Online): 2452-2562

ISSN (Print): 2452-2554

ISBN (Online): 978-1-68108-715-3

ISBN (Print): 978-1-68108-716-0

© 2018, Bentham eBooks imprint.

Published by Bentham Science Publishers – Sharjah, UAE. All Rights Reserved.

General:

1. Any dispute or claim arising out of or in connection with this License Agreement or the Work (including non-contractual disputes or claims) will be governed by and construed in accordance with the laws of the U.A.E. as applied in the Emirate of Dubai. Each party agrees that the courts of the Emirate of Dubai shall have exclusive jurisdiction to settle any dispute or claim arising out of or in connection with this License Agreement or the Work (including non-contractual disputes or claims).
2. Your rights under this License Agreement will automatically terminate without notice and without the need for a court order if at any point you breach any terms of this License Agreement. In no event will any delay or failure by Bentham Science Publishers in enforcing your compliance with this License Agreement constitute a waiver of any of its rights.
3. You acknowledge that you have read this License Agreement, and agree to be bound by its terms and conditions. To the extent that any other terms and conditions presented on any website of Bentham Science Publishers conflict with, or are inconsistent with, the terms and conditions set out in this License Agreement, you acknowledge that the terms and conditions set out in this License Agreement shall prevail.

Bentham Science Publishers Ltd.
Executive Suite Y - 2
PO Box 7917, Saif Zone
Sharjah, U.A.E.
Email: subscriptions@benthamscience.org

**BENTHAM
SCIENCE**

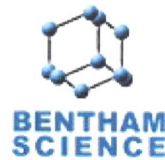

CONTENTS

FOREWORD

In 2015, according to statistics compiled by the Global Voice on Dementia produced by the Alzheimer's Disease International group, there were an estimated 46.8 million people worldwide living with dementia. Recent estimates for 2017 put this number closer to 50 million people. It is projected that this number will double every 20 years attaining 131.5 million people in 2050. In 2015, the worldwide estimated economic impact of dementia was roughly US$818 billion. While there are multiple pathological brain processes that can culminate in dementia, Alzheimer's disease (AD) accounts for 60 – 80% of all dementia cases making it imperative to understand the root causes.

In 1901, Alois Alzheimer observed a patient at the Frankfurt Asylum named Mrs. Auguste Deter. The 51-year-old patient had strange behavioral symptoms, including a loss of short-term memory. In April 1906, Mrs. Deter died and Alzheimer had the patient records and the brain sent to Munich. He identified amyloid plaques and neurofibrillary tangles which represented the first time the pathology and clinical symptoms of presenile dementia (later renamed Alzheimer's Disease; AD) were presented together.

Since that initial discovery, much has been gained with respect to the cellular pathologies indicative of AD. Accumulation of the beta-amyloid protein (β-amyloid, or A-beta [$A\beta$]) outside neurons results in the formation of amyloid plaques (protein aggregates). $A\beta$ is formed by the sequential cleavage of amyloid precursor protein (APP) by β-secretase and γ-secretase. Cleavage of APP by β-secretase and γ-secretase releases the $A\beta$ fragment and under suitable conditions (high concentration, oxidizing environment), begins to self-aggregate. $A\beta$ aggregates can induce membrane lipid peroxidation (MLP), which impairs the function of membrane ion-motive ATPases (Na^+ and Ca^{2+} pumps) and glucose transporters making neurons and synapses vulnerable to degeneration.

A second pathological feature of AD occurs when tau proteins are hyperphosphorylated causing it to dissociate from microtubules. The hyperphosphorylated tau proteins accumulate in the axoplasm and eventually aggregate into paired helical filaments, coalescing to form tangles. These insoluble aggregates, called neurofibrillary tangles (NFTs), form and destabilize microtubules ultimately disrupting axon function. As the microtubules break down, axonal transport of vesicles and other organelles to the synapse becomes disrupted, leading to impaired synaptic function.

While these pathological features have been intensively explored, there are newly discovered molecular processes at work that culminate in the neurodegenerative and behavioural features indicative of AD. This ebook presents these newly discovered molecular pathways that are at play during the neurodegenerative progression underlying AD. Developing an appropriate animal model of this human disease is of critical importance and the appropriate design of a valid animal model may be key in gaining a more complete understanding of the complexities of the disease process as well as in the development of therapeutics aimed at slowing, daresay, reversing the progression of the degeneration. This ebook also presents an update on the structural changes that are associated with AD pathology including synaptic and neural changes as well as alterations in lipid composition that may be a key mediating factor in the over-all deterioration of the brain. The final four chapters provide an update on how the emergence of plaques and tangles can lead to neurodegeneration with a focus on membrane breakdown, impaired intracellular transport, oxidative stress and calcium dysregulation.

With a clearer picture of the molecular cascades that mediate the pathological processes associated with AD, we will be in a better position to develop more effective therapeutics in staving off this ever-increasing global disease. This will not only have beneficial outcomes at the global level but also at a more personal level enhancing quality of life for the elderly and those that take care of them. This ebook aims to update our understanding of the molecular pathology of AD in hopes of providing the foundation for an effective cure.

Matthew Holahan
Department of Neuroscience
Carleton University, Ottawa
Canada

PREFACE

Alzheimer's disease (AD) is the most common cause of dementia worldwide, several groups are involved in studying the predisposition and disease development sought to understand and treat all its consequences.

AD is the product of the slow and progressive degenerative alteration that develops in the adult brain and can remain asymptomatic for a considerable time before the cognitive deficit becomes evident. The main challenge is to identify markers of this degenerative process, in this sense, data have been generated in the field bringing new mechanisms and hypothesis to explain its pathophysiology. This book intends to review the most recent studies in AD and get new perspectives to explain some aspects of this neurodegenerative disease.

The focus of this book is to discuss the cellular mechanisms in AD including well known theories and new perspectives in the main neuronal signaling pathophysiology (β-amyloid and phosphorylate tau). Current concepts on AD will be presented, bringing the more actual information about the cellular mechanisms and new views to explain the disease progress.

Fernando A. Oliveira
Center for Mathematics, Computing and Cognition
Federal University of ABC – UFABC, São Paulo
Brazil
&
Department of Neuroscience
Carleton University, Ottawa
Canada

List of Contributors

Andrea R. Vasconcelos	Pharmacology Department, Institute of Biomedical Sciences, University of São Paulo, São Paulo, Brazil
Cristoforo Scavone	Pharmacology Department, Institute of Biomedical Sciences, University of São Paulo, São Paulo, Brazil
Daniel C. Carrettiero	Center of Natural and Human Sciences, Federal University of ABC (UFABC), São Bernardo do Campo, São Paulo, Brazil
Daniel M. Silva	Center for Mathematics, Computation and Cognition, Federal University of ABC (UFABC), São Bernardo do Campo, São Paulo, Brazil
Daniela R. de Oliveira	Center for Mathematics, Computation and Cognition, Federal University of ABC (UFABC), São Bernardo do Campo, São Paulo, Brazil
Elisa M. Kawamoto	Pharmacology Department, Institute of Biomedical Sciences, University of São Paulo, São Paulo, Brazil
Fernanda L. Ribeiro	Center for Mathematics, Computation and Cognition, Federal University of ABC (UFABC), São Bernardo do Campo, São Paulo, Brazil
Fernando A. Oliveira	Center for Mathematics, Computation and Cognition, Federal University of ABC (UFABC), São Bernardo do Campo, São Paulo, Brazil
João C. dos Santos Silva	Center for Mathematics, Computation and Cognition, Federal University of ABC (UFABC), São Bernardo do Campo, São Paulo, Brazil
Laíz C. Silva-Gonçalves	Department of Biophysics, Federal University of São Paulo, São Paulo, Brazil
Luisa Ribeiro-Silva	Department of Biophysics, Federal University of São Paulo, São Paulo, Brazil
Manoel Arcisio-Miranda	Department of Biophysics, Federal University of São Paulo, São Paulo, Brazil
Marcela B. Echeverry	Center for Mathematics, Computation and Cognition, Federal University of ABC (UFABC), São Bernardo do Campo, São Paulo, Brazil
Maria C. Almeida	Center of Natural and Human Sciences, Federal University of ABC (UFABC), São Bernardo do Campo, São Paulo, Brazil
Merari F. R. Ferrari	Department of Genetics and Evolutionary Biology, Institute for Biosciences, University of Sao Paulo, Sao Paulo, Brazil
Paula F. Kinoshita	Pharmacology Department, Institute of Biomedical Sciences, University of São Paulo, São Paulo, Brazil
Rolf M. Paninka	Department of Biophysics, Federal University of São Paulo, São Paulo, Brazil
Samanta Rodrigues	Center for Mathematics, Computation and Cognition, Federal University of ABC (UFABC), São Bernardo do Campo, São Paulo, Brazil
Sonia G. Prieto	Center for Mathematics, Computation and Cognition, Federal University of ABC (UFABC), São Bernardo do Campo, São Paulo, Brazil
Tatiana L. Ferreira	Center for Mathematics, Computation and Cognition, Federal University of ABC (UFABC), São Bernardo do Campo, São Paulo, Brazil
Vitor S. Alves	Center for Mathematics, Computation and Cognition, Federal University of ABC (UFABC), São Bernardo do Campo, São Paulo, Brazil

CHAPTER 1

Differences and Implications of Animal Models for the Study of Alzheimer's Disease

Marcela Bermudez Echeverry[1,2,*], **Sonia Guerrero Prieto**[1], **João Carlos dos Santos Silva**[1], **Maria Camila Almeida**[1] and **Daniel Carneiro Carrettiero**[3]

[1] Center of Mathematics, Computation and Cognition, Federal University of ABC, São Bernardo do Campo – SP, Brazil

[2] Neuroscience Laboratory – School of Medicine, Universidad de Santander (UDES), Bucaramanga – Santander, Colombia, USA

[3] Center of Natural and Human Sciences, Federal University of ABC (UFABC), São Bernardo do Campo, São Paulo, Brazil

Abstract: In behavioural neurosciences, animal models are aimed at providing insights into normal and pathological human behaviour and its underlying neuronal processes. Alzheimer's disease (AD) is the most common origin of dementia in the elderly. Several factors have been identified, such as the amyloid precursor protein (APP), hyperphosphorylation of tau protein, and the secretase enzymes. Animal models are important for elucidation of mechanistic aspects of AD. Transgenic models recapitulate expression of human β-APP and tau hyperphosphorylation to understand the pathogenesis of AD. In this chapter, some animal models are reviewed and discussed briefly in order to elucidate some criteria that an animal model should fulfil to mimic human neurodegenerative diseases.

Keywords: Alzheimer's disease, Amyloid beta-protein, Animal models, *Octodon degu*, Transgenic models.

INTRODUCTION - ALZHEIMER'S DISEASE

The chronic or progressive dysfunction of cortical and subcortical function that results in complex cognitive decline that extends beyond normal cognitive decline, is usually described as dementia. These cognitive changes include symptoms affecting memory, impaired judgment or language, thinking, and are commonly accompanied by disturbances in social abilities that may eventually result in impairment of daily functioning, such as becoming lost at a usual path, or paying bills (Mayo Clinic on Alzheimer's Disease). Alzheimer's disease (AD),

* **Corresponding author Marcela Bermudez Echeverry:** Center for Mathematics, Computation and Cognition, Federal University of ABC, Rua Arcturus, 03, Jardim Antares, CEP 09606-070, São Bernardo do Campo – SP, Brazil; Tel +55 11 2320 6286; E-mail: marcela.echeverry@ufabc.edu.br

Fernando A. Oliveira (Ed.)

frontotemporal dementia (FTD), dementia with Lewy bodies, are usually referred as primary degenerative dementias, while secondary dementia might be the ones that occur as a consequence of another disease process [1].

Overall dementia incidence increases with age. For instance, 1.5% prevalence in patients over 65 years is described in developed countries, with the ratio doubling every 4 years reaching 30% of prevalence in patients with 80 years [2], being lower in men and in individuals of African or Asian origin [3]. Life expectancy is substantially shortened in dementia patients with 8 years of survival in average from the time of the diagnosis [4], with longer survival for women patients with AD and vascular dementia [5]. It is expected that the number of people living with dementia will double every 20 years, reaching 115.4 million by 2050 [6], being estimated that by 2050, 1 in 85 adults will be diagnosed with AD and a new case of AD is expected to develop every 33 seconds [6].

Current treatments with Acetylcholinesterase inhibitors (AChEIs) and memantine are well established in AD, but the effectiveness of the treatment varies across the population. Nevertheless, current drugs help mask the symptoms of AD, but do not treat the underlying disease or delay its progression, which makes the new developments to treat AD as an important topic. On the other hand, AChEIs use in the daily clinical routine cannot be recommended, with severe side-effects in patients with 'frontal lobe dementia' or FTD [7]. Extensive exploration of possible risk factors could give some clue, but so far no conclusive result has been obtained. Fig. (**1**) shows main risk factors identified in AD [8].

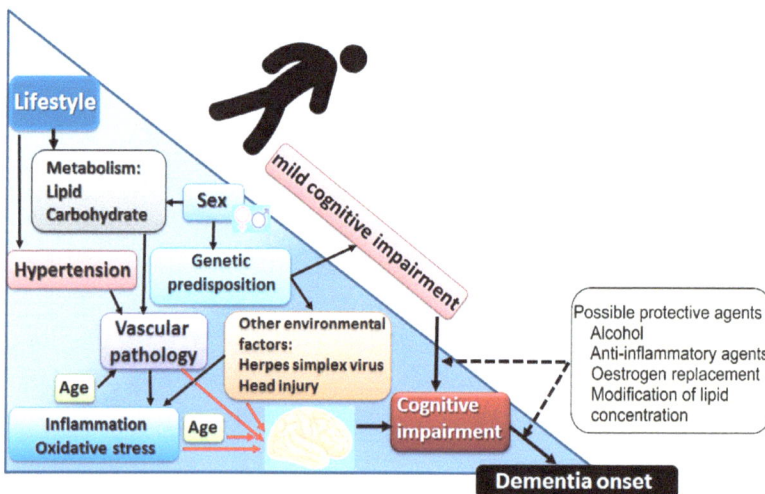

Fig. (1). Hypothetical scenarios for the onset of Alzheimer's disease (modified from [9]).

Risk Factors

• *Alcohol Use* - There is uncertainty under the effect of alcohol consumption and the incidence of dementia and cognitive decline [10]. Moderate amounts of alcohol has been shown to have a protective effect, however the risk of developing dementia may increase due to alcohol abuse [11].

• *Atherosclerosis* - It is a fairly common problem associated with aging. The stroke and reduced blood flow as a consequence of accumulation of fats, cholesterol and other substances on artery walls can also cause vascular dementia. Besides, studies have shown that conditions associated to blood vessels (vascular, stroke) may also be associated with AD [12].

• *Blood Pressure* - Both low (associated with hypometabolism) and high blood pressures have been quoted to serve as factor risk for dementia development [12, 13].

• *Depression* - Mood alterations may lead to cognitive dysfunctions and specially in men, late-life depression can be a indicative of dementia development [12, 14].

• *Diabetes* - An increased risk of developing AD and vascular dementia is associated with diabetes [12]. Furthermore, depending on their medial temporal lobe atrophy, long-term users of insulin have been shown to present significantly increased levels of plasma Amyloid β (Aβ) [15].

• *High Estrogen Levels* - Estrogen-alpha receptor is highly expressed in hippocampus, basal forebrain and cerebral cortex. Several studies have showed mechanisms underlying estrogen neuroprotection in cellular culture, consistent with a lower risk of AD described for women treated with steroid hormone estrogen compared to those who had not [16]. However, AD and depression has been shown to be affected by estrogen levels. Besides, a greater risk of developing dementia has been described for women on estrogen and progesterone replacement treatment for menopause [17]. Contradictory research findings have raised the hypothesis that there is a critical period during the perimenopause or just after menopause, in which hormonal replacement therapy could exert cognitive benefits [16].

• *Homocysteine Blood Levels* - Homocysteine, a type of aminoacid produced by the body has been described to increase the risk of developing vascular dementia [18].

• *Obesity* - The risk of developing dementia at older ages seems to be increased in obese and overweighed individuals at middle ages [19].

• *Smoking* - Both dementia and vascular diseases risk increase due to smoking [12]. A probable nicotine protected effect is with treatment delivered separately from tobacco, and activation of the alpha7 nACh receptors [20]

• *Aging* - Aging is for sure one of the major risk factor for AD. Aging is generally associated with telomere and HTERT (human telomerase reverse transcriptase). Functionally, the telomere, a sequence of DNA chains protects the end of chromosome from deterioration. Telomere length seems to be a possible cause for AD, where its shortening plays an important role in cognitive impairment, and pathogenesis of AD involved with oxidative stress and inflammation [21]. With advancing age, HTERT methylation frequency is also described to be involved in the AD pathogenesis [22] with decreased gene expression in CA1 hippocampal region [23], a neuronal population vulnerable in AD. Besides, the process of human aging also comprises an array of changes associated to metabolic state and thermal homeostasis, which has also been suggested as factors contributing to development of AD.

• *Cerebrovascular Damage* - While clinical findings between vascular dementia and AD are distinguishable, AD-associated cognitive decline can emerge after acute or chronic ischemia, hemorrhagic stroke or hypoperfusion episode, resulting in accumulative oxidative stress mediating neuronal and glial insults [24]. Thus, cerebrovascular pathology affecting the CNS could progress to a cognitive decline, taking several years to impact in the performance of cognitive functions, where the impairment of brain blood irrigation can superimposed on the mild cognitive impairment syndrome viewed as prodromal stage of AD.

• *Epigenetics* - A significant decrease of global DNA and RNA methylation have been described specifically in entorhinal cortex layer II of AD brain samples [25], and a loss of methylation control of two important genes, *BACE* and *presenelin 1*, is directly involved in AD [26]. Molecular derangements in methylation stabilizing factors were identified and associated with neurodegeneration, in special PHF1 (paired helical filaments) and PS396 immunoreactivity, both considered markers for neurofibrillary tangle formation [25, 27]. In addition, a disturbance of cell cycle events, with aberrant re-entry of neurons into the cell cycle (*e.g.* apoptosis) was also observed in AD [25].

• *Genetics* - The most prevalent form of AD, known as late-onset or sporadic AD, occurs later in life, with no evident inheritance pattern. However, a risk factor gene identified so far for sporadic AD is the apolipoprotein E (apoE), specifically ApoE4 with a ~16% prevalence in AD patients. Familial AD or early-onset AD, which is rarer (less than 1% of the total number cases), usually starts at age 30-60, is an autosomal dominant mutation with three genes identified: *APP, presenilin 1*

(PSEN1) and *presenilin 2* (PSEN2).

AD involves severe neuropathological changes in the hippocampus, followed by the association cortices and subcortical structures, including the amygdala and nucleus basalis of Meynert [20] (Fig. **2**).

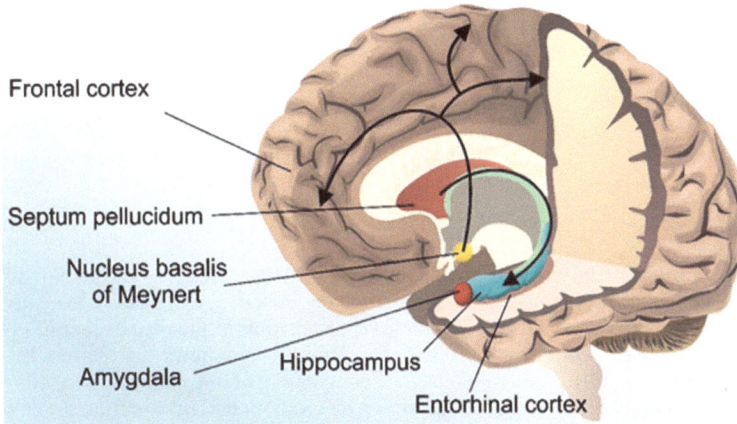

Fig. (2). The nucleus basalis of Meynert innervates the entire cerebral mantle with prominent afferents to limbic areas such as the hippocampus, entorhinal cortex and amygdala.

Synapse loss and massive neuronal cell death are characteristics of the AD brain, as well as Aβ (also known as Abeta) plaques and neurofibrillary lesions. The neurofibrillary lesions, also described as neurofibrillary tangles (NFTs) are characterized by hyperphosphorylated aggregates of the microtubule-associated protein tau (Fig. **3A**) and can be found in cell bodies and apical and distal dendrites, as well as in the abnormal neurites that are associated with some Aβ plaques [20, 28]. A*β* peptides are typically ~ 4kDa β-pleated sheet peptides with different N- and C-terminal endings that are derived from amyloid precursor protein (APP). β-secretase cleaves the APP, *via* the endosomal-lysosomal pathway to generate the amino terminus of A*β* [29]. *γ*-secretase further process the peptide at positions 40, 42, and 43 to generate the A*β* peptide [30] (Fig. **3C**). Different N-terminally truncated A*β* has been detected in post-mortem AD brain tissue [31].

Neuropathological diagnosis is confirmed by the presence of neurofibrillary tangles and neuropil threads [36]. The propagation of the disease can be classified into six different stages depending on the location of the tangle-bearing neurons and the severity of changes (transentorhinal stages I-II: clinically silent cases; limbic stages III-IV: incipient Alzheimer's disease; neocortical stages V-VI: fully developed Alzheimer's disease) (Fig. **4**).

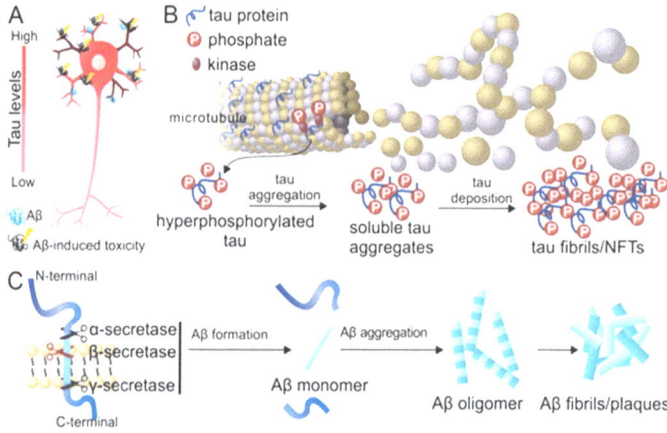

Fig. (3). Hallmarks of AD and pathological features. (**A**) Hyperphosphorylated tau dissociates from microtubule (MT)-associated protein tau, causing them to depolymerize, while tau is deposited in aggregates such as neurofibrillary tangles (NFTs). (**B**) Graphical representation of the distribution of high and low tau levels, associated with NFTs (intra-neuronal), and Aβ. This picture shows the relation between amyloid plaques and Tau-pathology. (**C**) The major protein component of the plaques is a 40–42 amino acid polypeptide termed Aβ (Aβ40 and Aβ42), that is derived by proteolytic cleavage from the amyloid precursor protein, APP. B-Secretase activity has been attributed to a single protein, BACE, whereas γ-Secretase activity depends on four molecules, presenilin, nicastrin, anterior pharynx-defective 1 (APH1) and presenilin enhancer 2 (PEN2). γ-Secretase dictates its length, with Aβ40 being the more common and Aβ42 the more fibrillogenic and neurotoxic species (modified from Götz and Ittner, 2008 [32]). On the other hands, cognitive decline in humans is not proportional to Aβ plaque load [33, 34], but does correlate with soluble Aβ species [33, 35].

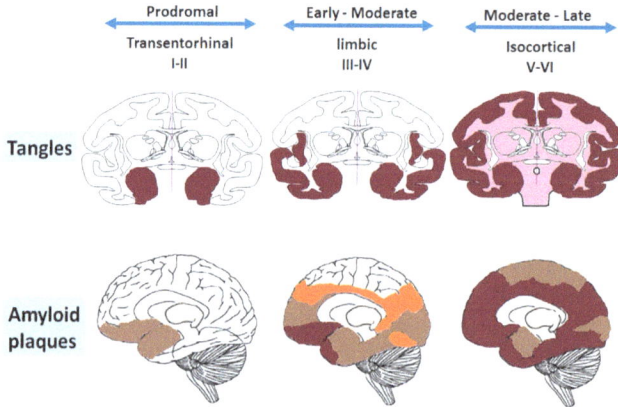

Fig. (4). Temporospatial spreading of tau-positive neurofibrillary lesions (tangles) in the process of AD and Amyloid plaques-positive lesions. According to the study [37], stages I–II refers to alterations mainly confined to the upper layers of the transentorhinal cortex (transentorhinal stages). Stages III–IV presents a severe involvement of the transentorhinal and entorhinal regions, with a less severe involvement of the hippocampus and several subcortical nuclei (limbic stages). Stages V–VI presents a massive development of neurofibrillary pathology in neocortical association areas (isocortical stages), and a further increase in pathology in the brain regions affected during stages I–IV. The red areas are proportional to the severity of tau pathology (modified from [37]).

ANIMALS MODELS OF AD – DIFFERENCES AND IMPLICATIONS

"An animal model with biological and/or clinical relevance in the behavioral neurosciences is a living organism used to study brain–behavior relations under controlled conditions, with the final goal to gain insight into, and to enable predictions about, these relations in humans and/or a species other than the one studied, or in the same species under conditions different from those under which the study was performed" cited in [38].

The most thoughtful challenges faced by medical research can be at least partially solved with the help of the tools like animal models. Indeed in dementia research, animal models have become crucial tools [28]. The following definitions found on the web emphasize two important attributes of a model: the open-source platform Wikipedia states that an animal model is *"a non-human animal that has a disease or injury that is similar to a human condition"* [39]. This definition illustrates that models are valuable as they represent a certain stage of disease and because processes that lead to that stage can be monitored longitudinally. In AD research, animal models have been useful in dissecting the pathogenic mechanisms of the pathology, as well as preclinical drug development. Yet, AD includes several aspects that still require a better biochemical and molecular characterization, and therefore it is imperative to develop tools in order to facilitate translational research.

In the web, Research models (http://www.alzforum.org/research-models) contain information about various animal models of Alzheimer's disease (see http://www.alzforum.org/res/com/tra) with causative genes as well as other proteins involved in the pathogenic process.

Invertebrate Models

Different animal models have been used to study neurodegenerative diseases. The majority genes of AD are evolutionarily conserved in simple organisms such as Drosophila and *C. elegans*, allowing the manipulation of orthologous genes and pathways *in vivo* to better understand of pathogenesis of AD and others disorders.

Caenorhabditis Elegans

It is estimate that at least 83% of the nematode *C. elegans* (*Caenorhabditis elegans*, Fig. **5**) proteome have human orthologous proteins [40], being an important model to study aging, protein aggregation (proteotoxicity) and other issues. For instance, similarity between the nematode and mammalian aging includes muscle atrophy and lipofuscin accumulation [41].

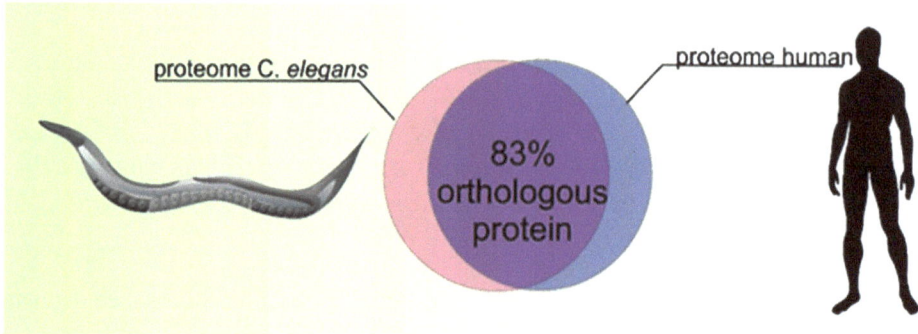

Fig. (5). Image of *C. elegans* adult hermaphrodite.

Other charactheristics of the nematode that are considered an advantage in biological research includes high fertility, a short life span and low cost maintenance. On the other hand, the worm does not present the complex behavior and cognitive responses that can be evaluated in vertebrates or mammalian models. Nevertheless, the nematode is considered a good model for the study of molecular pathways in neurodegenerative disease.

In *C. elegans,* the apl-1, is orthologous to the human APP involved in AD. However, it does not produce the Aβ peptides because it lacks the cleavage by β-secretase [42]. On the other hand, in the transgenic model of *C. elegans* expressing human- Aβ, accumulation of Aβ3-42 peptide [43] and Aβ1-42 [43] lead to progressive paralysis in the worm [44]. In addition, it has been found three presenilin genesin *C. elegans*: sel-12, hop-1 and spe-4. The sel-12 and hop-1 mutation results in memory deficits and morphological alterations in cholinergic interneurons [45].

Although complex behaviors are not possible to assess in *C. elegans,* motor behavior can be tested by three simple analyses: 1) "Chemotaxis", which corresponds to the movement of crawling in the presence of food stimuli. 2) "Trashing" or the swimming that the nematode exhibit in a liquid medium. 3) "Pharyngeal pumping", which is the muscular contraction as a result of food ingestion [46]. In addition to motor behavior, simple cognitive functions such as memory and learning are easily assessed in the *C. elegans* model, by looking at the negative olfactory associative conditioning or long-term associative memory [47] (Fig. **6**).

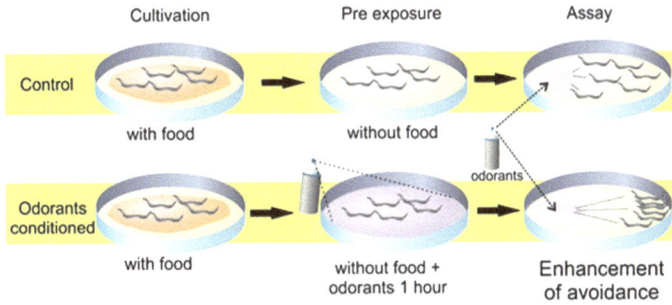

Fig. (6). The enhancement of avoidance behavior after the exposure to odorants in *C. elegans* (modified from experimental design [48]).

Drosophila

Genetic research has been using the fruit fly (*Drosophila melanogaster*) for more than hundred years. It was the first organism with fully sequenced genome [49]. The Drosophila is able to provide important insights into for experimental studies of multicellular organisms in genetic, anatomic and behavior fields [50]. The anatomical organization of the Drosophila brain (proto, deuto, and tritocerebrum) is homologous with the human brain, which is divided into forebrain, midbrain and hindbrain [51].

The main advantage of Drosophila is the possibility of gene manipulation. Besides, the short lifespan, with average of 120 days depending of stress or others stimulus, also makes this model an interesting one [50] (Fig. **7**). The range of possible behaviors possible to study in Drosophila includes olfactory learning, grooming, courtship, aggression, circadian rhythms and locomotor behavior [48].

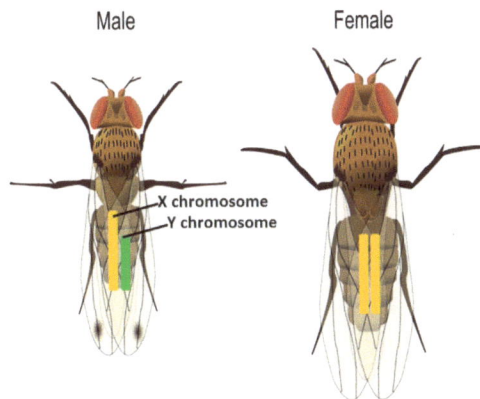

Fig. (7). Drosophila melanogaster with brick-red eyes and transverse black rings across the abdomen. Males are slightly smaller than female with darker backs and easily distinguished from females based on a distinct black patch at the abdomen [52].

About 70% of human genes responsible for diseases in humans are conserved in the Drosophila, including the orthologue of the human APP protein, the *Appl*, which is mainly localized in the cortical region of the fly´s brain [53] (Fig. **8**). An orthologue of the α-secretase, the *kuzbanian* gene, the homologous of BACE, the *dBACE*, and the functional orthologue of TAU, the *dtau* have also been described [43]. Additionally, the fruit fly also presented the ɣ-secretase complex.

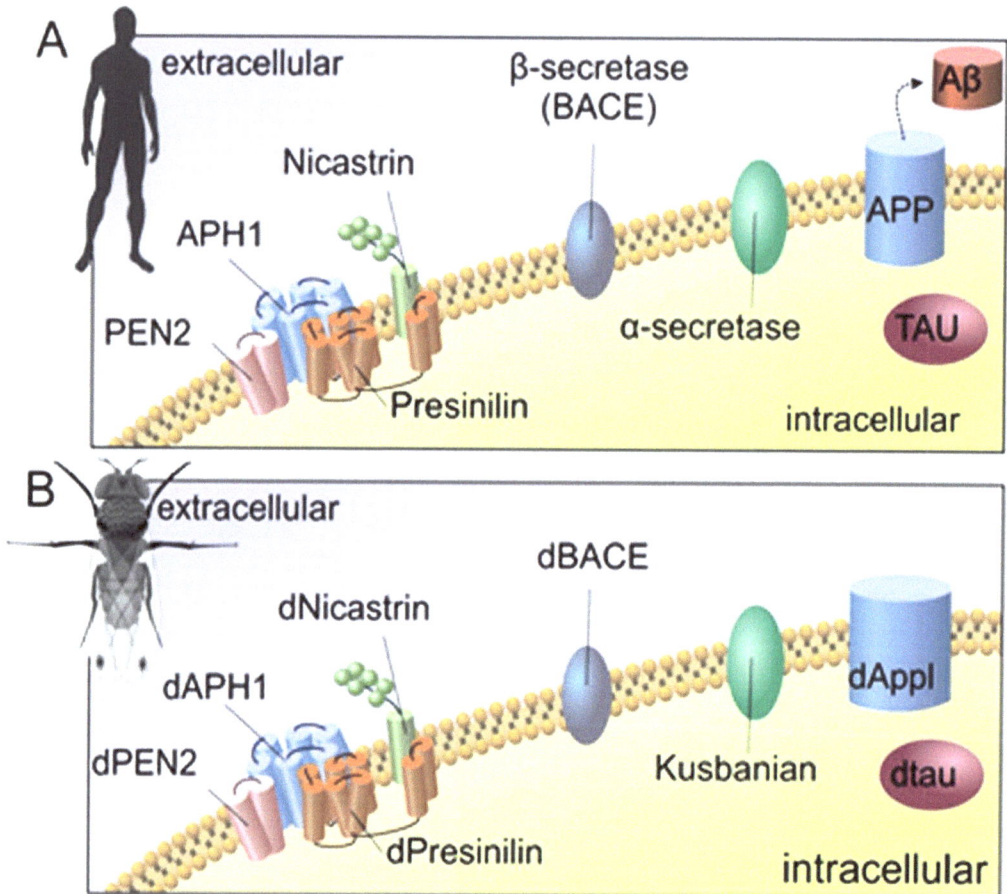

Fig. (8). Schematic illustration of proteins in human (A) and orthologous in drosophila (B) correlated with AD (modified from [54]).

The drosophila APP orthologous, *Appl*, have similar domains with the APP of vertebrate organisms, by deleting the Appl gene in the drosophila, researchers have found flies viable, fertile, and morphologically normal, yet they exhibit subtle behavioral deficits [54]. Furthermore, the overexpression of the β-secretase protein responsible for the cleavage of *Appl*, results in Aβ-like fragment aggregates leading to toxicity and neurodegeneration [55].

In a triple transgenic Drosophila model, combining expression of human APP (hAPP), human β-secretase (hBACE) and Drosophila γ-secretase presenilin (dPsn) [56, 57], it was observed Aβ40 and Aβ42 aggregation and the formation of plaques. These flies presented age-dependent neurodegenerative processes such as degenerated axons projections and increased in early fatality rate [58]. Similarly, the Aβ Drosophila transgenic, also presented accumulation of Aβ40 and Aβ42 peptides in the fly brain [59]. It has also been reported that the co-expression of presenilin mutants, APP and BACE accelerated the accumulation process of neurotoxic Aβ aggregates in [57].

In addition, studies assessing the mitochondrial loss in the axon resulting from the aberrant phosphorylation of the Tau are also available. Knockdown model has been used to study the Miro and Milton proteins which regulate mitochondrial attachment to microtubules in fruit fly (Fig. **9**), showing that mitochondrial loss produced by Milton increases Tau phosphorylation and enhances neurode-generation regulated by Tau [60, 61].

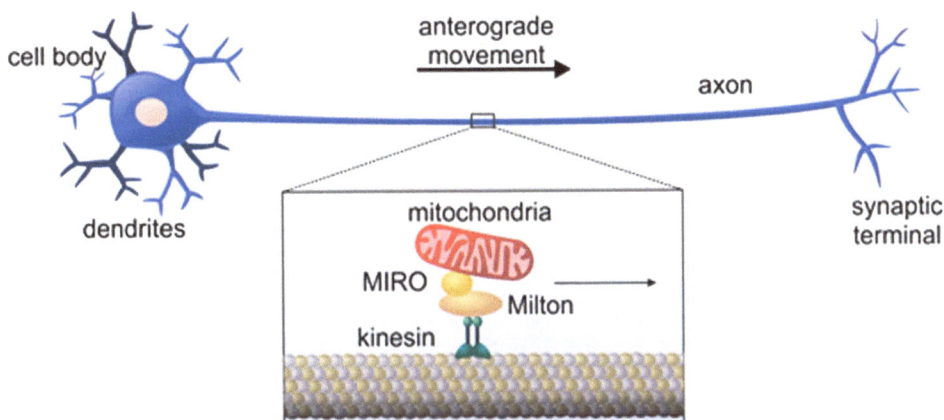

Fig. (9). Schematic representation of the protein complex that mediates anterograde mitochondrial movement. Miro is anchored to the outer membrane. The association of Milton with the mitochondrion is caused, at least in part, by the interaction of Milton and Miro (modified from [62]).

Different behavioral tests can be performed in the Drosophila model. Motor behavior is evaluated using the geotaxis response assay test [57] or climbing assay [63]. These tests allow evaluating the oriented movement toward a gravitational force (Fig. **10A**). The principal differences between the two tests are the number of tubes in the apparatus and analyzed results. Another test is the Pavlovian olfactory associative learning [60] (Fig. **10B**). The flies are trained with electroshock paired with one odor and after are exposed to a second odor without shock. Subsequently, the learning is measure allowing that flies choose between the two odors. The courtship behavior can also be analyzed [64] by checking the orientation, tapping, wing extension, courtship song, licking and copulation (Fig. **10C**).

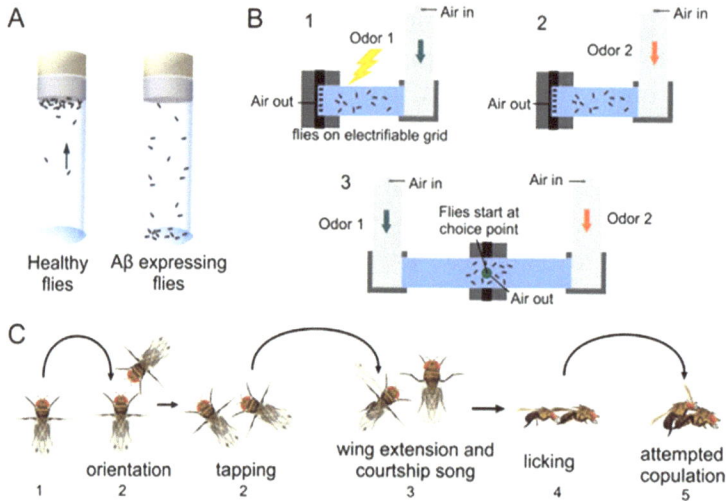

Fig. (10). Possible behavioral tests in Drosophila. (**A**) Oriented movement toward a gravitational force. The flies that express Aβ cannot fly against gravity force. (**B**) Pavlovian olfactory associative learning. (**B1**) The flies are exposed to electroshock and odor, and after are tested with other odor without electroshock stimuli. (**B2**) The drosophila chooses the preferential odor. (**C**). Courtship behavior is evaluate by looking at features such as orientation, tapping, wing extension, courtship song, licking and attempted copulation (modified from experimental design [55]).

Vertebrate Models

Rodents are the dominant model for the study of AD, but non-mammalian organisms also have been used to investigate neurodegenerative diseases. One example is the zebra fish.

Zebrafish

The zebrafish has the genome fully characterized, and is described to share 50- 80% homologous genes with human sequence [43]. The rapid development, large productivity capacity, easy and cheap maintenance are some of the major advantages of this model besides the facility to introduce genetic changes and the easiness to observe the changes. Although this model has lower cognitive behavior than rodent model, the zebrafish shows conditioned responses, memory and social behavior. In addition, their transparent embryos enable the manipulation of genes and proteins, allowing observing the embryogenesis and development of central nervous system (CNS) (Fig. **11**).

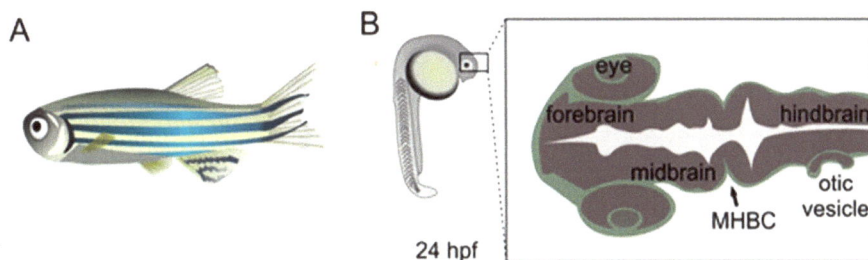

Fig. (11). Zebrafish, an animal model using in research. Twenty-four hours post fertilization (hpf), CNS of zebrafish embryo was stained with laminin antibody which outlines the neural tube in green and counterstained with propidium iodide to label the nuclei in red. MHBC: midbrain-hindbrain boundary constriction (modified from [65, 66] and https://www.nc3rs.org.uk/news/five-reasons-why-zebrafish--ake-excellent-research-models).

The Zebrafish orthologous genes to human known involved in the AD are shown in Table **1**. The appa and appb have differential expression patterns in the embryonic period with the appb mRNA found in telencephalon, midbrain, hindbrain, spinal cord and dorsal aorta [67]. On the other hand, the appa expression is observed in telencephalon, ventral diencephalon, terminal ganglia, lens, otic vesicles and somites [68].

Table 1. Zebrafish orthologues genes involved in AD (modified [43].

Human	Zebrafish orthologue
Mutations in FAD	
Amyloid Precursor Protein (APP)	*appa - appb*
Presenilin 1 (PSEN1)	*psen1*
Presenilin 2 (PSEN2)	*psen2*
Associated with risk for AD	*mapta - maptb*
Microtubule-Associated Protein Tau (MAPT)	
Apolipoprotein E (APOE)	*apoea- apoeb*
Clusterin (CLU)	*Clu*
Phosphatidylinositol Binding Clathrin Assembly Protein (PICALM)	*picalm*
Complement Component (3b/4b) Receptor 1 (CR1)	*Unknown*
Associated with γ-secretase complex members	
Presenilin Enhancer 2 (PSENEN), Nicastrin (NCT)and Anterior Pharynx Defective 1 Homolog B (APH1b)	*psenen, ncstn and aph 1b*
Beta-secretase: BACE1 and BACE2	*bace 1 and bace 2*

One experimental approach used to induce the aggregation of Aβ in the Zebrafish is the hindbrain injection of Aβ-42 peptide in embryos. The Aβ injection results in specific cognitive deficits and increased of tau phosphorylation by GSK-3β [68]. However, no neurofibrillary tangles neither apoptosis markers are found, suggesting that this model can be used to study the early stage of AD, as it presents similar molecular markers found in human. Additional, in the literature there are studies showing that application of Aβ in the eyes of the zebrafish, results in blood vessel branching, suggesting that the Aβ have physiological effects in capillary density [69].

Transgenic zebrafish has been used for study the mechanism of the AD and other neurodegenerative diseases. The expression of green fluorescent protein (GFP) from appb promoter was found in the CNS and vascular tissue in zebrafish during development stages and also in the adult [67], suggesting that this model might elucidate the mechanism in APP gene expression in AD. The overexpression of the GPF with the γ-glutamylhydrolase (γGH) has been used as a tool to study the hypotheses of oxidative stress in the AD. The folate deficit can induce aggregation Aβ and phosphorylated Tau [70], suggesting a pathological mechanism that connect the Aβ and Tau pathways.

The transgenic human protein TAU-P301L in zebrafish neurons provided an important model, as it resulted in a fast neurodegeneration [71]. Moreover, GSK3β inhibitors treatment reduced the hyperphosphorylation of Tau in this transgenic zebrafish, providing an insight on a tool for the pharmacological assessment.

The presenilin 1 and 2 have been studied in zebrafish model by inhibiting translation of psen1 and psen2 mRNA through injection of antisense oligonucleotides. The inhibition of psen1 resulted in somitogenesis defect [72]; while inhibition of psen2 revealed an important role of this gene in the signaling and embryo development [73], and programmed death cell.

Knockdown is also possible in Zebrafish. In the literature, this technique allowed to demonstrate that appb is necessary for the axonal growth in motor neurons and cytoskeletal of embryos [74].

Regarding behavioral tests possible with the Zebrafish model, the object recognition memory is widely used [75]. To evaluate object preference, the zebrafish is acclimated to the environment and exposed to two identical objects at first and then to a different object, and, finally is exposed to a familiar and a novel object (Fig. 12).

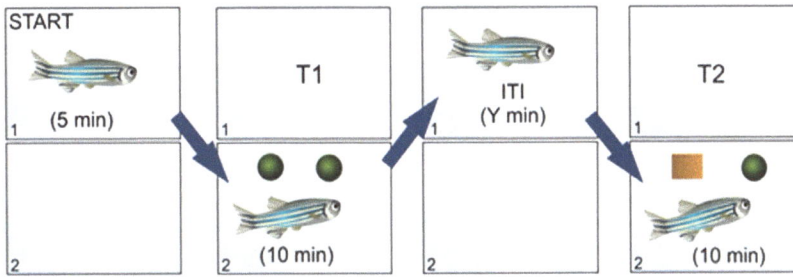

Fig. (12). Novel object preference test in Zebrafish. Test Object recognition memory. The first step is the acclimatization (5 min) in an identical experimental environmental. After, the fish is exposing to two identical objects for 10 min. During the inter-trial, the zebrafish is put back to the initial tank, and finally, put in the experimental tank for 10 min while exposed to a familiar and a novel object (modified from experimental design [75]

Another cognitive function that can be evaluated in zebrafish model is avoidance response [68]. This test consists of a visual stimulus (for example a ball) travelling in the half of tank (stimulus area) (**Fig. 13**). The number of fishes that are found in the non-stimulus area is considered that have cognitive avoidance ability. The locomotor activity can be evaluated in the zebra fish model through the exploration of new an environment (**Fig. 13**). The total distance travel, speed, time of mobile and absolute turn angle are possible parameters to be analyzed in this test [68, 76].

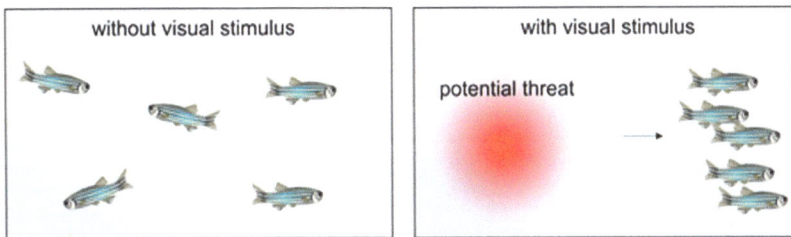

Fig. (13). Escape and avoidance behavior in zebrafish. Avoidance: a potential threat is anticipated by zebrafish that swim away to safety, by swimming to a protected area, diving to the bottom of the tank or joining a shoal of fish. Once the fish relax, they start to explore their surroundings. This way, quantitative data can be obtained for escape, avoidance, and exploratory behaviors (modified from experimental design [68])

Rodent Models

The whole aspects of the disease spectrum cannot be recapitulated by a single model. Nevertheless, each model are suitable for in-depth analysis of one or two components of the disease, which is not readily possible or ethical with human patients or samples [34].

Not only the cholinergic, beta-amyloid, and tau theories but also a genetic basis accounts for the multifactorial and complex molecular mechanisms of AD as well as the different symptomatology processes activation among human population which will progress into divergent neuropathological characteristics underlying behavior and cognitive changes [77]. Genetic models have still been invaluable in determining the molecular mechanisms of familial AD (fAD) and molecular events similar with idiopathic or sporadic form of AD.

Study of AD Risk Factors in Rodents

The autosomal-dominant early-onset familial AD are a consequence of mutations that occur in the presenilin 1 (14q24.3), presenilin 2 (1q31-q42), and Aβ A4 precursor protein (APP; 21q21.3) [78], which results in premature onset for the production of soluble 40 or 42 amino acid Aβ peptide. Besides, inheritance of apolipoprotein E epsilon 4 (ApoE4; 19q13.2) allele constitutes a major genetic risk factor (Fig. **14**) for developing Early Onset AD as well as late-onset AD predisposition and hypercholesterolaemia. Even though this feature is not sufficient to cause the disease by itself [77], together with other factors such as by acting in synergy with other susceptible genes, for example, programmed cell death protein 4 (PDCD4) and in a complex interaction with environmental factors, could lead to disease development [79].

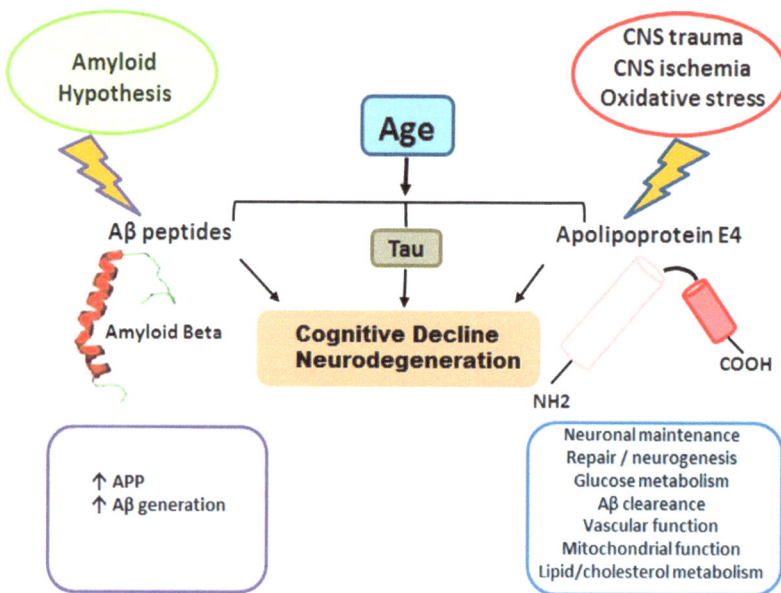

Fig. (14). Apolipoprotein E4 (ApoE4) and interaction with Aβ peptide to cause cognitive decline and neurodegeneration, as well converge on the amyloid. Also, ApoE4 can show a complex interaction with environmental factors (modified from [80]).

In transgenic mice and *in vitro*, the ApoE4 could be involved in cholesterol transport hindrance (Fig. **15**), diminished neuronal repair, Aβ deposition, fibrillisation, and plaque formation by acting as an Aβ interacting pathological chaperone [81, 82]. ApoE mRNA is found in cortical and hippocampal neurons in humans [83] and in transgenic mice expressing human ApoE under the control of the human ApoE promoter [84].

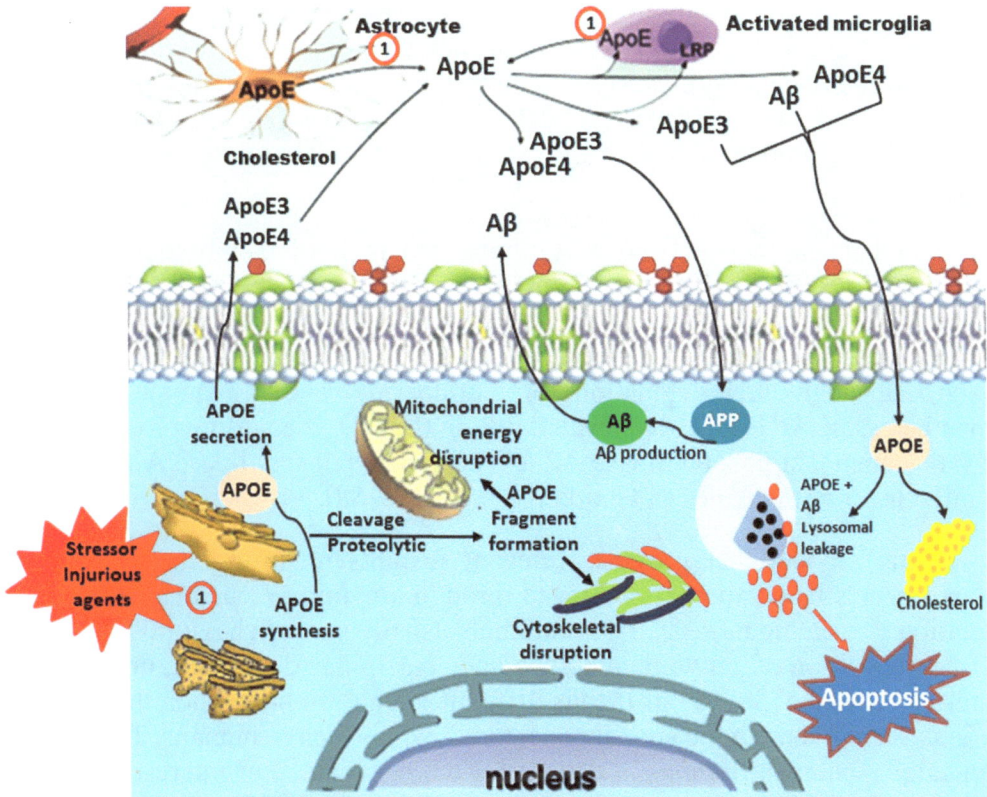

Fig. (15). ApoE isoforms in the CNS. ApoE is synthesized by astrocytes, activated microglia, and neurons express apoE under physiological and pathological conditions. Roles for apoE4: (1) enhanced Aβ production, (2) potentiation of Aβ1-42-induced lysosomal leakage and apoptosis, and (3) enhanced neuron-specific proteolysis resulting in translocation of neurotoxic apoE4 fragments in the cytosol, where they are associated with cytoskeletal disruption and mitochondrial dysfunction. Once produced APOE by astrocytes, or activated microglia or under pathological insults, neurotoxic effects are thought to be downstream of APOE 3 – APOE4-mediated toxicity (modified from [80]).

In the human and animal brain, staining using Thioflavin S but especially Congo red is the gold standard for diagnosing amyloid plaques because it only binds aggregated β- Sheets [34].

A simultaneous occurrence of hypocholinergic tone and Aβ accumulation in which Aβ and apolipoprotein E epsilon 4 (ApoE4) could interact with alpha7 nicotinic receptors leading to the repression of glycogen synthase 3β and downstream effects towards tau protein hyperphosphorylation has been hypothesized [76, 85]. Indeed, the first theory proposed to explain the etiology of AD was the cholinergic depletion hypothesis. This theory was founded on the studies showing that memory impairment, due to loss in cholinergic transmission, could be reversed following treatment of mild-to-moderate patients with cholinergic receptor agonist (*e.g.*, nicotinic acetylcholine receptors and muscarinic acetylcholine receptors), acetylcholinesterase inhibitors (*e.g.*, galantamine, donepezil, and rivastigmine), acetylcholine precursors (*e.g.*, L-alpha glyceryl-phosphorylcholine), and cholinergic enzymes (*e.g.*, choline acetyltransferase) [76, 86, 87].

Enzymes such as phospholipase A2, involved in lipid membrane metabolism connecting the cholinergic and glutamatergic systems could play a role in cognitive decline and neurodegenerative process in AD. Indeed, inhibition of phospholipase A2 both Ca^{+2} dependent but also independent can lead to formation of Aβ through downregulation of cholinergic and glutamate receptors. Nonetheless, if Aβ is already elevated during the AD, it could favor upregulation of Ca^{2+}-dependent phospholipase A2 and secretory phospholipase A2 implicated in inflammatory cytokines and oxidative stress [76, 88].

A "partial" model that provides relevant insights regarding the pathological related events listed above is achieved through amyloid precursor protein (APP) mutation transgenic models. Those animals usually show behavioral impairment before deposition of amyloid, and even once an Aβ has developed, neuronal loss tends to be minor [88, 89]. It is thus difficult to analyze how much the cognitive deficits seen in these mice are equivalent to the ones seen in humans. Thus, from a clinical perspective, findings in the animal models may be of interest in terms of understanding brain function but are of dubious significance in terms of understanding a specific human disease. Nonetheless, the partial nature of the model may also be a tool for furthering understanding of the elements important in disease.

In particular, in rodent models, APP, tau hyperphosphorylation, and the secretase enzymes, have become the pivotal point of current investigation. Several transgenic and non-transgenic animal models have been developed to clarify the mechanistic aspects of AD and to validate potential therapeutic targets.

The Rat Model

The rat has also been used as a model for AD pathogenesis. In particular, the effects of cortical Aβ accumulation on the cholinergic, noradrenergic and serotoninergic systems were extensively studied using rats [90, 91]. The AD-like brain insulin signaling impairment in rats are studied using the intracerebral injection of streptozotocin- icv (STZ) [90, 92]. These animals display reduced choline acetyltransferase activity [93], with high levels of oxidative stress and nitrative stress [94], astrogliosis, several inflammatory processes, and axonal neurotoxicity [95], changes in brain insulin signaling and alterations in Aβ homeostasis and higher levels of hyperphosphorylated Tau [96], as well as cognitive impairments as featured by deficits in learning, memory and cognitive behavior [96]. This model can represent sporadic AD.

Cerebral microinjection of a vehicle containing oligomers and Aβ monomers but not amyloid fibrils are commonly also used as a rat model for AD studies, as those injections have been shown to inhibited hippocampal long-term potentiation (LTP) in rats [97].

The Rabbit Model

Rabbits have become useful for modelling AD when validating the neuroprotective effects of metal chelators [98]. Adding copper to a group of cholesterol-fed rabbits can induce amyloid deposition and cognitive impairment, with Aβ aggregation related to redox activity of metals such as copper [99].

The role of Aluminum (Al) linked to AD remains controversial and the hypothesis has been abandoned by researchers. Previously, in 1965, Wisniewski, Terry, and Klatzo demonstrated the formation of NFTs after brain injection of Al into rabbits [100]. Al^{3+} administration also has been described to influence oligomerization and promotes conformational changes in Aβ, suggesting an effect on amyloid cascade [101]. Nevertheless, it was verified that excessive oral intake of Al does not accelerate AD pathophysiology in transgenic mouse for Aβ and tau phosphorylation accumulation (AβPP and AβPP/tau transgenic mice) [102], as such, in other AβPP mice model, Tg2576 mice, the start of plaques deposited at 9 months of age was also not modified after administration Al *via* diet from 6 to 9 months of age [103]. Thus, Al is associated with dialysis encephalopathy that differs from AD in presentation, clinical progression, and time course [104]. Yet, despite this clinical picture difference, Al is considered neurotoxic compound and it can induce decreased expression of neurofilament [105], neprilysin [106] and altered expression of β-APP secretase (BACE1 and BACE2) [107].

Transgenic AD models have been generated to investigate FAD mutation, thus the phenotype of transgenic strain, promoter used and the background mouse strain are very important points to consider when choosing a transgenic models to study AD clinical symptoms [33]. In Table **2** and Fig. **16**, a summary with the most used transgenic mouse models.

Transgenic Mice

The discovery that tau dysfunction and Aβ accumulation is the essential events leading to neurodegeneration in AD have led to the development of transgenic animal models. Most transgenic rodent models are based on the over-expression of three mutated genes: (i) amyloid precursor protein (APP) and/or (ii) Presenilins (PS1 and 2) and/or (iii) tau hyperphosphorylation and formation of NFTs (MAPT – microtubule-associated protein tau).

Götz & Ittner [32] had shown a schematic representation to study AD and FTD (Fig. **16**). FTD appear between the ages of 40 and 65, usually does not include formation of amyloid plaques, exhibit impolite and socially inappropriate behavior and is linked to a mutation in the tau gene FTDP-17, N279K, ΔK280, P301L, P301S, V337 and R406W [32]. Consistent with patients expressing early onset of FTD, P301S, where mouse prion protein (PrP) was used, it shows higher neuronal loss than in P301L tau transgenic mice, with changes prominent in brain areas and ventricular enlargement, as observed in patients with FTD [108].

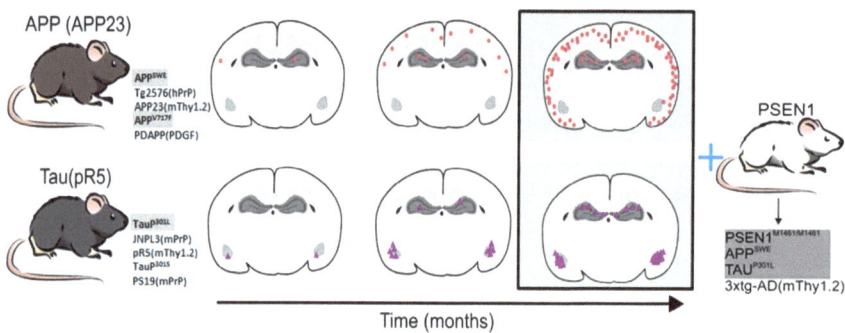

Fig. (16). Expression of plaques and NFTs in transgenic mice. Mutations are listed (grey boxes) together with their strain names and the promoters (in parenthesis) that were used for expression. Here, progression of the pathology in pR5 mice showed NFT formation in the amygdala and eventually found in the hippocampus, but the cortex is virtually spared. In APP23 mice, plaque formation is protuberant in the cortex and in the hippocampus. FTD, usually does not include formation of amyloid plaques and *tau* transgenic mice are used. This reflects, to some extent, the situation in the brain of patients with AD, in which plaques and NFTs are anatomically separated (modified from [32]).

The most commonly used transgenic mice in AD to study different neuro-pathological changes are challenged to behavioral test to assess hippocampus-dependent memory functions. Since AD is a neuropathology accompanied by cognitive failure, behavioral tests are critical requirements with well-established hippocampal-dependent learning and memory assessment correlates with biological mechanisms like resources for drugs discovery.

Overexpression of the Amyloid Precursor Protein (APP)

PDAPP mouse is generated from platelet derived growth factor-β (PDGF) promoter plus APP, which results in an 18-fold elevation of APP RNA and age-dependent amyloid deposition, with dystrophic neurites and reactive astrocytes. Aβ42 immunotherapy studies in young PDAPP mouse, resulted in amyloid pathology reduction in older mice, with ameliorated memory deficits [109]. However clinical trials of the same immunotherapy resulted in meningoencephalitis development in some individuals, even though a reduction in Aβ plaques and astrogliosis was observed in some areas of cortex [110].

Like PDAPP mice, the Tg2576 mice, the most widely transgenic model used, express a 5-fold increase in human APP levels in cortical and limbic structures, with spatial memory impaired in 9- to 10- month-old mice [111]. This transgenic express increased Aβ40 and Aβ42 more or less proportionately.

After PDAPP and Tg2576 mice many other transgenic lines were developed with difference in region and temporal profile of plaque deposition. TgCRND8 mice expressing multiple APP mutations, exhibits amyloid deposition at 3 month of age. APP23 mice is used because the Thy-1 promoter results in prominent vascular amyloid deposition. Similarly, Tg2576 mice also show huge vascular amyloid plaques, whereas this feature is absent in PDAPP mice [112].

Other difference among APP transgenic is the genetic background. PDAPP mice have been maintained on a mixed C57BL6/DBA/Swiss-Webster background, whereas, Tg2576 mice are studied on a hybrid C57BL6/SJL background [113].

Presenilin Mutations Transgenic

Mutations in PS1 is the most recognized cause of early-onset FAD, with ~160 mutations already described. PS1 has a locus on chromosome 14, and PS2 on chromosome 1. There is more PS1FAD than PS2 FAD mutant transgenic lines. PS1 FAD has been generated with the same promoters used for PDGF and PrP (APP transgenic mice). Although PS FAD mutant shows increase in Aβ42, single transgenic PS1 or PS2 mice do not develop plaques. However, PS when crossed with APP lines, mutations cause earlier and widespread plaque formation. The PS1/APP mice are frequently used. Besides, PS1 or PS2 FAD mutant lines shown excessive neuronal loss in the entorhinal cortex, with impaired hippocampal neurogenesis, age-related neurodegenerative changes [114, 115]. Combined mutations of 3 APP and PS1 FAD created a 5X FAD mutant mouse with neuronal loss sufficient to cause AD similar to humans [116].

Tau Models and Aβ–tau Association

As aforementioned NFTs containing hyperphosphorylated forms of tau can be studied with thioflavin-S and Congo red histological dyes, and they are recognized by specific antibodies. Although, phosphorylated tau accumulates within dystrophic neurites in PDAPP mice, these alterations cannot be recognized by histological dyes as in humans [117]. Then, the first crossed transgenic line known as JPNL3 to develop NFT-like lesions, expresses the P301L mutation (transgenic line that reproduce aggregation and NFT-formation in mice [118, 119], associated with FTDP-17, and Tg2576 mice. A triple transgenic model, 3xTg-AD, was generated (2 transgenes containing APP-Swedish and P301L FTDP-17 mutations), where mice had increased Aβ40 and Aβ42 levels, accumulated intraneuronal Aβ, amyloid plaques and NFT-like lesions [120]. In addition, in 3xTg-AD mice, amyloid plaques preceded tau pathology evident until about 1 year of age, with altered synaptic dysfunction and deficits in spatial memory [120]. A reduced Aβ accumulation is described in this animal model after anti-Aβ antibodies applied intra-hippocampal, with clearance of early-stage tau pathology [121].

Yet, modelling Aβ–tau association, NFTs formation can be aggravated by intracerebral injection of $Aβ_{42}$ form in the P301L tau transgenic pR5 model, or by crossing APP23 and JNPL3 transgenic mice [122]. These processes could be mediated by GSK3β (tau kinase glycogen synthase kinase 3β), which is also involved in APP processing [123]. For ApoE models, the ABCA1, a protein that removes cholesterol and phospholipids from cells, has been proposed, and studies showed significant reduced Aβ levels and plaque burden, when an overexpression of ABCA1 in PDAPP mice was induced [124].

Non-transgenic Mammalian Animal

Chicken Embryo

The chicken neuronal cultures are a useful model for studies at the cellular level where access to human neuronal tissue is unavailable [130]. The chicken embryo, during prenatal development, contains BACE-1, BACE-, PS1 and PS2, niastrin, and neprilysin, which is required for the degradation and clearance of the Aβ peptide [131]. But, a critical question is if adult-aged chicken has assembly machineries related to pathological lesions in AD. So far, one study showed no significantly difference in old chicken [132].

Table 2. Transgenic mice and pathology (modified from [26, 113]).

Line	Promoter	Pathology	Cognitive Impairment described
APP23	Murine *Thy1*	- Neuropathology Plaques: Yes - P-tau: Yes - NFT: no [125]	Yes
PSAPP mice	Hamster *PrP,* *PDGFβ*	- Neuropathology Plaques: Yes - P-tau: Yes - NFT: not reported [126]	Yes
TgCRND8 mice	Syrian hamster *PrP*	- Neuropathology Plaques: Yes - P-tau: not reported - NFT: no [127]	Yes
pR5 mice Promoter driven P301L	Murine *Thy1*	- Neuropathology Plaques: no - P-tau: Yes - NFT: Yes [128]	not reported
3xTg-AD	*Murine Thy1* (PS1 knockin)	- Neuropathology Plaques: Yes - P-tau: Yes - NFT: Yes [121	not reported
Tg2576 mice	Hamster *PrP*	- Neuropathology Plaques: Yes - P-tau: Yes - NFT: no [122]	Yes
Triple transgenic Mice Tg2576		- Neuropathology Plaques: Yes. Aβ deposits Mutant PS1, PS2, and ApoE Senile plaques - P-tau: Yes - NFT: Yes [123]	Yes
PDAPP mice	*PDGFβ*	- Neuropathology Plaques: Yes - P-tau: Yes - NFT: no [129]	Yes
TAPP mice	Hamster *PrP,* Murine *PrP*	- Neuropathology Plaques: Yes - P-tau: Yes - NFT: Yes [130]	not reported

Primates

Although the production and handling of transgenic mice is relatively easy, fundamental differences between rodents and humans cannot be ignored. Thus, it becomes important then that nonhuman primates share many structural and functional features with humans, such as longer average life spans. Interestingly, the most challenging questions about longevity, as well as the complexity of brain networks or social intelligence can practically only be examined in nonhuman primates. In this sense, the importance of nonhumans primates models resides no only on the opportunity to better understand the pathophysiology of aging unique to primates, but also for testing intervention strategies to improve healthy and avoid or counteract cognitive decline and neurodegenerative diseases [133, 134].

Indeed, comparative studies on the evolution of aging in mammalian brain has shown that only a small subset of age-related genes are conserved from mouse to human, rhesus macaques shows a similarity of up to 80% of genes detected in the human prefrontal cortex [135, 136]

Despite their biological closeness to humans, AD has never been described in nonhuman primate species [137, 138], although the age-associated neuro-degeneration in primates is associated with brain atrophy, amyloid plaques, tau pathology and a loss of cholinergic neurons [139]. The frequency of amyloid pathology in 695-Aβ peptide (APP$_{695}$) in macaque monkey characterizes an animal model to study human neurodegenerative diseases [140]. In aged monkeys [141] and aged rhesus monkeys [142], contrary to humans, Aβ40 and Aβ42 are present in senile plaques, suggesting that primates exhibit differences in amyloid processing and deposition during the aging process. Hence, nonhuman primates are a good model of brain aging and Aβ-amyloidosis, even in the absence of neurodegenerative disease. These the incomplete manifestation of AD-like changes in simians may indicate the unique susceptibility of the human brain to AD [137, 138].

In addition, in aged chimpanzee, the hippocampus was described to be obviously free of tauopathy and neuronal loss, and the NFTs were described mainly in cortical neurons [143]. On the other hand, apolipoprotein E and complement factors C1q and C3c in macaques are homologous to the isoforms identified in human AD [144]. Interestingly, a study showed that all nonhuman primates tested to date were homozygous for ApoE4 according to the human nomenclature. However, an amino acid substitution at position 61 distinguishes simian ApoE from human ApoE, causing nonhuman primate ApoE4 to interact with lipoproteins similarly to ApoE3 in humans [145].

Dogs

Due to an elaborate social life being closely associated with humans, dogs are commonly used for cognitive and behavioral studies [146]. Several APP processing genes, such as ApoE and presenilin detectable in the humans are also presented in dogs, that also share the amino acid sequence of Aβ42 with humans [147]. Cortex and hippocampus are the two first brain regions that presents deposition of Aβ in dogs [148], and dense neuritic plaques and neurofibrillary tangles are observed [149]. The Aβ plaques are formed as a result of endogenous/exogenous factors, but do not occur in all aged dogs, suggesting individual vulnerability [150].

Tau Phosphorylation in Hibernating Mammals

Studies on hibernating animals, including the arctic ground squirrel (*Spermaphilus parryii*), Syrian hamsters (*Mesocricetus auratus*) and black bears (*Ursus americanus*), has revealed a temperature-dependent phosphorylation of tau, with more intense phospho-tau levels reported in torpid animals compared to euthermic animals [151]. Temperaure-induced tau hyperphosphorylation has been described to be influenced by tau kinase glycogen synthase kinase 3 beta (GSK3-beta) cyclin-dependent kinase 5 (cdk5), stress activated protein kinase/Jun-amin--terminal kinase (SAPK/JNK) and mitogen-activated protein kinases/extracellular regulated protein kinase (MAPK/ERK) in these species [151]. Although this pattern of tau phosphorylation in hibernating animals is completely reversible after arousal, hibernating animals revealed of great importance to study the pathways regulating tau phosphorylation, and may play a vital role to test new therapeutics for the treatment of AD, especially those related to tau phosphorylation and formation of NFTs [90].

Natural Model - Octodon Degus

In recent years, a rodent endogenous to Chile, the *Octodon degus* (O. degus - Sciurus degus) (Fig. **17**) has gained importance as a valuable model for many different diseases, including those related with neurodegeneration. This rodent seems to naturally develop several symptoms that can be linked to a similar number of pathological conditions (Fig. **18**).

Several characteristics of *Octodon degus* (Fig. **19** and **20**) makes is an interesting model for the study of several pathologies, including preclinical research of Aβ accumulation [153], cataracts [155], hormone dysregulation [156], and tau tangles [93, 157] (Fig. **19**). This rodent has been shown [153], in its natural environment, to spontaneously (after 34 months of age) produce plaques in different brain areas, including extracellular (all cortical layers) and intracellular (second and the third cortical layers) frontal cortex, and dorsal hippocampus, neuropathological hallmarks of AD.

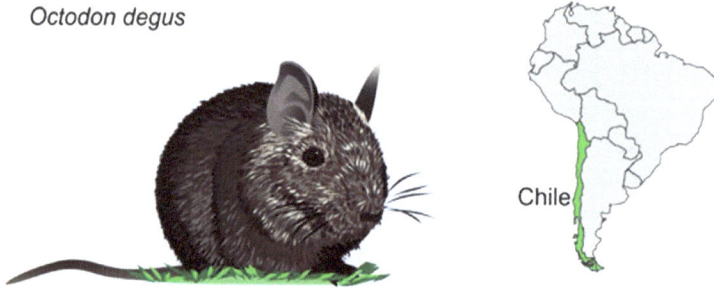

Fig. (17). *Octodon degus* inhabits the lower slopes of the Andes [152]. It is often used in laboratory studies outside of its native range, for example, neurodegeneration pathological conditions [153].

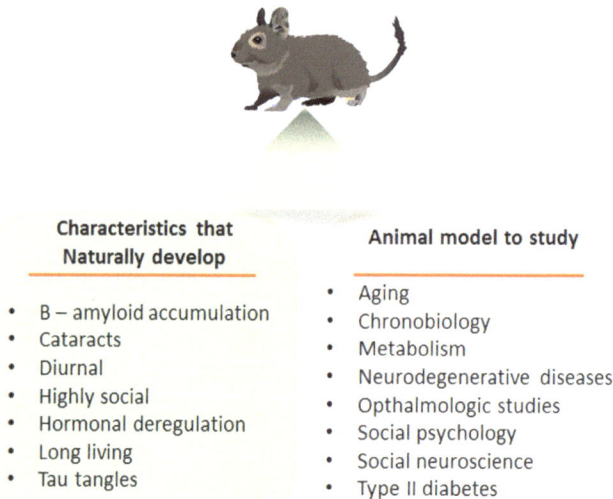

Fig. (18). several characteristics that naturally develop in the *Octodon degus*. A good animal model to study several physiologic, psychologic, and pathological conditions (modified from [154]).

Moreover, both immunohistochemical and genetic analyses performed on the *Octodon degus* exposed a high degree of similarity between human deposits and the APP, with the Aβ peptide sequence being highly homologous to human´s (97.5%). Only a single amino acid substitution with respect to the human is found in the *Octodon degus*, representing a greater advantage when compared to other models (Fig. **19**). Another advantage is that overexpression of human APP are not necessary in this model to generate significant levels of amyloid protein.

Exon 17-18

Mice/Rat   D A E F G H D S G F - E V R H Q K L V F F A - E D V G S N K G A I - ...

Human   D A E F R H D S G Y - E V H H Q K L V F F A - E D V G S N K G A I - ...

O. degus   D A E F R H D S G Y - E V R H Q K L V F F A - E D V G S N K G A I - ...

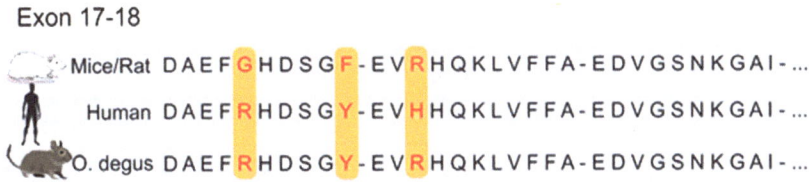

Fig. (19). Differences and similarities between mice/rat, human, and *Octodon degus* amino acid Aβ sequence [144] (modified from [154]).

The cerebral cortex of adult *Octodon degus* is rich in cholinergic neurons, which are known to be lost during progression of AD. Cortex and hippocampus of aged *Octodon degus* also show intense astrogliosis [90] as well as memory impairment with age [158]. *Octodon degus* may be considered the first wild-type rodent model for the study of AD pathology [153] (Fig. **20**), being then, an interesting tool that might allow researchers to dramatically widen the range of experimental manipulation [159].

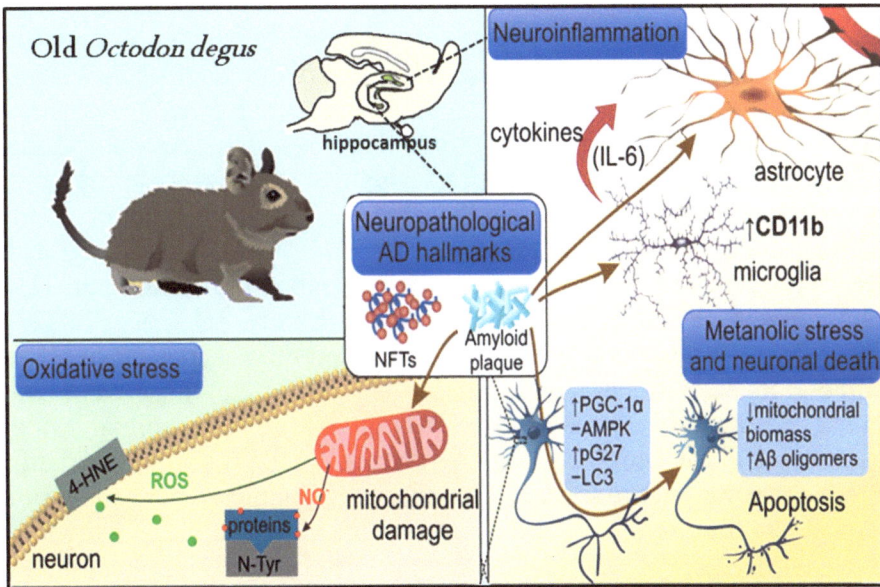

Fig. (20). In this diagram, Inestrosa *et al.* 2015 [160] summarize the mechanisms that are responsible for the neuropathological lesions previously described in his studies [153]. Briefly, neuroinflamation, after amyloid plaques and neurofibrillary tangles production, can active glial cells. Interleukin 6 mediate the cross talk between glial and microglial cells. Reactive oxygen species induced by mitochondrial damage can enhance the formation of 4-hydroxynonenal and nitrotyrosine. Finally, metabolic stress and neuronal death increase in peroxisome proliferative-activated receptor γ coactivator-1α and possible p62 might protect against the neuronal damage and in parallel, it shows the apoptotic hallmarks of AD (condensed nuclei and activation of the caspase pathway) (modified from [160]).

CONCLUSION

- Animal models developed in species ranging from worms to rodents will continue to be essential for accessing AD-type pathology *in vivo*, specifically genetic modifications underlying pathophysiology and the disease course. Transgenic models have allowed reproducing many critical aspects of the AD. Although there is no single model that recapitulates the complete disease process, and their analogy to human cognition is not completely accurate, animal models are essential as they allow for testing of therapeutic strategies that are impractical or unethical in humans.

- Although there is no such a perfect model, some animal models are suitable for its capacity to reproduce both pathophysiological conditions and behavioral outcomes. Several studies have demonstrated that Alzheimer´s pathology markers are absent in wild-type rodents, which lead to the development of transgenic animals overexpressing human APP, harboring familial AD mutations or to perform intracerebral injections of Aβ aggregates and other drugs (such as STZ) to achieve homologous states of the disease.

- Nonetheless, *Octodom degus* may be considered as the first natural rodent model for the study of AD pathology, especially because it presents two of the major histopathological markers for this disorder (A*β* plaques and NFTs containing hyperphosphorylated tau).

- For further directions, workshops about Translation of Animal Models for Nervous System Disorders discuss promising successes that can be built upon (http://www.ncbi.nlm.nih.gov/books/NBK158937/). In neuroscience there is translational success of animal models in six areas of research: Alzheimer's disease, neurodegeneration, stroke, addiction, schizophrenia, and pain. Usually, groups focused their discussions on three key questions: (i) Would this research area benefit from a new or improved standardized animal model? (ii) How well do animal model and human clinical endpoints correlate in this area of research? (iii) What is needed to bridge the translational gap between animal models and clinical science in this area? Conversely, there is a need for more standardization of models reflecting neurodegenerative disease in patients, with main points of discussion: (a) the scientific approach to neurodegeneration research (*e.g.*, target-centric *versus* systems-based) may need to be updated; (b) animal model studies might be replaced with more Phase 0 clinical trials in humans.; (c) there is a need for pharmacodynamic markers and biomarkers that clearly reflect the disease.

- Finally, the Table **3** shows an outlook of the characteristics and disadvantages of different models to study AD.

Table 3. Characteristics and disadvantages of some invertebrate and vertebrate models used in AD research [110, 120, 152].

CHARACTERISTICS	DISADVANTAGES
Drosophila	
Genetic modifications with genes overexpressed for NFT and neurodegeneration (huTau and GSK-3 homolog), axonal transport phenotype (APPL or huAPP), neuronal apoptosis (huAPP).	Difficult to produce neuropathology plaques, P-tau, NFTs and neuronal loss in unique model
C. elegans	
Genetic modifications with genes overexpressed for neurodegeneration synaptic and behavioral (huTau), paralysis (Aβ in bodywall). High fertility, low costly to maintenance, short life span, easily available techniques for genetic manipulation	Difficult to produce neuropathology plaques, P-tau, NFTs and neuronal loss in unique model
Chicken embryo	
Chicken embryo contains molecules to clearance of the Aβ peptide	In adult-aged chicken could be more difficult to identify these molecules
Murine	
Triple transgenic: Aβ deposits Mutant PS1, PS2, and ApoE senile plaques; with P-tau and NFTs formation	Difficulty of producing neuronal loss. Neuronal loss can only be induced by the combination of multiple mutations different to humans
Octodon degus	
A good animal model to study several physiologic, psychologic, and pathological conditions. Aβ only a single amino acid substitution with respect to the human.	Inhabits the lower slopes of the Andes and degus need a little more care. Non-transgenic
Dogs	
Commonly used for cognitive and behavioral studies. ApoE and presenilin detectable like in human	Aβ plaques do not occur in all aged dogs
Primates	
Share features with humans and longer average life spans. ApoE similar to human	AD has never been described. Senile plaques with Aβ40 and Aβ42, even in the absence of neurodegenerative disease. Hippocampus free of taupathy

CONSENT FOR PUBLICATION

Not applicable.

CONFLICT OF INTERESTS

The authors declare no conflict of interests.

ACKNOWLEDGEMENT

Declared none.

REFERENCES

[1]   Pérez-Trallero E, Cilla G, Urbieta M. Rubella immunisation of men: advantages of herd immunity. Lancet 1996; 348(9024): 413.
[http://dx.doi.org/10.1016/S0140-6736(05)65039-8] [PMID: 8709765]

[2]   Ritchie K, Kildea D. Is senile dementia "age-related" or "ageing-related"? evidence from meta-analysis of dementia prevalence in the oldest old. Lancet 1995; 346(8980): 931-4.
[http://dx.doi.org/10.1016/S0140-6736(95)91556-7] [PMID: 7564727]

[3]   Zhang Y, Marcillat O, Giulivi C, Ernster L, Davies KJ. The oxidative inactivation of mitochondrial electron transport chain components and ATPase. J Biol Chem 1990; 265(27): 16330-6.
[PMID: 2168888]

[4]   Fitzpatrick AL, Kuller LH, Lopez OL, Kawas CH, Jagust W. Survival following dementia onset: Alzheimer's disease and vascular dementia. J Neurol Sci 2005; 229-230: 43-9.
[http://dx.doi.org/10.1016/j.jns.2004.11.022] [PMID: 15760618]

[5]   World Health Organization. Dementia: a public health priority. Alzheimer's Disease International 2012.

[6]   Brookmeyer R, Johnson E, Ziegler-Graham K, Arrighi HM. Forecasting the global burden of Alzheimer's disease. Alzheimers Dement 2007; 3(3): 186-91.
[http://dx.doi.org/10.1016/j.jalz.2007.04.381] [PMID: 19595937]

[7]   J.L. C, S. A-E. Evidence for psychotropic effects of acetylcholinesterase inhibitors. CNS Drugs 2000; 13(6): 385-95.
[http://dx.doi.org/10.2165/00023210-200013060-00001]

[8]   Ilomaki J, Jokanovic N, Tan EC, Lonnroos E. Alcohol Consumption, Dementia and Cognitive Decline: An Overview of Systematic Reviews. Curr Clin Pharmacol 2015; 10(3): 204-12.
[http://dx.doi.org/10.2174/1574884710031508201455339] [PMID: 26338173]

[9]   Ritchie K, Lovestone S. The dementias. Lancet 2002; 360(9347): 1759-66.
[http://dx.doi.org/10.1016/S0140-6736(02)11667-9] [PMID: 12480441]

[10]   Ilomaki J, Jokanovic N, Tan EC, Lonnroos E. Alcohol consumption, dementia and cognitive decline: an overview of systematic reviews. Curr Clin Pharmacol 2015; 10(3): 204-12.
[http://dx.doi.org/10.2174/1574884710031508201455339] [PMID: 26338173]

[11]   Handing EP, Andel R, Kadlecova P, Gatz M, Pedersen NL. Midlife alcohol consumption and risk of dementia over 43 years of follow-Uup: a population-based study from the swedish twin registry. J Gerontol - Ser A Biol Sci Med Sci 2014; 70(10): 1248-54.

[12]   Xu W, Tan L, Wang H-F, *et al.* Meta-analysis of modifiable risk factors for Alzheimer's disease. J Neurol Neurosurg Psychiatry 2015; 86(12): 1299-306.
[PMID: 26294005]

[13]   Landin K, Blennow K, Wallin A, Gottfries C-G. Low blood pressure and blood glucose levels in Alzheimer's disease. Evidence for a hypometabolic disorder? J Intern Med 1993; 233(4): 357-63. [http://dx.doi.org/10.1111/j.1365-2796.1993.tb00684.x] [PMID: 8463769]

[14]   Zhao Q-F, Tan L, Wang H-F, *et al.* The prevalence of neuropsychiatric symptoms in Alzheimer's disease: Systematic review and meta-analysis. J Affect Disord 2016; 190: 264-71. [http://dx.doi.org/10.1016/j.jad.2015.09.069] [PMID: 26540080]

[15]   Blasko I, Kemmler G, Krampla W, *et al.* Plasma amyloid beta protein 42 in non-demented persons aged 75 years: effects of concomitant medication and medial temporal lobe atrophy. Neurobiol Aging 2005; 26(8): 1135-43. [http://dx.doi.org/10.1016/j.neurobiolaging.2005.03.006] [PMID: 15917096]

[16]   Janicki SC, Schupf N. Hormonal influences on cognition ans risk for alzheimer disease. Curr Neurol Neurosci 2010; 5(10): 359-66. [http://dx.doi.org/10.1007/s11910-010-0122-6]

[17]   Zhang S, Shi C, Mao C, *et al.* Plasma homocysteine, vitamin B12 and folate levels in multiple system atrophy: A case-control study. PLoS One 2015; 10(8): e0136468. [http://dx.doi.org/10.1371/journal.pone.0136468] [PMID: 26291976]

[18]   Ishii M, Iadecola C. Adipocyte-derived factors in age-related dementia and their contribution to vascular and Alzheimer pathology. Biochim Biophys Acta 2015. [PMID: 26546479]

[19]   Arnold SE, Hyman BT, Flory J, Damasio AR, Van Hoesen GW, Van Hoesen GW. The topographical and neuroanatomical distribution of neurofibrillary tangles and neuritic plaques in the cerebral cortex of patients with Alzheimer's disease. Cereb Cortex 1991; 1(1): 103-16. [http://dx.doi.org/10.1093/cercor/1.1.103] [PMID: 1822725]

[20]   Glenner GG, Wong CW. Alzheimer's disease: initial report of the purification and characterization of a novel cerebrovascular amyloid protein. Biochem Biophys Res Commun 1984; 120(3): 885-90. [http://dx.doi.org/10.1016/S0006-291X(84)80190-4] [PMID: 6375662]

[21]   Cai Z, Yan L-J, Ratka A. Telomere shortening and Alzheimer's disease. Neuromolecular Med 2013; 15(1): 25-48. [http://dx.doi.org/10.1007/s12017-012-8207-9] [PMID: 23161153]

[22]   Silva PNO, Gigek CO, Leal MF, *et al.* Promoter methylation analysis of SIRT3, SMARCA5, HTERT and CDH1 genes in aging and Alzheimer's disease. J Alzheimers Dis 2008; 13(2): 173-6. [http://dx.doi.org/10.3233/JAD-2008-13207] [PMID: 18376059]

[23]   Franco S, Blasco MA, Siedlak SL, *et al.* Telomeres and telomerase in Alzheimer's disease: epiphenomena or a new focus for therapeutic strategy? Alzheimers Dement 2006; 2(3): 164-8. [http://dx.doi.org/10.1016/j.jalz.2006.03.001] [PMID: 19595878]

[24]   Marlatt MW, Lucassen PJ, Perry G, Smith MA, Zhu X. Alzheimer's disease: cerebrovascular dysfunction, oxidative stress, and advanced clinical therapies. J Alzheimers Dis 2008; 15(2): 199-210. [http://dx.doi.org/10.3233/JAD-2008-15206] [PMID: 18953109]

[25]   Mastroeni D, Grover A, Delvaux E, Whiteside C, Coleman PD, Rogers J. Epigenetic changes in Alzheimer's disease: decrements in DNA methylation. Neurobiol Aging 2010; 31(12): 2025-37. [Internet]. [http://dx.doi.org/10.1016/j.neurobiolaging.2008.12.005] [PMID: 19117641]

[26]   Scarpa S, Fuso A, D'Anselmi F, Cavallaro RA. Presenilin 1 gene silencing by S-adenosylmethionine: a treatment for Alzheimer disease? FEBS Lett 2003; 541(1-3): 145-8. [http://dx.doi.org/10.1016/S0014-5793(03)00277-1] [PMID: 12706835]

[27]   Augustinack JC, Schneider A, Mandelkow EM, Hyman BT. Specific tau phosphorylation sites correlate with severity of neuronal cytopathology in Alzheimer's disease. Acta Neuropathol 2002; 103(1): 26-35.

[http://dx.doi.org/10.1007/s004010100423] [PMID: 11837744]

[28]   Götz J, Götz NN. Animal models for Alzheimer's disease and frontotemporal dementia: a perspective. ASN Neuro 2009; 1(4): 251-64.
[http://dx.doi.org/10.1042/AN20090042] [PMID: 19839939]

[29]   Masters CL, Multhaup G, Simms G, Pottgiesser J, Martins RN, Beyreuther K. Neuronal origin of a cerebral amyloid: neurofibrillary tangles of Alzheimer's disease contain the same protein as the amyloid of plaque cores and blood vessels. EMBO J 1985; 4(11): 2757-63.
[PMID: 4065091]

[30]   Vassar R, Bennett BD, Babu-Khan S, *et al.* Beta-secretase cleavage of Alzheimer's amyloid precursor protein by the transmembrane aspartic protease BACE. Science 1999; 286(5440): 735-41.
[http://dx.doi.org/10.1126/science.286.5440.735] [PMID: 10531052]

[31]   Härtig W, Goldhammer S, Bauer U, *et al.* Concomitant detection of β-amyloid peptides with N-terminal truncation and different C-terminal endings in cortical plaques from cases with Alzheimer's disease, senile monkeys and triple transgenic mice. J Chem Neuroanat 2010; 40(1): 82-92.
[http://dx.doi.org/10.1016/j.jchemneu.2010.03.006] [PMID: 20347032]

[32]   Götz J, Ittner LM. Animal models of Alzheimer's disease and frontotemporal dementia. Nat Rev Neurosci 2008; 9(7): 532-44.
[http://dx.doi.org/10.1038/nrn2420] [PMID: 18568014]

[33]   Terry RD, Masliah E, Salmon DP, *et al.* Physical basis of cognitive alterations in Alzheimer's disease: synapse loss is the major correlate of cognitive impairment. Ann Neurol 1991; 30(4): 572-80.
[http://dx.doi.org/10.1002/ana.410300410] [PMID: 1789684]

[34]   LaFerla FM, Green KN. Animal models of Alzheimer disease. Cold Spring Harb Perspect Med 2012; 2(11): 1-14.
[http://dx.doi.org/10.1101/cshperspect.a006320] [PMID: 23002015]

[35]   Wang J, Dickson DW, Trojanowski JQ, Lee VM. The levels of soluble *versus* insoluble brain Abeta distinguish Alzheimer's disease from normal and pathologic aging. Exp Neurol 1999; 158(2): 328-37.
[http://dx.doi.org/10.1006/exnr.1999.7085] [PMID: 10415140]

[36]   Braak H, Braak E. Evolution of neuronal changes in the course of Alzheimer's disease. J Neural Transm Suppl 1998; 53: 127-40.
[http://dx.doi.org/10.1007/978-3-7091-6467-9_11] [PMID: 9700651]

[37]   Braak H, Braak E. Staging of Alzheimer's disease-related neurofibrillary changes. Neurobiol Aging 1995; 16(3): 271-8.
[http://dx.doi.org/10.1016/0197-4580(95)00021-6] [PMID: 7566337]

[38]   van der Staay FJ. Animal models of behavioral dysfunctions: basic concepts and classifications, and an evaluation strategy. Brain Res Brain Res Rev 2006; 52(1): 131-59.
[http://dx.doi.org/10.1016/j.brainresrev.2006.01.006] [PMID: 16529820]

[39]   Model organism Wikipedia 2015 June; 1-13.

[40]   Lai CH, Chou CY, Ch'ang LY, Liu CS, Lin W. Identification of novel human genes evolutionarily conserved in *Caenorhabditis elegans* by comparative proteomics. Genome Res 2000; 10(5): 703-13.
[http://dx.doi.org/10.1101/gr.10.5.703] [PMID: 10810093]

[41]   Klass MR. Aging in the nematode *Caenorhabditis elegans*: major biological and environmental factors influencing life span. Mech Ageing Dev 1977; 6(6): 413-29.
[http://dx.doi.org/10.1016/0047-6374(77)90043-4] [PMID: 926867]

[42]   Wentzell J, Kretzschmar D. Alzheimer's disease and tauopathy studies in flies and worms. Neurobiol Dis 2010; 40(1): 21-8.
[http://dx.doi.org/10.1016/j.nbd.2010.03.007] [PMID: 20302939]

[43]   Saraceno C, Musardo S, Marcello E, Pelucchi S, Di Luca M. Modeling Alzheimer's disease: from past

to future 2013.
[http://dx.doi.org/10.3389/fphar.2013.00077]

[44] Ehud C, Jan B, Rhonda P, Jeffery K, Andrew D. Opposing Activities Protect Against Age-Onset Proteotoxicity. Science (80-) 2006; 313(1): 1-5.

[45] Calahorro F, Ruiz-Rubio M. *Caenorhabditis elegans* as an experimental tool for the study of complex neurological diseases: Parkinson's disease, Alzheimer's disease and autism spectrum disorder. Invert Neurosci 2011; 11(2): 73-83.
[http://dx.doi.org/10.1007/s10158-011-0126-1] [PMID: 22068627]

[46] Mulcahy P, O'Doherty A, Paucard A, O'Brien T, Kirik D, Dowd E. Development and characterisation of a novel rat model of Parkinson's disease induced by sequential intranigral administration of AAV-α-synuclein and the pesticide, rotenone. Neuroscience 2012; 203: 170-9.
[http://dx.doi.org/10.1016/j.neuroscience.2011.12.011] [PMID: 22198020]

[47] Gyurkó MD, Csermely P, Sőti C, Sztétak A. Distinct roles of the RasGAP family proteins in C. elegans associative learning and memory. Sci Rep 2015; 5: 15084.
[http://dx.doi.org/10.1038/srep15084] [PMID: 26469632]

[48] Fernandez-funez P, Mena L, Rincon-limas DE. Modeling the complex pathology of Alzheimer's disease in Drosophila 2015.

[49] Adams MD, Celniker SE, Holt RA, *et al.* The genome sequence of drosophila melanogaster 2000; 287(March): 2185-96.
[http://dx.doi.org/10.1126/science.287.5461.2185]

[50] Prüßing K, Voigt A, Schulz JB. *Drosophila melanogaster* as a model organism for Alzheimer's disease Drosophila melanogaster as a model organism for Alzheimer ' s disease. Mol Neurodegener 2013; 8: 35.

[51] Reichert H. A tripartite organization of the urbilaterian brain: developmental genetic evidence from Drosophila 2005.
[http://dx.doi.org/10.1016/j.brainresbull.2004.11.028]

[52] Ng CS, Kopp A. Sex combs are important for male mating success in Drosophila melanogaster. Behav Genet 2008; 38(2): 195-201.
[http://dx.doi.org/10.1007/s10519-008-9190-7] [PMID: 18213513]

[53] Chien S, Reiter LT, Bier E, Gribskov M. Homophila: human disease gene cognates in Drosophila. Nucleic Acids Res 2002; 30(1): 149-51.
[http://dx.doi.org/10.1093/nar/30.1.149] [PMID: 11752278]

[54] Iijima-Ando K, Iijima K. Transgenic Drosophila models of Alzheimer's disease and tauopathies 2010.
[http://dx.doi.org/10.1007/s00429-009-0234-4]

[55] Luo L, Tully T, White K. Human amyloid precursor protein ameliorates behavioral deficit of flies deleted for Appl gene. Neuron 1992; 9(4): 595-605.
[http://dx.doi.org/10.1016/0896-6273(92)90024-8] [PMID: 1389179]

[56] Carmine-Simmen K, Proctor T, Tschäpe J, *et al.* Neurotoxic effects induced by the Drosophila amyloid-beta peptide suggest a conserved toxic function. Neurobiol Dis 2009; 33(2): 274-81.

[57] Boyles RS, Lantz KM, Poertner S, Georges SJ, Andres AJ. Presenilin controls CBP levels in the adult Drosophila central nervous system. PLoS One [Internet] , 2010 Jan; [cited 2015 Nov 30];5(12): e14332.

[58] Greeve I, Kretzschmar D, Tschäpe J-A, *et al.* Age-dependent neurodegeneration and Alzheimer-amyloid plaque formation in transgenic Drosophila. J Neurosci 2004; 24(16): 3899-906.

[59] Ye Y, Fortini ME. Apoptotic activities of wild-type and Alzheimer's disease-related mutant presenilins in Drosophila melanogaster. J Cell Biol 1999; 146(6): 1351-64.
[http://dx.doi.org/10.1083/jcb.146.6.1351] [PMID: 10491396]

[60]   Iijima K, Liu HP, Chiang AS, Hearn SA, Konsolaki M, Zhong Y. Dissecting the pathological effects of human Abeta40 and Abeta42 in Drosophila: a potential model for Alzheimer's disease. Proc Natl Acad Sci USA 2004; 101(17): 6623-8.
[http://dx.doi.org/10.1073/pnas.0400895101] [PMID: 15069204]

[61]   Iijima-Ando K, Sekiya M, Maruko-Otake A, *et al.* Loss of axonal mitochondria promotes tau-mediated neurodegeneration and Alzheimer's disease-related tau phosphorylation *via* PAR-1. PLoS Genet 2012; 8(8): e1002918.

[62]   Glater EE, Megeath LJ, Stowers RS, Schwarz TL. Axonal transport of mitochondria requires milton to recruit kinesin heavy chain and is light chain independent. J Cell Biol 2006; 173(4): 545-57.
[http://dx.doi.org/10.1083/jcb.200601067] [PMID: 16717129]

[63]   Crowther DC, Kinghorn KJ, Miranda E, *et al.* Intraneuronal Aβ, non-amyloid aggregates and neurodegeneration in a Drosophila model of Alzheimer's disease. Neuroscience 2005; 132(1): 123-35.

[64]   Chakraborty R, Vepuri V, Mhatre SD, *et al.* Characterization of a Drosophila Alzheimer's disease model: pharmacological rescue of cognitive defects. PLoS One 2011; 6(6): e20799.

[65]   Gutzman JH, Graeden EG, Lowery LA, Holley HS, Sive H. Formation of the zebrafish midbrain-hindbrain boundary constriction requires laminin-dependent basal constriction. Mech Dev 2008; 125(11-12): 974-83.
[http://dx.doi.org/10.1016/j.mod.2008.07.004] [PMID: 18682291]

[66]   Lowery LA, De Rienzo G, Gutzman JH, Sive H. Characterization and classification of zebrafish brain morphology mutants. Anat Rec (Hoboken) 2009; 292(1): 94-106.
[http://dx.doi.org/10.1002/ar.20768] [PMID: 19051268]

[67]   Lee JA, Cole GJ. Generation of transgenic zebrafish expressing green fluorescent protein under control of zebrafish amyloid precursor protein gene regulatory elements. Zebrafish 2007; 4(4): 277-86.
[http://dx.doi.org/10.1089/zeb.2007.0516] [PMID: 18284334]

[68]   Nery LR, Eltz NS, Hackman C, *et al.* Brain intraventricular injection of amyloid-β in zebrafish embryo impairs cognition and increases tau phosphorylation, effects reversed by lithium. PLoS One 2014; 9(9): e105862.

[69]   Cunvong K, Huffmire D, Ethell DW, Cameron DJ. Amyloid-β increases capillary bed density in the adult zebrafish retina. Invest Ophthalmol Vis Sci 2013; 54(2): 1516-21.
[http://dx.doi.org/10.1167/iovs.12-10821]

[70]   Kao T-T, Chu C-Y, Lee G-H, *et al.* Folate deficiency-induced oxidative stress contributes to neuropathy in young and aged zebrafish--implication in neural tube defects and Alzheimer's diseases. Neurobiol Dis 2014; 71: 234-44.

[71]   Paquet D, Bhat R, Sydow A, *et al.* A zebrafish model of tauopathy allows *in vivo* imaging of neuronal cell death and drug evaluation. J Clin Invest 2009; 119(5): 1382-95.
[http://dx.doi.org/10.1172/JCI37537] [PMID: 19363289]

[72]   Nornes S, Groth C, Camp E, Ey P, Lardelli M. Developmental control of Presenilin1 expression, endoproteolysis, and interaction in zebrafish embryos. Exp Cell Res 2003; 289(1): 124-32.
[http://dx.doi.org/10.1016/S0014-4827(03)00257-X]

[73]   Nornes S, Newman M, Wells S, Verdile G, Martins RN, Lardelli M. Independent and cooperative action of Psen2 with Psen1 in zebrafish embryos. Exp Cell Res 2009; 315(16): 2791-801.
[http://dx.doi.org/10.1016/j.yexcr.2009.06.023]

[74]   Song P, Pimplikar SW. Knockdown of amyloid precursor protein in zebrafish causes defects in motor axon outgrowth. PLoS One 2012; 7(4): e34209.

[75]   May Z, Morrill A, Holcombe A, *et al.* Object recognition memory in zebrafish. Behav Brain Res 2016; 296: 199-210.
[http://dx.doi.org/10.1016/j.bbr.2015.09.016] [PMID: 26376244]

[76]   Leclerc B, Abulrob A. Perspectives in molecular imaging using staging biomarkers and immunotherapies in alzheimer's disease. Sci World J 2013.
[http://dx.doi.org/10.1155/2013/589308]

[77]   Reiman EM, Chen K, Langbaum JBS, *et al.* Higher serum total cholesterol levels in late middle age are associated with glucose hypometabolism in brain regions affected by Alzheimer's disease and normal aging. Neuroimage 2010; 49(1): 169-76.
[http://dx.doi.org/10.1016/j.neuroimage.2009.07.025] [PMID: 19631758]

[78]   Sorbi S, Forleo P, Tedde A, *et al.* Genetic risk factors in familial Alzheimer's disease. Mech Ageing Dev 2001; 122(16): 1951-60.
[http://dx.doi.org/10.1016/S0047-6374(01)00308-6] [PMID: 11589913]

[79]   Ghebranious N, Mukesh B, Giampietro PF, *et al.* A pilot study of gene/gene and gene/environment interactions in Alzheimer disease. Clin Med Res 2011; 9(1): 17-25.
[http://dx.doi.org/10.3121/cmr.2010.894] [PMID: 20682755]

[80]   Mahley RW, Weisgraber KH, Huang Y. Apolipoprotein E4: a causative factor and therapeutic target in neuropathology, including Alzheimer's disease. Proc Natl Acad Sci USA 2006; 103(15): 5644-51.
[http://dx.doi.org/10.1073/pnas.0600549103] [PMID: 16567625]

[81]   Sadowski M, Pankiewicz J, Scholtzova H, *et al.* A synthetic peptide blocking the apolipoprotein E/beta-amyloid binding mitigates beta-amyloid toxicity and fibril formation *In vitro* and reduces beta-amyloid plaques in transgenic mice. Am J Pathol 2004; 165(3): 937-48.
[http://dx.doi.org/10.1016/S0002-9440(10)63355-X] [PMID: 15331417]

[82]   Zhong N, Scearce-Levie K, Ramaswamy G, Weisgraber KH. Apolipoprotein E4 domain interaction: synaptic and cognitive deficits in mice. Alzheimers Dement 2008; 4(3): 179-92.
[http://dx.doi.org/10.1016/j.jalz.2008.01.006] [PMID: 18631967]

[83]   Xu P-T, Gilbert JR, Qiu H-L, *et al.* Specific regional transcription of apolipoprotein E in human brain neurons. Am J Pathol 1999; 154(2): 601-11.
[http://dx.doi.org/10.1016/S0002-9440(10)65305-9] [PMID: 10027417]

[84]   Boschert U, Merlo-Pich E, Higgins G, Roses AD, Catsicas S. Apolipoprotein E expression by neurons surviving excitotoxic stress. Neurobiol Dis 1999; 6(6): 508-14.
[http://dx.doi.org/10.1006/nbdi.1999.0251] [PMID: 10600406]

[85]   Bencherif M, Lippiello PM. Alpha7 neuronal nicotinic receptors: the missing link to understanding Alzheimer's etiopathology? Med Hypotheses 2010; 74(2): 281-5. [Internet].
[http://dx.doi.org/10.1016/j.mehy.2009.09.011] [PMID: 19800174]

[86]   Moreno Moreno M de J. Cognitive improvement in mild to moderate alzheimer's dementia after treatment with the acetylcholine precursor choline. Clin Ther 2002; 178-94.

[87]   Prvulovic D, Hampel H, Pantel J. Galantamine for Alzheimer's disease. Expert Opin Drug Metab Toxicol 2010; 6(3): 345-54.
[http://dx.doi.org/10.1517/17425251003592137] [PMID: 20113148]

[88]   Ashe KH. Learning and memory in transgenic mice modeling Alzheimer's disease. Learn Mem 2001; 8(6): 301-8.
[http://dx.doi.org/10.1101/lm.43701] [PMID: 11773429]

[89]   Chen G, Chen KS, Knox JH, *et al.* A learning deficit related to age and b-amyloid plaques in a mouse model of Alzheimer's disease. Nature 1998; 2000(408): 975-9.

[90]   Braidy N, Muñoz P, Palacios AG, *et al.* Recent rodent models for Alzheimer's disease: clinical implications and basic research. J Neural Transm (Vienna) 2012; 119(2): 173-95.
[http://dx.doi.org/10.1007/s00702-011-0731-5] [PMID: 22086139]

[91]   Gonzalo-Ruiz A, González I, Sanz-Anquela JM. Effects of β-amyloid protein on serotoninergic, noradrenergic, and cholinergic markers in neurons of the pontomesencephalic tegmentum in the rat. J

Chem Neuroanat 2003; 26(3): 153-69.
[http://dx.doi.org/10.1016/S0891-0618(03)00046-2] [PMID: 14615025]

[92]   Hoyer S. Glucose metabolism and insulin receptor signal transduction in Alzheimer disease. Eur J Pharmacol 2004; 490(1-3): 115-25.
[http://dx.doi.org/10.1016/j.ejphar.2004.02.049] [PMID: 15094078]

[93]   Ardiles AO, Tapia-Rojas CC, Mandal M, *et al.* Postsynaptic dysfunction is associated with spatial and object recognition memory loss in a natural model of Alzheimer's disease. Proc Natl Acad Sci USA 2012; 109(34): 13835-40.
[http://dx.doi.org/10.1073/pnas.1201209109] [PMID: 22869717]

[94]   Pathan AR, Viswanad B, Sonkusare SK, Ramarao P. Chronic administration of pioglitazone attenuates intracerebroventricular streptozotocin induced-memory impairment in rats. Life Sci 2006; 79(23): 2209-16.
[http://dx.doi.org/10.1016/j.lfs.2006.07.018] [PMID: 16904700]

[95]   Prickaerts J, Fahrig T, Blokland A. Cognitive performance and biochemical markers in septum, hippocampus and striatum of rats after an i.c.v. injection of streptozotocin: a correlation analysis. Behav Brain Res 1999; 102(1-2): 73-88.
[http://dx.doi.org/10.1016/S0166-4328(98)00158-2] [PMID: 10403017]

[96]   Salkovic-Petrisic M, Tribl F, Schmidt M, Hoyer S, Riederer P. Alzheimer-like changes in protein kinase B and glycogen synthase kinase-3 in rat frontal cortex and hippocampus after damage to the insulin signalling pathway. J Neurochem 2006; 96(4): 1005-15.
[http://dx.doi.org/10.1111/j.1471-4159.2005.03637.x] [PMID: 16412093]

[97]   Walsh DM, Klyubin I, Fadeeva JV, *et al.* Naturally secreted oligomers of amyloid β protein potently inhibit hippocampal long-term potentiation *in vivo*. Nature 2002; 416(6880): 535-9.
[http://dx.doi.org/10.1038/416535a] [PMID: 11932745]

[98]   Woodruff-Pak DS, Agelan A, Del Valle L. A rabbit model of Alzheimer's disease: Valid at neuropathological, cognitive, and therapeutic levels. Adv Alzheimer Dis 2011; 1: 77-88.

[99]   Sparks DL, Friedland R, Petanceska S, *et al.* Trace copper levels in the drinking water, but not zinc or aluminum influence CNS Alzheimer-like pathology. J Nutr Health Aging 2006; 10(4): 247-54.
[PMID: 16886094]

[100] Terry R, Peña C. Experiemntal productions of neurofibrillary degenerations. Neuropathol Exp Neurol 1965; 24(2): 200-10.
[http://dx.doi.org/10.1097/00005072-196504000-00003]

[101] Kawahara M, Kato-Negishi M. Link between aluminum and the pathogenesis of alzheimer's disease: the integration of the aluminum and amyloid cascade hypotheses. Int J Alzheimers Dis 2011; 2011: 276393.
[http://dx.doi.org/10.4061/2011/276393] [PMID: 21423554]

[102] Akiyama H, Hosokawa M, Kametani F, *et al.* Long-term oral intake of aluminium or zinc does not accelerate Alzheimer pathology in AβPP and AβPP/tau transgenic mice. Neuropathology 2012; 32(4): 390-7.
[http://dx.doi.org/10.1111/j.1440-1789.2011.01274.x] [PMID: 22118300]

[103] Ribes D, Torrente M, Vicens P, Colomina MT, Gómez M, Domingo JL. Recognition memory and β-amyloid plaques in adult Tg2576 mice are not modified after oral exposure to aluminum. Alzheimer Dis Assoc Disord 2012; 26(2): 179-85.
[http://dx.doi.org/10.1097/WAD.0b013e3182211ab1] [PMID: 21642811]

[104] Lidsky TI. Is the aluminum hypothesis dead? J Occup Environ Med 2014; 56(5) (Suppl.): S73-9.
[http://dx.doi.org/10.1097/JOM.0000000000000063] [PMID: 24806729]

[105] Muma NA, Singer SM. Aluminum-induced neuropathology: transient changes in microtubule-associated proteins. Neurotoxicol Teratol 1996; 18(6): 679-90.

[http://dx.doi.org/10.1016/S0892-0362(96)00126-2] [PMID: 8947945]

[106] Luo Y, Niu F, Sun Z, *et al.* Altered expression of Abeta metabolism-associated molecules from D-galactose/AlCl(3) induced mouse brain. Mech Ageing Dev 2009; 130(4): 248-52.
[http://dx.doi.org/10.1016/j.mad.2008.12.005] [PMID: 19150622]

[107] Castorina A, Tiralongo A, Giunta S, Carnazza ML, Scapagnini G, D'Agata V. Early effects of aluminum chloride on beta-secretase mRNA expression in a neuronal model of beta-amyloid toxicity. Cell Biol Toxicol 2010; 26(4): 367-77.
[http://dx.doi.org/10.1007/s10565-009-9149-3] [PMID: 20111991]

[108] Yoshiyama Y, Higuchi M, Zhang B, *et al.* Synapse loss and microglial activation precede tangles in a P301S tauopathy mouse model. Neuron 2007; 53(3): 337-51.
[http://dx.doi.org/10.1016/j.neuron.2007.01.010] [PMID: 17270732]

[109] Schenk D, Barbour R, Dunn W, *et al.* Immunization with amyloid-beta attenuates Alzheimer-diseas--like pathology in the PDAPP mouse. Nature 1999; 400(6740): 173-7.
[http://dx.doi.org/10.1038/22124] [PMID: 10408445]

[110] Ferrer I, Boada Rovira M, Sánchez Guerra ML, Rey MJ, Costa-Jussá F. Neuropathology and pathogenesis of encephalitis following amyloid-β immunization in Alzheimer's disease. Brain Pathol 2004; 14(1): 11-20.
[http://dx.doi.org/10.1111/j.1750-3639.2004.tb00493.x] [PMID: 14997933]

[111] Hsiao K, Chapman P, Nilsen S, *et al.* Correlative memory deficits, Aβ elevation, and amyloid plaques in transgenic mice. Science (80-) 1996; 274(5284): 99-102.

[112] Sasaki A, Shoji M, Harigaya Y, *et al.* Amyloid cored plaques in Tg2576 transgenic mice are characterized by giant plaques, slightly activated microglia, and the lack of paired helical filament-typed, dystrophic neurites. Virchows Arch 2002; 441(4): 358-67.
[http://dx.doi.org/10.1007/s00428-002-0643-8] [PMID: 12404061]

[113] Elder GA, Gama Sosa MA, De Gasperi R. Transgenic mouse models of Alzheimer's disease. Mt Sinai J Med 2010; 77(1): 69-81.
[http://dx.doi.org/10.1002/msj.20159] [PMID: 20101721]

[114] Lazarov O, Peterson LD, Peterson DA, Sisodia SS. Expression of a familial Alzheimer's disease-linked presenilin-1 variant enhances perforant pathway lesion-induced neuronal loss in the entorhinal cortex. J Neurosci 2006; 26(2): 429-34.
[http://dx.doi.org/10.1523/JNEUROSCI.3961-05.2006] [PMID: 16407539]

[115] Chevallier NL, Soriano S, Kang DE, Masliah E, Hu G, Koo EH. Perturbed neurogenesis in the adult hippocampus associated with presenilin-1 A246E mutation. Am J Pathol 2005; 167(1): 151-9. [Internet].
[http://dx.doi.org/10.1016/S0002-9440(10)62962-8] [PMID: 15972961]

[116] Oakley H, Cole SL, Logan S, *et al.* Intraneuronal beta-amyloid aggregates, neurodegeneration, and neuron loss in transgenic mice with five familial Alzheimer's disease mutations: potential factors in amyloid plaque formation. J Neurosci 2006; 26(40): 10129-40.
[http://dx.doi.org/10.1523/JNEUROSCI.1202-06.2006] [PMID: 17021169]

[117] Masliah E, Sisk A, Mallory M, Games D. Neurofibrillary pathology in transgenic mice overexpressing V717F beta-amyloid precursor protein. J Neuropathol Exp Neurol 2001; 60(4): 357-68.
[http://dx.doi.org/10.1093/jnen/60.4.357] [PMID: 11305871]

[118] Götz J, Chen F, Van Dorpe J, Nitsch RM. Formation of neurofibrillary tangles in P301L tau transgenic mice induced by Aβ42 fibrils. Science (80-) 2001; 293(5534): 1491-5.

[119] Lewis J, Dickson DW, Lin WL, Chisholm L, Corral A, Jones G, *et al.* Enhanced neurofibrillary degeneration in transgenic mice expressing mutant tau and APP. Science (80-) 2001; 293(5534): 1487-91.
[http://dx.doi.org/10.1126/science.1058189]

[120] Oddo S, Caccamo A, Shepherd JD, *et al.* Triple-transgenic model of Alzheimer's disease with plaques and tangles: intracellular Abeta and synaptic dysfunction. Neuron 2003; 39(3): 409-21.
[http://dx.doi.org/10.1016/S0896-6273(03)00434-3] [PMID: 12895417]

[121] Oddo S, Billings L, Kesslak JP, Cribbs DH, LaFerla FM. Abeta immunotherapy leads to clearance of early, but not late, hyperphosphorylated tau aggregates *via* the proteasome. Neuron 2004; 43(3): 321-32.
[http://dx.doi.org/10.1016/j.neuron.2004.07.003] [PMID: 15294141]

[122] Bolmont T, Clavaguera F, Meyer-Luehmann M, *et al.* Induction of tau pathology by intracerebral infusion of amyloid-β -containing brain extract and by amyloid-β deposition in APP x Tau transgenic mice. Am J Pathol 2007; 171(6): 2012-20.
[http://dx.doi.org/10.2353/ajpath.2007.070403] [PMID: 18055549]

[123] Terwel D, Muyllaert D, Dewachter I, *et al.* Amyloid activates GSK-3β to aggravate neuronal tauopathy in bigenic mice. Am J Pathol 2008; 172(3): 786-98.
[http://dx.doi.org/10.2353/ajpath.2008.070904] [PMID: 18258852]

[124] Wahrle SE, Jiang H, Parsadanian M, *et al.* Overexpression of ABCA1 reduces amyloid deposition in the PDAPP mouse model of Alzheimer disease. J Clin Invest 2008; 118(2): 671-82.
[PMID: 18202749]

[125] Van Dam D, D'Hooge R, Staufenbiel M, Van Ginneken C, Van Meir F, De Deyn PP. Age-dependent cognitive decline in the APP23 model precedes amyloid deposition. Eur J Neurosci 2003; 17(2): 388-96.
[http://dx.doi.org/10.1046/j.1460-9568.2003.02444.x] [PMID: 12542676]

[126] Richards JG, Higgins GA, Ouagazzal AM, *et al.* PS2APP transgenic mice, coexpressing hPS2mut and hAPPswe, show age-related cognitive deficits associated with discrete brain amyloid deposition and inflammation. J Neurosci 2003; 23(26): 8989-9003.
[http://dx.doi.org/10.1523/JNEUROSCI.23-26-08989.2003] [PMID: 14523101]

[127] Chishti MA, Yang D-S, Janus C, *et al.* Early-onset amyloid deposition and cognitive deficits in transgenic mice expressing a double mutant form of amyloid precursor protein 695. J Biol Chem 2001; 276(24): 21562-70.
[http://dx.doi.org/10.1074/jbc.M100710200] [PMID: 11279122]

[128] Lewis J, McGowan E, Rockwood J, *et al.* Neurofibrillary tangles, amyotrophy and progressive motor disturbance in mice expressing mutant (P301L) tau protein. Nat Genet 2000; 25(4): 402-5.
[http://dx.doi.org/10.1038/78078] [PMID: 10932182]

[129] Games D, Adams D, Alessandrini R, *et al.* Alzheimer-type neuropathology in transgenic mice overexpressing V717F beta-amyloid precursor protein. Nature 1995; 373(6514): 523-7.
[http://dx.doi.org/10.1038/373523a0] [PMID: 7845465]

[130] Whiteman IT, Gervasio OL, Cullen KM, *et al.* Activated actin-depolymerizing factor/cofilin sequesters phosphorylated microtubule-associated protein during the assembly of alzheimer-like neuritic cytoskeletal striations. J Neurosci 2009; 29(41): 12994-3005.
[http://dx.doi.org/10.1523/JNEUROSCI.3531-09.2009] [PMID: 19828813]

[131] Carrodeguas JA, Rodolosse A, Garza MV, *et al.* The chick embryo appears as a natural model for research in beta-amyloid precursor protein processing. Neuroscience 2005; 134(4): 1285-300.
[http://dx.doi.org/10.1016/j.neuroscience.2005.05.020] [PMID: 16039787]

[132] Dani SU, Pittella JEH, Boehme A, Hori A, Schneider B. Progressive formation of neuritic plaques and neurofibrillary tangles is exponentially related to age and neuronal size. A morphometric study of three geographically distinct series of aging people. Dement Geriatr Cogn Disord 1997; 8(4): 217-27.
[http://dx.doi.org/10.1159/000106634] [PMID: 9213066]

[133] Joly M, Ammersdörfer S, Schmidtke D, Zimmermann E. Touchscreen-based cognitive tasks reveal age-related impairment in a primate aging model, the grey mouse lemur (*Microcebus murinus*). PLoS

One 2014; 9(10): e109393.
[http://dx.doi.org/10.1371/journal.pone.0109393] [PMID: 25299046]

[134] Zürcher NR, Rodriguez JS, Jenkins SL, *et al.* Performance of juvenile baboons on neuropsychological tests assessing associative learning, motivation and attention. J Neurosci Methods 2010; 188(2): 219-25.
[http://dx.doi.org/10.1016/j.jneumeth.2010.02.011] [PMID: 20170676]

[135] Marvanová M, Ménager J, Bezard E, Bontrop RE, Pradier L, Wong G. Microarray analysis of nonhuman primates: validation of experimental models in neurological disorders. FASEB J 2003; 17 (8): 929-31.
[http://dx.doi.org/10.1096/fj.02-0681fje] [PMID: 12626435]

[136] Loerch PM, Lu T, Dakin KA, *et al.* Evolution of the aging brain transcriptome and synaptic regulation. PLoS One 2008; 3(10): e3329.
[http://dx.doi.org/10.1371/journal.pone.0003329] [PMID: 18830410]

[137] Levine H III, Walker LC. Molecular polymorphism of Abeta in Alzheimer's disease. Neurobiol Aging 2010; 31(4): 542-8.
[http://dx.doi.org/10.1016/j.neurobiolaging.2008.05.026] [PMID: 18619711]

[138] Jucker M. The benefits and limitations of animal models for translational research in neurodegenerative diseases. Nat Med 2010; 16(11): 1210-4. [Internet].
[http://dx.doi.org/10.1038/nm.2224] [PMID: 21052075]

[139] Voytko ML. Nonhuman primates as models for aging and Alzheimer's disease. Lab Anim Sci 1998; 48(6): 611-7.
[PMID: 10090085]

[140] Gearing M, Tigges J, Mori H, Mirra SS. β-Amyloid (A β) deposition in the brains of aged orangutans. Neurobiol Aging 1997; 18(2): 139-46.
[http://dx.doi.org/10.1016/S0197-4580(97)00012-2] [PMID: 9258890]

[141] Kanemaru K, Iwatsubo T, Ihara Y. Comparable amyloid beta-protein (A beta) 42(43) and A beta 40 deposition in the aged monkey brain. Neurosci Lett 1996; 214(2-3): 196-8.
[http://dx.doi.org/10.1016/0304-3940(96)12893-7] [PMID: 8878117]

[142] Gearing M, Tigges J, Mori H, Mirra SS. A beta40 is a major form of beta-amyloid in nonhuman primates. Neurobiol Aging 1996; 17(6): 903-8.
[http://dx.doi.org/10.1016/S0197-4580(96)00164-9] [PMID: 9363802]

[143] Rosen RF, Farberg AS, Gearing M, *et al.* Tauopathy with paired helical filaments in an aged chimpanzee. J Comp Neurol 2008; 509(3): 259-70.
[http://dx.doi.org/10.1002/cne.21744] [PMID: 18481275]

[144] Härtig W, Brückner G, Schmidt C, *et al.* Co-localization of β-amyloid peptides, apolipoprotein E and glial markers in senile plaques in the prefrontal cortex of old rhesus monkeys. Brain Res 1997; 751(2): 315-22.
[http://dx.doi.org/10.1016/S0006-8993(96)01423-0] [PMID: 9099821]

[145] Morelli L, Wei L, Amorim A, *et al.* Cerebrovascular amyloidosis in squirrel monkeys and rhesus monkeys: apolipoprotein E genotype. FEBS Lett 1996; 379(2): 132-4.
[http://dx.doi.org/10.1016/0014-5793(95)01491-8] [PMID: 8635577]

[146] Hare B, Brown M, Williamson C, Tomasello M. The domestication of social cognition in dogs. Science (80-) 2002; 298(5598): 1634-6.
[http://dx.doi.org/10.1126/science.1072702]

[147] Johnstone EM, Chaney MO, Norris FH, Pascual R, Little SP. Conservation of the sequence of the Alzheimer's disease amyloid peptide in dog, polar bear and five other mammals by cross-species polymerase chain reaction analysis. Brain Res Mol Brain Res 1991; 10(4): 299-305.
[http://dx.doi.org/10.1016/0169-328X(91)90088-F] [PMID: 1656157]

[148] Rofina J, van Andel I, van Ederen AM, Papaioannou N, Yamaguchi H, Gruys E. Canine counterpart of senile dementia of the Alzheimer type: amyloid plaques near capillaries but lack of spatial relationship with activated microglia and macrophages. Amyloid 2003; 10(2): 86-96.
[http://dx.doi.org/10.3109/13506120309041730] [PMID: 12964416]

[149] Pugliese M, Mascort J, Mahy N, Ferrer I. Diffuse beta-amyloid plaques and hyperphosphorylated tau are unrelated processes in aged dogs with behavioral deficits. Acta Neuropathol 2006; 112(2): 175-83.
[http://dx.doi.org/10.1007/s00401-006-0087-3] [PMID: 16775693]

[150] Russell MJ, White R, Patel E, Markesbery WR, Watson CR, Geddes JW. Familial influence on plaque formation in the beagle brain. Neuroreport 1992; 3(12): 1093-6.
[http://dx.doi.org/10.1097/00001756-199212000-00015] [PMID: 1493222]

[151] Stieler JT, Bullmann T, Kohl F, *et al.* The physiological link between metabolic rate depression and tau phosphorylation in mammalian hibernation. PLoS One 2011; 6(1): e14530.
[http://dx.doi.org/10.1371/journal.pone.0014530] [PMID: 21267079]

[152] Contreras LC, Gutiérrez JR. Effects of the subterranean herbivorous rodent Spalacopus cyanus on herbaceous vegetation in arid coastal Chile. Oecologia 1991; 87(1): 106-9.
[http://dx.doi.org/10.1007/BF00323787] [PMID: 28313359]

[153] Inestrosa NC, Reyes AE, Chacón MA, *et al.* Human-like rodent amyloid-β-peptide determines Alzheimer pathology in aged wild-type Octodon degu. Neurobiol Aging 2005; 26(7): 1023-8.
[http://dx.doi.org/10.1016/j.neurobiolaging.2004.09.016] [PMID: 15748782]

[154] Tarragon E, Lopez D, Estrada C, *et al. Octodon degus*: a model for the cognitive impairment associated with Alzheimer's disease. CNS Neurosci Ther 2013; 19(9): 643-8.
[http://dx.doi.org/10.1111/cns.12125] [PMID: 23710760]

[155] Brown C, Donnelly TM. Cataracts and reduced fertility in degus (Octodon degus). Contracts secondary to spontaneous diabetes mellitus. Lab Anim (NY) 2001; 30(6): 25-6.
[PMID: 11395944]

[156] Ebensperger LA, Ramírez-Estrada J, León C, *et al.* Sociality, glucocorticoids and direct fitness in the communally rearing rodent, Octodon degus. Horm Behav 2011; 60(4): 346-52. [Internet].
[http://dx.doi.org/10.1016/j.yhbeh.2011.07.002] [PMID: 21777588]

[157] Spires TL, Hyman BT. Transgenic models of Alzheimer's disease: learning from animals. NeuroRx 2005; 2(3): 423-37.
[http://dx.doi.org/10.1602/neurorx.2.3.423] [PMID: 16389306]

[158] Popović N, Baño-Otálora B, Rol MÁ, Caballero-Bleda M, Madrid JA, Popović M. Aging and time-o--day effects on anxiety in female Octodon degus. Behav Brain Res 2009; 200(1): 117-21.
[http://dx.doi.org/10.1016/j.bbr.2009.01.001] [PMID: 19162080]

[159] Okanoya K, Tokimoto N, Kumazawa N, Hihara S, Iriki A. Tool-use training in a species of rodent: the emergence of an optimal motor strategy and functional understanding. PLoS One 2008; 3(3): e1860.
[http://dx.doi.org/10.1371/journal.pone.0001860] [PMID: 18365015]

[160] Inestrosa NC, Ríos JA, Cisternas P, *et al.* Age progression of neuropathological markers in the brain of the chilean rodent octodon degus, a natural model of alzheimer's disease. Brain Pathol 2015; 25(6): 679-91.
[http://dx.doi.org/10.1111/bpa.12226] [PMID: 25351914]

Recent Advances in Alzheimer Research, 2018, Vol. 2, 41-74

CHAPTER 2

Micro and Macro Morphologic Changes in Alzheimer's Disease

Daniel Moreira-Silva, Samanta Rodrigues and **Tatiana L. Ferreira**[*]

Center for Mathematics, Computation and Cognition, Federal University of ABC (UFABC), São Bernardo do Campo, São Paulo, Brazil

Abstract: A normal development of the central nervous system is an essential process to a healthy the adult brain. After birth, some brain areas are still maturing and, even in the adulthood, the brain networks are in constant reorganization. The physiological and morphological changes that occur during nervous system maturation can be the key to the insurgence of neurodegenerative diseases such Alzheimer's disease (AD). AD is the most common cause of severe cognitive decline in elderly. The set of neuronal morphological changes presented even before clinical symptoms onset is strongly correlated with future cognitive impairments. However, it is not clear yet which morphofunctional features are more accurate to distinguish the healthy and the abnormal brain as well as its future susceptibility in developing AD. In this chapter, we described the neuroanatomic aspects of AD. Specifically, we focused on the progression of affected areas throughout AD stages and on the selective aspects that make several neuronal populations and brain areas more vulnerable to pathological changes. External and internal factors that might influence morphological features are also addressed. While intrinsic characteristics such as myelination and pigmentation could help to predict the pattern of anatomic advance of AD, on the other hand, cognitive reserve is an example of how external input and lifestyle can delay the appearance of clinical symptoms even when morphologic changes are already pronounced. The early diagnosis and staging are fundamental steps to provide information for more specific therapeutic approaches. Ultimately, some of the advances and techniques for this challenging diagnosis are also detailed.

Keywords: AD diagnosis, AD stages, Cognitive reserve, Dementia, Elderly, Entorhinal cortex, Medial temporal lobe, Myelination, Neurodegeneration, Neuronal susceptibility, Pigmentation.

---

[*] **Corresponding author Tatiana Lima Ferreira:** Center for Mathematics, Computation and Cognition, Federal University of ABC (UFABC), São Bernardo do Campo, São Paulo, Brazil; Tel: +55 11 2320-6271; E-mail: tatiana.ferreira@ufabc.edu.br

Fernando A. Oliveira (Ed.)

INTRODUCTION

Nervous system is topographically classified in two main categories: peripheral nervous system (PNS) and central nervous system (CNS). PNS is the part outside the skull and spine and it is related with the capability to interact with the environment by sensory and motor systems and to maintain the state of the internal milieu by autonomic nervous system. On the other hand, CNS is the nervous tissue comprised into skull and spine composed by spinal cord and brain. Cranial and spinal nerves connect these two systems carrying environmental or internal information and transmitting back the effector response (autonomic or behavioral) from brain and spine [1 - 3].

Brain development initiates when the neurulation occurs shortly after conception. Approximately between the 2nd and 4th week of gestation, a portion of the embryo tissue (ectoderm) becomes thick and forms neural grooves that merge later shaping the neural tube. At the end of this period, some ectoderm cells start to migrate laterally to form cranial and spinal nerves, and the neural tube fuse. Then, the posterior end of neural tube develops and forms spinal cord, and the anterior end of the tube gives rise to 3 brain vesicles. These vesicles develop later into the brain major structures (5 stages vesicles: myelencephalon, metencephalon, mesencephalon, diencephalon and telencephalon). During brain development, each of these areas support different functions with different patterns of activation in a hierarchical fashion. Until birth, the brain continues to grow in an accelerated rhythm changing in function and morphology. At the end of this time, the brain is totally formed and functionally active with billions of neurons and glial cells [1, 3].

Even after birth, innumerous processes continue to ensure brain maturation such as cell proliferation, migration and differentiation, synaptogenesis, synaptic pruning and apoptosis [4]. Neurons establish their synaptic connections during the first 1-2 years of life and lose connections to puberty until thirty age [5]. Neuronal growth and synapse formation are processes of brain ontogeny that can also be influenced by genetic and environmental factors [6 - 10]. As different regions develop in different rates, any mistake on these development steps that cause malformation of the neural tube might lead to a poor development or erroneous maturation of major brain structures and consequently affect the brain activity critically [11, 12].

Nervous system damages promoted by mechanical injury or stroke can also affect its functionality. The specific impairments of behavioral responses depending on the involved region and severity of trauma. However, the brain has the fantastic capability to reorganize its connections at cortical and subcortical levels, starting to use new pathways in the unaffected hemisphere and developing new networks [13]. This ability is called neuroplasticity and the young brain is more plastic than an adult one because it is still in development [4, 14]. A large number of factors during and after damage recovery outcome: the early age, the beginning of treatment shortly after the injury and a substantial time of therapy are factors that contribute to a better rehabilitation [13, 15].

In parallel with brain mechanical injury and stroke, the elderly brain also suffers changes by natural physiological and morphological processes. It is not very clear yet how these patterns are established across individuals. Thus, to separate the healthy morphological changes of the pathological conditions remains challenging.

AD is the most common cause of pathological cognitive decline. The patterns of neuronal death in the AD patient are accompanied by symptoms such as the progressive failure of language, memory and visuospatial abilities. Some authors hypothesize that these symptoms can be generated by an exacerbated aging process induced by AD progression [16 - 18]. To address this question, Ohnishi and colleagues (2001) conducted a study using magnetic resonance image (MRI) to compare the regional morphological brain changes in healthy normal aging and AD patients . The voxel-by-voxel analysis showed a distinct region-dependent vulnerability especially in the polymodal association areas of limbic cortices during normal aging and of medial temporal structures in AD patients. According to this study, the elderly and the AD brain morphological changes are dichotomous and not a continuous spectrum. Even considering only AD subjects, Byun and co-workers found heterogeneity of regional brain atrophy patterns associated with distinct progression rates in AD [19], which may be related to different susceptibility to neuronal degeneration.

AD PATHOLOGICAL CHANGES IN NEURONAL POPULATIONS

Neuronal Morphology and Degree of Maturation

The different propensity to develop AD anatomical markers is observed in distinctive neuronal populations. Some neurons have different inclination to resist or to be affected by CNS deterioration started by AD. Although AD degeneration has the predisposition to commit regions involved in high-order cognitive processes, some neuronal types remain morphologically and functionally intact even in the neighborhood of these damaged areas [20, 21]. Some factors may influence the neuronal resistance to AD such cumulative oxidative, ionic and metabolic stress; protein malfunctions; cell size, shape and location and the stage of differentiation and myelination [22].

In cortical areas, neurodegeneration firstly reaches a type of projection neuron in the transentorhinal region and, just then, other types of projection cells less vulnerable are affected [23]. While pyramidal neurons in the hippocampus and in the frontal lobe die during early stages of AD, granule neurons from dentate gyrus and cortical interneurons seems to remain intact a little longer [22].

Large neurons with myelinated axons that project to long distances are typically more vulnerable, such hippocampal and cortical pyramidal cells in layers III and V [22, 24]. Nevertheless, projection neurons with short axons just became damaged in late stages of AD, such smaller pyramidal neurons in the layers II and IV and spiny stellate cells in the layer IV of the neocortex [24, 25].

In the hippocampus, the same logic can be applied: efferent neurons in the CA1 region, subiculum and in the layers II and V of entorhinal cortex are preferentially damaged. However, large pyramidal cells in the CA3 region and the neurons of the dentate hilus demonstrated to be resistant in form neurofibrillary tangles (NFTs), suggesting that other cell characteristics, besides morphology and size, are involved with the inclination to neurodegenerative processes [24].

One of these characteristics is the stage of neuronal maturation and connectivity stabilization. Neurodegeneration in AD seems to occur prior in a set of neurons with a higher degree of plasticity and susceptibility to alterations of the regular cell-cycle [21]. Brain areas tend to have most of their connections stabilized after development. Nevertheless, some neuron subsets especially from limbic and cortical areas remain labile. They are related with functions such memory, learning and consciousness and suffer a life-long permanent synaptic restructuring in order to adapt to environmental demands [21, 26]. The constant destabilization of previous synaptic connections could underlie the possibility of cumulative failures in a lifetime. This increase can be the critical primary mechanism that would trigger AD pathology [27].

In general, brain areas which have a high degree of plasticity during life – that are responsible cognitive functions (see Fig. **1a**) – are also the last ones to get completely mature during the ontogenesis: neocortex, hippocampus and cholinergic basal forebrain neurons. Not surprisingly, these regions are more vulnerable to AD neurodegeneration, as shown in Fig. (**1b**) [21, 28 - 31].

Recent studies demonstrated that the maintenance of these immature features in healthy elderly keeps hippocampal neurons in a not fully differentiated stage. They stuck at G_0 phase, expressing cyclins E and B [35]. These "immature" neurons have more intense changes in membrane fluidity, axonal disturbs and dendritic reorganization and are consequently more susceptible to accumulate failures of their morpho-regulatory proteins. The accumulation of damage in cell

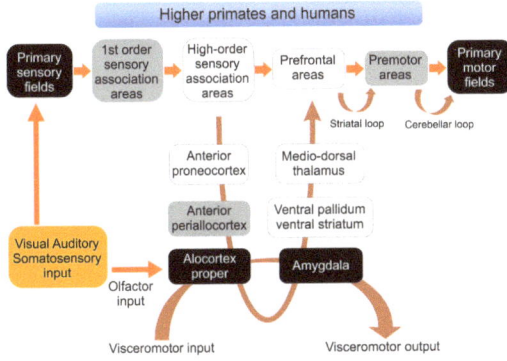

(a)

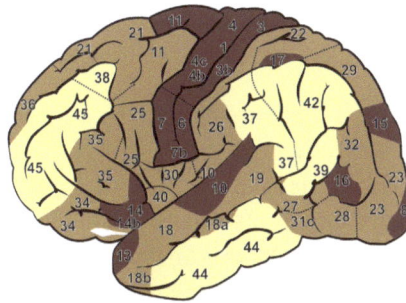

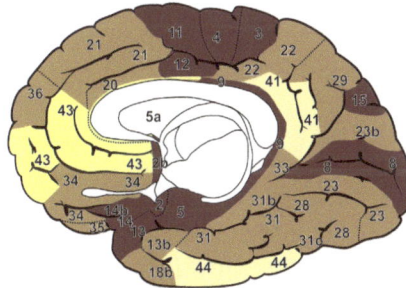

(b)

Fig. (1). (a) Hierarchical subdivision of information flow in the cerebral cortex. Late myelinated areas, generally responsible for processing high order cognitive functions, such working memory and decision making, in white. Intermediate myelinated areas in grey and early myelinated areas in black, adapted from Braak [32]. **(b)** Ontogenic map of the brain cortex, (adapted from Fuster, 2003 [33], originally published by Flechsig, 1901 [34]). The numeration indicates the sequence of the myelination in the areas as well as the colors. First myelinated areas in dark brown, intermediate in light brown and late myelinated areas in yellow/beige.

adhesion molecules and junctional molecules, which are critical to establish intercellular interactions, would contribute to the insurgence of neuronal dysfunction and the histopatological hallmarks of AD. Subclinical AD and clinical AD patients present increased expression of collagen IV, pertecan and fibronectin (components of extracellular matrix) in frontal and temporal cortex when compared to controls, correlating with the levels of amyloid deposition [21, 36, 37].

Another class of molecules that regulates neuronal resistance against AD is the calcium-binding proteins like parvalbumin, calbindin and calretinin. These proteins promote an intracellular calcium buffering and enzymatic regulation. Their functions are deeply studied in the hippocampus and the neocortex. Some authors have reported that interneurons containing calcium-binding proteins rarely present NFT formation [25]. There are parvalbumin-positive neurons distributed throughout the temporal polar, hippocampal formation, perirhinal and entorhinal cortices [38].

Parvalbumin-immunoreative interneurons in the neocortex display very preserved morphologic aspects even in the advanced stages of AD and are also more resistant to cell death [39]. However, in the hippocampus, parvalbumin-immunoreactive neurons are not resistant to AD. It has been reported neuronal loss and reduction of the dendritic arborization of parvalbumin-positive cells from CA1 field, as well as morphologic changes of neurons in the enthorhinal cortex [25, 40]. Chandelier cells of human temporal cortex that displayed parvalbumin-immunoreactivity have also showed a reduction in the amount of their terminals in the layer II of brains with people with AD [41].

Myelination as a Central Process Underlying Susceptibility to Neurodegeneration in AD

After the onset of degeneration in brain areas and neuronal populations that are more vulnerable to AD, the damage throughout the cortex does not spread in a random and indiscriminate way. Actually, the chronologic pattern of distribution of neuropathological alterations is generally the inverse of myelination process and parallel in relation to pigmentation. In other words, neurons with late myelination and early pigmentation are primarily affected [24, 31, 42].

Dr. Bartzokis is one of the investigators that most contributed to establish a development model of cognitive decline and Alzheimer's disease based on myelination. Bartzokis and co-workers argue that the protracted myelination of cortical areas vulnerable to AD would occur due to oligodendrocytes that keeps differentiating in cells that produce myelin even until 50 years old [42]. Oligodendrocytes are under intense metabolic activity in order to produces all the cholesterol used by human brain and maintain myelin sheaths. It makes this type of cell very susceptible to many stressing conditions such inflammatory cytokines and excitotoxic neurotransmitters, that leads to cell death [43]. Cell loss occurs particularly when these cells are supplying thick and long myelinated axons of neurons that are generally fully differentiated just late in the life and have a continuous expanding number of segments. The accumulation of failures in the metabolism of oligodendrocytes leads to a progressive pattern of myelin breakdown that mimics the physiological process of myelination, but in reverse. The gradual decrease in the velocity of synaptic transmission drives to a loss of synchrony into neuronal networks, affecting primarily high-order cognitive functions like the formation of new memories. In studies with primates, Peters and Sethares found out that the process of myelin breakdown is associated with impaired cognitive performance in advanced age. These myelination dysfunction initiate even when the increase of myelination is still active and white matter volume is expanding, in consonance to Bartzokis' ideas [44, 45].

The major hallmarks of AD – accumulation of hyperphosphorylated tau protein and amyloid aggregation – would be also correlated to the myelination process. More recent studies showed that the breakdown of myelination contributes to produce toxic Aβ fibrils, that thereafter will deposit and participate of the generation of amyloid plaques [46 - 48]. On the other hand, Aβ plaques increase the proliferation of oligodendrocytes precursor cells and, consequently, the number of failures in their reaction against brain damages. In addition, the toxicity induced by Aβ- promotes myelin break during the earlier stages of AD. The pattern of this myelin disruption is correlated with the spatial and temporal progression of the cognitive impairment in the disease [48].

Concerning to the familial Alzheimer s' disease (FAD), subjects with mutation in PS1 gene, compared to non-carriers family members of the PS1 mutation, showed lower white matter volume and integrity in the late myelinated regions at the presymptomatic stage of the disease [47, 49].

The processes of myelination and formation of fibrillary lesions also seem to influence each other in a two-way interaction. Oligodendrocytes express tau-positive fibrillary tangles in their cytoplasm similarly to neuronal NFTs. Mutations in tau protein are responsible for oligodendroglial fibrillary lesions as well. It is suggested that NFTs would contribute to oligodendrocyte dysfunction *via* oxidative stress and neuroinflammation [50, 51].

Bartzoki's ideas can be expanded to pathologic processes seen in other progressive neurodegenerative diseases. Quantifying myelin breakdown throughout life advance using magnetic resonance imaging might be a new promising diagnostic tool for AD and other neurodegenerative disorders [51, 52].

Pigmentation

The degree of neuronal pigmentation is other important cellular characteristic that is suggested to influence the susceptibility to develop AD. Studies report that NFTs appear early and in higher densities in late myelinating brain regions. These areas start to become pigmented earlier, previously of early myelinated neurons, in which pigmentation is usually delayed and merged. All neurons that remain without lipofuscin or neuromelanin aggregations – or those which present just a few granules – in advanced age are not affected by AD neurodegeneration in any stage of the disease. The solitary cells of Cajal and projection neurons from the lateral mammillary nucleus of hypothalamus are examples of these cells with lack of pigmentation that resist to neurodegeneration lesions, such NFTs [20, 24].

Cognitive Reserve: An Eminent Influencing Factor on Selective Morphologic Brain Changes Delaying the Onset of Cognitive Decline in AD

Besides morphological and molecular factors, lifestyle has a considerable influence on brain resilience to AD development. Particularly those factors related to cognitive processes such as the level of education and bilingualism [53]. Activities that improve the cognitive performance throughout life are reflected in brain morphologic alteration. Cognitive reserve concept was introduced in order to explain the inconsistencies between the degree of brain damage and clinical symptoms among different AD patients. Studies suggest that life exposures such as education, occupation, and leisure activity can provide reserve against age-or AD related pathology This reserve is supposed to act in a compensatory way, preventing the accumulation of cell damages in pre-clinical stages and probably delaying the onset of the dementia. People with a higher cognitive reserve would manifest cognitive deficits only in an advanced staging of neuronal pathologic alterations in AD [54, 55]. A cohort study carried by Serra and colleagues, using MRI technique, is a good example of how cognitive reserve can be related to brain morphology and early cognitive failures. In this study, subjects with amnesic mild cognitive impairment (MCI) that had a higher level of formal education performed better in some cognitive tasks that involved visuo-spatial abilities compared to subjects with a lower level of education. They also had greater volumes of grey matter in some brain areas such as the supramarginal gyus, the frontal opercular cortex and the right posterior cingulate/precuneus. In contrast, these same subjects – with a higher level of education – showed reduced volumes of the grey matter in the temporal poles and entorhinal cortices. These data suggest that cognitive reserve is more based on some specific located "brain" reserves than in a general enhancement of the neuroplasticity in the whole brain [56].

Imaging studies performed by Gold and colleagues showed that lifelong bilingualism indeed increases cognitive reserve. Elderly bilingual subjects with similar levels of cognitive performance presented a higher microstructural white matter integrity compared to monolingual subjects. Particularly, in brain areas such the fornix, inferior longitudinal fasciculus and corpus callosum. The cognitive reserve of the bilingual subjects would contribute to protects against the reduction of white matter integrity during aging and prevent more severe cognitive deficits [53].

The following schematic graphic (Fig. **2**) illustrates how the cognitive reserve could interfere in the relation between pathology alterations in AD and its clinical outcome. Besides having a late onset of AD proper dementia, Yaakov Stern group showed that after the first signal of cognitive symptoms, people with higher cognitive reserves show more rapid decline in cognitive functions [57].

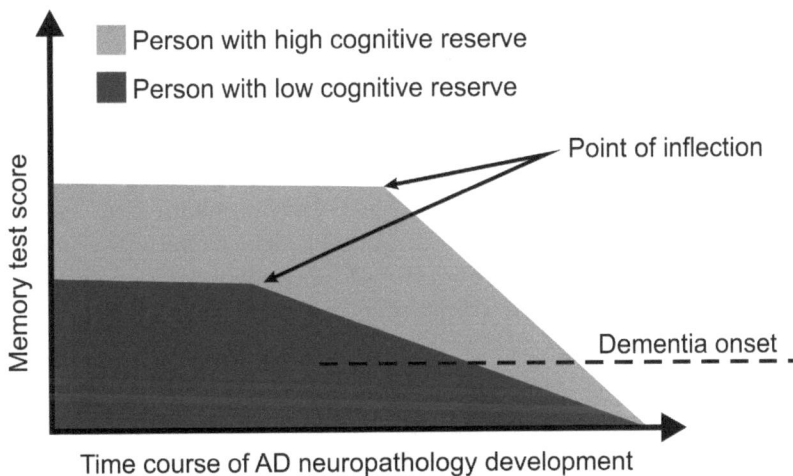

Fig. (2). The relation between cognitive reserve and AD neuropathology (adapted from Stern) [57].

Pathological Changes from One Neuron to Another

There is a growing interest in the investigation of the mechanisms that underlie the early and pre-symptomatic phase of AD. The vulnerability of neurons subsets, in specific brain areas, does not fully explain the cellular damage dissemination through the brain in AD course. For example, the same cell type, cortical pyramidal cells, are susceptible to develop lesions in the layer Va while those in the layer IV are resistant. Although morphological individual characteristics between cells subpopulations are taken into account, the assumption of different vulnerabilities does not consider that all of the affected brain regions and subpopulations are, in a higher or lower level, anatomically interconnected [58].

It has been postulated a recent theory that aggregates of misfolded or hyperphosphorylated tau protein of the pretangle material could be transmitted through the axons transynaptically like a viral particle as prion-like protein. These pathological molecules would be released in the synaptic cleft, probably mediated by structures such exosomes, and somehow would be absorbed by the postsynaptic neuron. Once in the postsynaptic site, these damaged protein aggregates are supposed to function as a template to induce the generation of more misfolded and truncated proteins, triggering the accumulation of abnormal tau protein in the recipient neuron [20, 58].

This theory of neuron-to-neuron propagation is congruent to recent findings that AD pathology begins in the locus coeruleus even prior to reach the cerebral cortex. In a cohort study with under 30 years old subjects, with no evidence of tau pathology, it was observed that most of them had tau protein pretangles in subcortical regions such brainstem and did not presented pretangles or NFTs in the transentorhinal area. In theory, the last one is more vulnerable to degeneration. Thus, subcortical nuclei could send abnormal molecules to the cortical nerve cells nerve cells given that they are interconnected synaptically by ascending projections. It would stimulate the pathological alterations into the pyramidal cells of transentorhinal or entorhinal areas. From there, dissemination would follow the perforant pathway in the direction of hippocampal formation. From transentorhinal region, damaged molecules are transmitted toward neocortical association areas, such adjacent high order association regions of the basal temporal neocortex and prefrontal cortex. These regions are generally more affected in the late stages of AD. In parallel to the pathologic dissemination during AD development, it is suggested that the proper locus coeruleus accumulates pathologic damages inside itself. It could explain why this area becomes gradually intensely affected by NFTs until advanced stages of AD. These findings highlight a potential field for therapeutically designed studies focusing in the early phase of AD, when pathologic damage is still restricted to the brainstem, before to disseminate through cortical areas [20, 58].

ANATOMICAL PATTERNS OF ALTERATION THROUGHOUT AD STAGES

Although the brain degeneration is the major factor underlying dementia, it is not required for AD diagnosis. A possible reason is the fact that brain volume is hard to be measured by imaging techniques. The difficulty to determine atrophy with great accuracy is due to the big differences regarding to brain size and shape among individuals. In addition, the aging process *per se* promotes a gradual atrophy of the white matter, what makes the differences among healthy and AD individuals even more diffuse. Nevertheless, there is a well-established rate of brain atrophy as soon as AD is clinically diagnosed – about 2.4% a year. The loss of volume is more accentuated in the inferior and fusiform gyri, amygdala, superior and middle frontal gyri, hippocampus and entorhinal cortex. Brain atrophy can be caused by both cell shrinkage and/or synaptic loss. It is believed that the main reason that could trigger neuronal atrophy is the development of neurofibrillary tangles with abnormal tau protein. Yet, several other factors may influence such oxidative stress, inflammation, vascular changes and amyloid deposition [59].

While AD pathology progresses, the cognitive symptoms appear and are accentuated, the neurofibrillary lesions gradually extend from transentorhinal region to hippocampal formation, amygdala, neocortex associative areas and motor and sensory regions. This expansion of neurofribrillary lesions accompanies most of the pattern of brain atrophy. The sequence of the neurodegeneration process is relatively similar among patients and is discriminated into six phases based on the evolution of neurofibrillary changes over the brain. Previous to the six stages of NFTs development and dissemination, there is still two earlier phases designed 1a and 1b. They are characterized by the formation of tau pretangles [60, 61].

Initial Stages Ia and Ib – Pretangle Formation

A special attention has been dedicated to investigate the mechanisms underlying the earlier stages of AD. Inasmuch as throughout the pretangle phases there are only abnormalities in respect to tau protein and absence of β-amyloid pathologic alterations. The study of therapies that target specific action against prefibrillar changes of tau and prevent the onset of clinical symptoms is a promising field. The early product of the pathological processes of phosphorylation is a form of tau protein that is still soluble and non-argyrophilic. It is still obscure how long the pretangle stage can last. The second hallmark in the progress of the neurofibrillary pathology is the aggregation of tau in insoluble and argyrophilic precipitates. As mentioned before, after appearing initially in subcortical regions such the locus coeruleus, the pretangle pathologic processes in AD are spread through the cerebral cortex, primarily to the transentorhinal region. The phase when occurs this transition to cortical areas is designated "cortical stage 1a" of tau pathology. During the cortical stage 1b, the initial subcortical lesions are accompanied by inclusions of abnormal tau protein in the pyramidal cells of transentorhinal region. However, at the second stage, the abnormal material appears in dendrites and, after then, reaches the soma and the axon. In locus coeruleus, instead, the lesions appear initially in the axon [20, 61, 62]. Afterwards, the pyramidal cells have their dendrites morphology altered. They are filled by tau aggregates in the course of AD, acquiring a swollen, curled and twisted aspect. With the advance of AD, due to the insurgence of structures that look like short appendages, the distal segments of these modified dendrites become detached from the proximal regions. Hereafter, the isolated branches are completely degraded. The distal segments are developed just when there is a high degree of neuronal maturation and are responsible to make contact to late-maturing pyramidal cells. These facts just corroborate how interesting and efficient can be the use of maturation as a tool to predict neuron resistance to AD. Not only the degree of the whole neuron maturation, but also of the neuronal cell structures – according to its emergence stage, onto and phylogenetically – can protect or enhance neuronal susceptibility to AD [20, 61, 62]. The mechanisms by which neuronal axon from brainstem transmits aggregates of tau protein to the transentorhinal region are still not completely clear. It is probable that, just a small part of the abnormal material would find sites to bind in the somatodendritic compartment of the recipient neuron and thereat most of it would exist in the cytosol in a hyperphosphorylated and aggregated state. In the progress of AD, all these affected cells could live through the pretangle phase without developing insoluble neuropil threads (NTs) and NFTs for years, although their functional integrity can be prejudiced along the time advance. The abnormal tau material forms a viscous mass, which is slowly distributed along all the portions of the long axon of neurons from corpus coeruleus until reach more distal parts of the axon and be disseminated [20, 60 - 64].

Stages 1 and 2 – The Onset of NFTs Dissemination

In stages I and II, the lesions are still restricted to a few outputs from transentorhinal region. The entorhinal region and CA1 and CA2 fields are generally affected only late in the stage II. The entorhinal region proper remains unchanged or is just minimally affected. Although this mild deterioration might be harmful enough to affect the outflow of information to neocortex, these pathologic changes are generally not sufficient to trigger the manifestation of clinical symptoms [20, 61].

In the stage I, there is also probably a dissemination of lesions to the spinal cord and olfactory bulb such as most of the non-thalamic nuclei with diffuse cortical projection, which have developed at this point at least some degree of tau pathology. Cholinergic projections cells from the basal forebrain and neurons of the hypothalamic tuberomamillary nucleus present also abnormal tau material. Some studies suggested that abnormal tau material would be transmitted *via* descending projections from nucleus subcoeruleus and the caudal raphe nuclei to the lower brainstem and spinal cord, extending from cervical to sacral segments of the brain [20, 65].

A study performed by Dugger and collaborators, comparing subjects with AD and non-demented (ND) individuals showed that the cervical segments are the part of spine cord most affected by tau phosphorylation (96% AD *vs*. 43% ND), followed by thoracic, lumbar and sacral. In addition, they found that the spinal cord was indeed affected in early stages of AD, before dementia. While 0% of AD cases presented p-tau in the spine at the Braak stage 0, 40% of subjects in stage I presented immunoreactivity for p-tau in some segment and all subjects with tau phosphorylation in the spine cord presented also p-tau in the brain. Following Braak stages II, III, IV, V and VI, phosphorylated tau protein was found in the spine cord of 60%, 64%, 89%, 93% and 100% of AD patients, respectively. Phosphorylated tau in the stage I is mostly present in the cervical segment of spine cord, followed by thoracic and lumbar segment. P-tau appears in the sacral segment only in the stage II [65].

Later, still at stage I, the entorhinal cellular layers pre-α, pri-α and occasionally also the deeper one pri-β are taken by neurofibrillary changes targeting the transition to the adjacent temporal neocortex. In parallel, areas involved in olfactory system are also affected *i.e.* the anterior olfactory nucleus and the mitral and tufted cells of olfactory bulb. In the subsequent stages of AD, other components of the olfactory system such the olfactory area of the amygdala and the ambient gyrus of the entorhinal region are also damaged by neurofibrillary lesions [20]. As consequence of the intense degeneration in the olfactory bulb and in the olfactory cortical structures, the olfactory tract is also damaged, losing their density. The moment when occurs the appearance of AD damages in the brain areas of the olfactory system can vary among different studies, depending on factors such the exact layer of olfactory bulb in which the histological analysis has been performed. Nevertheless, it is almost consensual that at the end of stage II, at least part of the olfactory system is compromised. Imaging investigations showed that even subjects with mild cognitive impairment have presented atrophy in the olfactory bulb and the olfactory tract and that this atrophy was correlated with the scores of cognitive performance, measured by the Mini Mental State Examination [66].

At the stage II, the presubiculum area is not involved yet, but in the hippocampal formation, pyramidal cells of CA1 and CA2 already commence to present positive immunoreactivity to tau protein phosphorylation. Meanwhile, despite the well-established dissemination of neurofibrillary changes, the β-amyloid deposition is only observed at the stage III [20].

Thus, phase I and II can still be considered preclinical stages, which are characterized by a silent advance of neurofibrillary alterations. There is a transition between pretangle phase and the formation of the proper NFTs and NTs, fully insoluble and argyrophilic. The argyrophilic material that was present before predominantly in dendritic branching is now extending to other portions and generates NTs. It still obscure why NTs precede the appearance of NFTs in the pyramidal cells [20, 63].

Stages III and IV – The Advance of AD Pathology Through Limbic Areas and the Beginning of Clinical Features

The stage III is highlighted by the increase of the degree of severity in the pathological involvement of transentorhinal and entorhinal regions. The hippocampal formation, temporal and insular cortical areas and also a few subcortical nuclei remain slightly affected by neurofibrillary changes [61]. In the stage IV, the neurodegeneration processes extend from the entorhinal area to the adjacent neocortex. The neocortex is involved at this point by tau pathology not only in the basal temporal fields as seen in previous stages, but as well in the insular, anterior cingulate, subgenual and anterogenual regions. The only neocortical area that remains intact or very subtly involved is the occipital neocortex [20].

Generally, the lesions disseminate through the brain in a symmetric way between the two lateral hemispheres. One hemisphere may be only one stage behind the other in the regular sequence of the progression of the pathologic changes. In the stages III and IV, the lesions are already able to promote the first consistent functional disturbs. The limbic system is compromised at multiples sites (stages III and IV are also designed limbic stages), affecting the interaction with the prefrontal cortex, reflecting in some cognitive deficits and personality alterations. At this point, some individuals may be still not have developed clinical symptoms depending on their cognitive reserve [61].

The neurofibrillary lesions present in the subcortical nuclei during the stage II worsen in stage III, reaching all the brainstem nuclei with diffuse cortical projections. In the stage III, lesions include the brainstem nuclei, that regulate the eye movements, including the Edingar Westphal nucleus, the interstitial nucleus of Cajal, the nucleus of Darkschewitsch and the rostral interstitial nucleus of the medial longitudinal fascicle. The last mentioned area is the most affected, presenting mild tau pathology since the earlier stages of AD and the degree of the severity grows in parallel to the development of the AD stages in the whole brain [20, 67]. In addition, the first abnormal tau material appears in the limbic nuclei of the thalamus (reuniens nucleus and anterodorsal nucleus) and the in anterodorsal portions of the reticulate nucleus of the thalamus. The central nucleus of the amygdala becomes damaged as well by tau abnormalities. Thus, besides the slowing of the vertical saccades caused by the damages in the visual processing regions, there is also an impairment of the high order processing of the autonomic system due to central amygdala lesions [20, 68].

In this stage of AD, it is common to notice agitation in the patients. This clinical feature is related to the dissemination of neurofibrillary tangles from areas earlier involved such the nucleus basalis of Meynert (which receives noradregenergic input from the locus coeruleus, affected even before), to regions where their cholinergic neurons project, such the amygdala and the cingulate cortex, which regulate emotional behavior [69]. The neurofibrillary damage into the amygdala becomes even more robust because of the serotoninergic afferents from raphe nuclei, which present at this point, higher capacity to transmit abnormal tau material [70].

Lesions in the limbic nuclei of the thalamus are more intensified and disseminated to the central nucleus of the amygdala, contributing for the enhancement of the amygdalar neurofibrillary changes. Neurofibrillary changes originated from thalamic nuclei might reach the cholinergic interneurons in the ventral and dorsal striatum (accumbens, putamen and caudate nuclei), without affecting the pallidum complex yet. At this point, the central and cortical amygdala nuclei have their lesions worsen and only the medial subnuclei are still unaffected. Abnormal tau material is also seen in the tectum and pars compacta of the substantia nigra and this presence can be related to the motor symptoms in AD [20].

Besides agitation, depression during AD is probably related to morphological alterations in the amygdala as well. Studies showed that patients with Lewy bodies in the amygdala are more susceptible to develop depression in the course of AD [71]. An exacerbation of β-amyloid deposition and neurofibrillary tangles in the amygdala could also trigger the development of behavioral symptoms in AD individuals, which are similar to Klüver-Bucy syndrome, such hypersexuality, hyperphagia, hyperorality and apathy [72].

In patients with AD, it was observed not only a reduced amygdalar volume compared to controls, but also a positive correlation between the cognitive performance and the amygdalar volume, measured by MRI. Although the general brain volume was reduced in AD patients, there was no correlation between the brain volume and cognitive performance [73]. Moreover, the amygdalar atrophy - as well as hippocampal - in healthy elderly presented potential to predict the risk of developing dementia in the next six years [74]. The volume of amygdala can be also used as a determinant factor to differentiate AD from other types of dementia like frontotemporal lobar degeneration (FTLD). Tests carried out by Barnes showed that hippocampal atrophy cannot be used to differentiate AD from FTLD, yet an asymmetrical atrophy of the amygdala suggests FTLD. In AD, as mentioned before, normally the neurodegeneration and cell loss follow a symmetric pattern between the two hemispheres [75].

Lesions that started to be disseminated along the components of the olfactory system at stage III reach not only the olfactory tract and bulb. The periamygdalar and piriform areas, as well as the regions of the entorhinal area and of the amygdala that participates of the olfactory information processing are lesioned. Imaging studies revealed that patients with MCI that posteriorly developed AD presented a greater volume loss in the olfactory network compared to those whose the MCI did not convert to AD [76]. The clinical symptoms seem to accompany the morphologic and molecular damage in the olfactory system. The presence of olfactory deficits in patients with MCI demonstrated to be determinant to predict the development of AD and it correlates with other features such hippocampal volume and the memory performance. Nevertheless, there was no correlation between alterations in the components of the olfactory system in the brain and β-amyloid burden [20, 66].

Meanwhile, in the stage III, more abnormal tau material accumulates in the neurits of the cells of more external layers of the entorhinal region, especially pre-α and pri- α layers, which play an important role in the exchange of information between the the entorhinal region, the neocortex and the hippocampal formation. Although the subiculum, presubiculum CA3 and CA4 are still not involved, the pyramidal cells of CA1 and CA2 become even more affected by pathologic changes. The dilations of dendritic branches, which started at stage II, are more pronounced during stage III, and ready to be eliminated from the cells mainly in the stages IV and V. Therefore, the neuronal interconnectivity, enhanced by synaptic plasticity, between the pyramidal cells of CA1 field and the perforant pathway are reduced. There is a partial disconnection between the hippocampus and the neocortex and consequently, an impairment of high-order cognitive processing. The peak of damages in the hippocampal formation is reached in the stage IV, when more external layers are involved and presented numerous neurofibrillary changes in the pre-β and pre-γ. The subiculum and presubiculum present their first tau aggregates and while CA1 and CA2 have intense neurofibrillary changes, driving to cell loss, CA3 and CA4 show their first tau lesions [20, 77].

With the advance of pathologic changes from transentorhinal region to adjacent neocortical areas, chandelier cells become involved. Chandelier cells are an exceptional case of neurons that remain free of lipofuscin granules or develop just a few granules and still become affected by tau pathology. Moreover, inhibitory cortical chandelier cells set a gabaergic local network and do not have a rich dendritic arborization, with many spine branches. This feature what was supposed to reduce even more the theoretical risk of developing AD. Chandelier cells, generally seen in the superficial layers of the basal temporal lobe, are the only type of cells under all these conditions that can present non-fibrillary tau material. For some reason, in this sort of local circuits, the non-argyrophilic inclusions never are converted to argyrophilic lesions. The appearance of abnormal tau material in chandelier cells probably leads to cell death quickly, without passing through NFT stage, because chandelier cells with abnormal tau are not seen in the stage IV. It is possible that their somatodendritic compartment fails in the conversion of abnormal tau to neurofibrillary filaments, which are supposed to be less toxic to the neurons. The death of specific chandelier cells in the same site may occur probably because only chandelier cells that are connected with the axons of pyramidal cells, containing abnormal tau material, would be affected. This material would be transferred in an axoaxonic way between the pyramidal and chandelier cells since the axon in chandelier cells is the first fraction affected by non-fibrillary inclusion, while soma and dendrites become rarely involved [20, 78].

Stages V and VI - Advanced AD

Along AD progression, the local lesions are extended reaching a larger number of brain regions. The apex of the injury extension is reached at the stages V and VI. As the lesions caused by the NFTs are spreading through the cortex, the cognitive symptoms are also getting worse. There is a correlation between clinical scores of dementia and the anatomical distribution of NFTs [20, 79] due to the fact that cortical amount of NFTs is related to mechanisms that promote cognitive deterioration [23, 60].

In the stage V, a great portion of motor cortex and sensory area is affected by neurodegenerative processes, including regions that had a mildly involvement until then. The occipital primary visual cortex (in the border of calcarine sulcus) is preserved, but the secondary and tertiary areas present crescent and severe damages. Besides the occipital cortex, lesions extend to prefrontal and polimodal areas of parietal and temporal neocortex. In the peristriate areas (belt regions) the damaged layers II and III have diffused NPs and a large number of AT8 immunoreactive (AT8-ir) pyramidal cells in layers IIIa, IIIb and V (most part of them containing argyrophilic NTs/NFTs). The lower border of IIIa and b layers blurs in the transition between these and IIIc and IV layers (outer line of Baillarger). On the other hand, the deep plexus of Vb layer (inner line of Baillarger) remains narrow and the injury does not tend to extend to layer VI and whiter matter. The parastriate areas are less affected, but exhibit the same pattern in the border field with predominance of NPs clusters [20].

The plaque amounts increase following the progressive accumulation of NFTs and PHF-τ to a maximum of types and components in NFT-stage V, and then it has a slightly decrease [20, 79]. The end-stage of pathological process is the stage VI when the primary sensory neocortex region and the premotor areas are also affected. Pyramidal cells of layers III, Va, and VI are the most damaged. Almost no layer remains intact with many AT8-ir neuronal processes that reach the layer Vb and the white substance. Later, many neocortical areas (most pronounced in the basal temporal region) display NPs with reduced immunoreactivity and Gallyas-positive argyrophilia that probably indicate neuronal degradation. The occipital lobe is gradually shaded by increases of NTs/NFTs density that were originated in primary visual field and parastriate areas and go through high order association ones. Layer V displays very dense networks of NTs, with Aβ deposition and NPs. The striate area shelters Aβ-plaques and dot-like deposits of A-β and the border of this region is interrupted by radially oriented AT8-ir axons. As result of all these deposits, the boundary between parastriate and peristriate regions becomes recognizable in the end-stage of AD cases. The AD progression is the same in allocortical and subcortical areas. In the entorhinal region, neurons of layers pre-α are almost completely lost, remaining only tombstone tangles. In dentate fascia, the granule cells are fully of argyrophilic globose NFTs. The colliculi is severe damaged by tau lesions and presents a large number of A---plaques, and NPs [20, 80]. Other subcortical nuclei suffer considerable aggregation of NFTs/NTs too. Striatum, amygdala, claustrum, reuniens and reticular nuclei of thalamus, tuberomammillary nucleus of hypothalamus and substantia nigra pars compacta are regions that present a lot of neurofibrillary processes, especially, in the end-stages of AD progression. However, for these areas, an individual variation must be considered [80]. Table **1** summarizes the pattern of spatial advance of the neurofibrillary lesions along the brain areas during AD development considering all stages (for more information, see Box **1** below).

Table 1. The gradual accumulation of neurofribrillary tangles (NFT) and neuropil threads (NT) throughout AD stages. Adapted from Braak & Braak, 1991.

Location	Stage					
	AD progression					
	I	II	III	IV	V	VI
Transentorhinal-Pre-α	i-+	+-++	++	+++g	+++g	+++g
Entorhinal-Pre-α	.-i	+	++	+++	+++g	+++g

(Table 1) contd.....

Location	Stage					
	AD progression					
	I	**II**	**III**	**IV**	**V**	**VI**
Anterodorsal nucleus of the thalamus	i	i-+	+-++	++	+++g	+++g
Entorhinal-Pri-α	.	i	+	+-++	++	+++g
Basal magnocellular complex	.	i	+	+-++	++	+++g
Amygdala	.	i	+	++	+++	+++g
Entorhinal-Pre-β	.	.	i	+	+-++	++
Association areas of the isocortex	.	.	i	+	+++	+++
Parastriate area of the isocortex	.	.	.-i	i-+	+	++
Striatum	.	.	i	i-+	+	++
Reuniens nucleus of the thalamus	.	.	i	+	++	+++
Tuberomamillary nucleus of the hypothalamus	.	.	i	+	++	+++
CA4: Non-pyramidal cells	.	.	.	i-+	+-++	+++g
Subiculum	.	.	.	i	+	+-++
Para-/Transsubiculum	.	.	.	.-i	+	++
Striate area of the isocortex	.	.	.	.-i	i-+	+
Claustrum	.	.	.	i	+	++
Reticular nucleus of the thalamus	.	.	.	i	+	++
Fascia dentata	.	.	.	.	.-i	+-++
CA4/CA3: Pyramidal cells	.	.	.	.	i-+	+-++
Presubiculum	.	.	.	.	.-i	+
Lateral tuberal nucleus of the hypothalamus	.	.	.	.	i	+
Substantia nigra *pars compacta*	.	.	.	.	i	+-++

The amount of altered molecules is labeled (.) when no aggregation is observable, (i) when there are isolated groups and (+) for few, (++) for moderate and (+++) for large agglomerates of NFT and NT. The presence of gost tangles is labeled with (g).

Cerebellum: A Special Case

For a long time, it had been thought that the cerebellum participated only of activities related to motor control. However, investigations about the cerebellum indicate that this encephalic structure has a cognitive role much bigger than merely being responsible for motoric function. Functional neuroimaging shows that cerebellum is activated during the execution of high order cognitive functions, which involve language, working memory, timing and prediction [81, 82]. Subjects with damaged cerebellum showed deficits in planning, learning, memory, judging and attention tasks. Therefore, the interest about the participation of cerebellum in AD, which was underrated before, started to grow.

Morphometric studies based on more accurate and sensitive techniques revealed alterations in cerebellum morphology, mostly during advanced stages of AD. The volume of cerebellum was 21% lower in the severe phase of AD, when compared to elderly control. This decrease was significant only in the cerebellar cortex (24% of volume reduction in the molecular layer and 22% in the granular layer) but not in the white matter. Also the amount of Purkinje cells was reduced in AD patients, 32% smaller than controls, correlating with the decreased volume in the molecular layer. The number of granular cells was also reduced and correlated to all the other decreases [83]. Yet, the loss of Purkinje cells is a phenomenon that occurs naturally during the ageing. Since healthy elderly and AD have a decrease in the number of Purkinje cells, it might be tricky to use this parameter to help in the diagnostic [84].

Despite all the morphologic changes that occurred in the cerebellum, this region, as well as the striatum, is known by remaining free of neuritic plaques. Diffuse plaques, which are present in the molecular layer of cerebellum, are immunopositive for A-β, but do not convert into neuritic plaques. Probably because it is necessary a sufficient density of cross-β sheet structures so that the primitive plaques become neuritic plaques. In regions early involved in AD pathology, such the transentorhinal area, there are high densities of neuritic plaques [20].

Differences in the Pattern of Morphologic Changes in Familial AD

In contrast to sporadic AD, which is normally developed late in the life and has a slow progression, the familial type of AD (FAD) can appear earlier, generally between 30 and 65 years of age, and promotes a rapid deterioration of the brain and behavior. In the same way as the cognitive clinical symptoms emerge in a different pattern when comparing sporadic and familial AD, the morphologic alterations throughout the brain are also distinct [85, 86]. Given that FAD can be originated from (one or more) mutations in different genes, such the presenilin or the apolipoprotein-E, the pattern of the pathology through the brain might be very distinct even among FAD individuals, depending on which mutations and genes are affected [87]. During FAD, PET imaging showed an atrophy of medial temporal structures (hippocampus and entorhinal cortex included), which is also reported in sporadic AD [88, 89]. However, in the FAD the advance of the amyloid plaques through the brain does not follow the same trends. Carriers of mutation in the presenilin 1 (PSEN1) gene in presymptomatic stages showed a greater amount of amyloid aggregates in the thalamus while patients with sporadic AD presented more amyloid retention in frontotemporal regions [90]. Other study with PET imaging reported an early amyloid presence in the striatum of PSEN1 carriers, which is not associated to cognitive symptoms. In addition, the carriers displayed less amyloid retention in cortical areas than sporadic AD patients [91]. Since carriers of mutations related to FAD generally have rapid cognitive deterioration and symptoms of alexia, agraphia and alexia, which associated to cortical damages, even presenting less amyloid aggregates in the cortex as described by the studies above, it is possible that the amyloid presence is less determinant to the onset of cognitive deficits in AD. This hypothesis is corroborated by the fact that sporadic AD patients present a slow progress of cognitive deterioration even though they have a greater cortical amyloid presence [86]. These cognitive deficits present in carriers of PSEN1 mutations are probably more related to the frontemporal tau pathology and cell loss [59].

However, in the both types of AD, the brain atrophy precedes the clinical symptoms onset. The concentration of β-1,42 in the CSF may decrease 25 years before the first symptoms of AD and amyloid plaques in the brain are displayed 15 years before clinical stages of AD [87, 92].

In a study comparing brain MR images of patients with early onset AD (EAD), generally corresponding to FAD, and late onset AD (LAD), generally corresponding to sporadic AD, it was noticed, after a correction for age, that the atrophy in the right and left temporal cortices, left amygdala, left posterior hippocampus and left posterior cingulate cortex was higher in EAD subjects. In addition, EAD group showed less intense atrophy in the anterior hippocampus and amygdala compared to LAD patients [86]. In relation to LAD, EAD patients showed also a greater atrophy in white matter, specifically of the splenium and genu of the corpus callosum and parahippocampal tract [93].

Even before the appearance of clinical cognitive symptoms, carriers of mutations associated to FAD (PS1 and APP genes) demonstrated a lower cortical thickness in six brain regions (entorhinal cortex, inferior parietal cortex, superior parietal cortex, superior parietal cortex, superior frontal cortex, supramarginal gyrus and precuneus) compared to non-carriers. The thickness in the presymptomatic phase was correlated to preclinical cognitive deficits and the subsequent cortical thinning. There were significant differences especially in the precuneus of ApoE4 carriers, which was thinner than in control subjects 4 years before the onset of clinical features of AD [94].

Generally, genetic forms of AD promote a greater cell loss compared to sporadic AD. It is still not very clear the reasons of this variability but it is speculated that mutations in the APP and PSEN1 genes lead to initial formation of NFTs in the CA fields of the hippocampus. On the other hand, NFTs in sporadic AD have their initial onset site preferentially in the entorhinal region [95]. In the AD type associated to PSEN1 mutations, the atrophy in the frontal and temporal areas seems to be even bigger than in FAD associated to APP mutations or sporadic AD. It probably occurs because mutations in PSEN1 trigger alterations in other substrates crucial to the development of AD pathology, such tau and Bcl2 proteins [59, 96]. Mutations in PSEN1 also stimulate the amyloid deposition, which may lead to amyloid angiopathy, particularly in the cerebellum [97]. Carriers of mutations in genes such APP and PSEN1 presented molecular alterations not only in the brain but also in the cerebrospinal liquid. Compared to non-carriers, carriers had significant lower levels of Aβ-42 and higher levels of total tau and p-tau, accompanied by a reduction in the volume of the left precuneus, the superior temporal gyrus and the fusiform gyrus [98]. Changes in the ApoE gene also strongly influence the alterations of the AD development pattern, in either sporadic or familial AD [99]. ApoE demonstrated to be a major factor for enhancing the susceptibility to neuronal death under AD conditions, especially the presence of an ApoE ε4 allele (ApoE4). In a context with pathological accumulation of tau protein, ApoE4 makes the neurons less resistant to degeneration, while its absence was protective against neuronal death. ApoE4 positive neurons have a greater innate immune reactivity, inducing more neuroinflammatory processes during neurodegenerative conditions, exacerbating damaging responses promoted by p-tau accumulation. Besides to enhance p-tau neuroinflammatory and neurotoxic capacity, ApoE4 presence also changes the pattern of abnormal p-tau spreading throughout the brain, altering the pattern of brain atrophy during AD course [100].

The presence of ApoE4, besides to increase to risk of developing AD, enhances the presence of p-tau [101] and reduces the thickness of the cortex in the left rostral, superior frontal and right caudal midfrontal regions, comparing to individuals ε3/3. Otherwise, the presence of the allele ε2 is neuroprotective, increasing the thickness of the cortex in a few areas of the temporal lobe and orbitofrontal region, compared to subjects ε3/3 and ε3/4 [102]. A study carried out by Manning and colleagues corroborates the pathologic role of the ApoE ε4 allele. Individuals ε4+ with AD or mild cognitive impairment presented a more intense atrophy of the temporal lobe, in particular of the hippocampus, than non-carriers of ε4 [103]. Lehtovirta and colleagues [104] reported before that ε4 could reduce the volume of right hippocampus and of the right hippocampus and of the right amygdala. The atrophy of these areas was associated to lower scores in memory tests than subjects with absence of ε4. Changes in the frontal lobe among carriers of ε2, ε3 or ε4 were not observed [104]. Nonetheless, in a MR study with non-demented individuals aging between 39 and 80 years, although it has been also found a lower volume of the right hippocampus in subjects ε4/4, ε4/3 and ε4/2 compared to ε3/, ε3/2 and ε2/2, it was not found any difference in the cognitive performance between the groups. In other words, in healthy subjects, the atrophy of the right hippocampus, even before late life stages and cognitive decline, might be a warning signal of the high risk to develop AD [105]. In healthy individuals with average age of 57 years, it was not noticed changes in the hippocampal volume were noticed, while the thickness of the cortices of entorhinal region and subiculum was reduced [106]. An investigation that studied individuals with similar age (61 years) reported that ε4 carriers besides to present reduced thickness in the subiculum and entorhinal region, had the general volume of the temporal lobe also reduced [107].

The variations described in the susceptibility of people with ε4 may be influenced not only by technical factors such the type of imaging analysis that was performed, but also by extra individual differences in family history. Subjects with previous cases of AD in the family and carrying ε4 showed tendency to present greater atrophy in the right posterior hippocampus, compared to ε4 carriers without family history of AD [108]. Besides the morphologic changes, MR analysis showed also alterations in the functionality of the hippocampus during memory tasks in subjects ε4+. The allele carriers presented a higher activation of cortical regions to compensate a subtle reduction of CA1, CA2, CA3 and dentate gyrus, despite of having any cognitive deficits. Therefore, the increase of extrahippocampal activation during memory processes is possibly a signal prior to morphologic and cognitive damages, which could be interesting to the early diagnosis of FAD associated to ε4 [109, 110].

Box 1. The five stages of β-amyloid deposition through the brain.

The development of β-amyloid plaques generally starts late in AD course and before A-β can be detected in the cerebrospinal fluid, brain regions such the amygdala, insula, precuneus e hippocampus are already suffering atrophy [120]. Although the distribution of the plaques throughout the brain follows a less predictable pattern compared to the appearance of tau abnormalities, the gradual deposition of β-amyloid can be divided in five phases. In the phase 1 of the Aβ dissemination (still in the form of diffuse plaques) appear initially into the less myelinated basal areas of the frontal and temporal neocortex. Next, during phase 2, the entorhinals layers pre- β and pre-γ and the CA1 field present their first amyloid deposits. Moreover, the amygdala and the insular and cingulate cortices can also present addition plaques during this phase yet. Phase 3 is characterized by the deposition of A-β in the dentate gyrus of the hippocampus and in the basal temporal neocortical areas, which are especially involved with memory processes. The striatum, magnocellular nuclei of the basal forebrain and part of thalamus and hypothalamus are also affected during phase 3. In phase 4, A-β deposits are expanded along other hippocampal and neocortical areas. At this point, brainstem has been also reached by A-β deposits, which are evident in the red nucleus and in the inferior colliculi of the mesencephalon. Finally, in the phase 5, A-β depositions are spread along the reticular formation (medulla) and the cerebellar cortex [20].

ADVANCES IN MORPHOLOGY STUDIES OF AD: NEW TECHNIQUES AND EXPERIMENTAL APPROACHES

Although thousands of studies aiming to understand better the mechanisms of AD are produced every year, there is currently no therapy to prevent, heal or even slow the progression of the AD pathology and clinical symptoms. At the same time, life expectation is growing in the whole world and consequently, the number of elderly people is rapidly increasing. Thus, there is a pressing need to find more advanced techniques to AD therapy as well as more precise diagnosis to avoid the huge financial burden demanded by AD patients (estimated in about US$ 600 billion in 2010). In general, the studies mostly focus the earlier phases of AD. These studies aim to find biomarkers to predict future clinical decline, discover crucial agents of the pathological mechanisms at this stages and neutralize their effects with innovative drugs [111].

As it is known, AD pathology does not promote a random pattern of degeneration in the brain. So, it becomes essential to establish an accurate map of the anatomical sequence of alterations along the years for understanding and tracking the dissemination of AD throughout the brain. The comprehension of these complex alterations would help to predict the course of cognitive decline, agitation, depression and other symptoms [112].

The most used tool to help in the diagnosis of AD is MR imaging, that contributes to the clinical cognitive evaluation. However, there are several variations of this technique, such functional MR, DTI-MR and others. Some studies try also to predict the risk of an individual to develop AD by developing computational analysis that convert the biological data obtained from MR imaging into equations and formulas. However, there are only few algorithms that now recreate the pattern of deterioration of cortical gray matter and the presence of amyloid and tau alterations [113]. A study conducted by Morra and colleagues originated an automated hippocampal segmentation, which they called the auto context model (ACM). After analyzing MR scans of 400 subjects (100 AD patients, 200 with MCI and 100 elderly controls), it was created binary maps of the hippocampus were created and normalized by age and gender. The statistical analysis showed that atrophy of the right hippocampus is associated with geriatric depression but not with cognitive decline or educational level [114]. Using MRI data from children and adolescents, Gogtay and Thompson [115] applied detailed 3D and 4D models to achieve the dynamic pattern of changes during the cortical maturation. Their constructed time-lapse maps were used to compare the grey matter in normal development and illness. The authors found that the trajectory of the changes in the healthy brain is the opposite from the neurodegenerative pattern seen in AD *i.e.*, the deficits appear first in the last maturated areas. The results support the hypothesis that the early myelination during cortical development protected the neuron from degeneration.

Differently from the typical MR, the functional MR allows to evaluate physiological parameters of the brain correlated to performance in cognitive tasks during AD. A new model of analysis proposed by Binnewijzend and colleagues, using resting-state functional MR was able to differentiate the patterns of functional connectivity among healthy elderly and subjects with AD or MCI. AD patients presented lower functional connectivity in the precuneus and the posterior cingulate cortex in relation to the controls and MCI subjects demonstrated intermediary levels of functional connectivity in these brain areas [116].

The proton magnetic resonance spectroscopy (MRS) deeps even further in the brain physiology, it allows a molecular approach by the assessment of cerebral metabolites. For example, this technique permits to measure glutamate and creatine by a non-invasive manner *in vivo*. An investigation carried out by Herminghaus (2003), using MRS, differentiated healthy subjects from AD patients analysing their levels of a few metabolites. In the same study, it was also observed a different pattern between patients with probable AD and the patients with probable vascular dementia. Metabolites attributed to cell loss and to atrophy were increased in both probable AD and vascular dementia subjects. Inositol was enhanced as well, suggesting the occurrence of gliosis. Yet, AD patients presented a pattern of alterations that was predominantly observed in frontotemporal areas while vascular dementia patients showed a subcortical pattern of alterations. This study demonstrates a potential contribution of MRS as a tool for more precise diagnostic classification of dementias [117].

With the advent of positron emission tomography (PET), it becomes possible to extrapolate the morphologic evaluations from a macro to a micro level. Based on changes in cerebral blood flow and metabolism, PET promotes a more accurate and detailed analysis. For example, using fluoro-deoxyglucose PET (FDG-PET) scanning, hypometabolism was detected in the posterior cingulate cortex during an AD stage when no atrophy evidence was observed by MR imaging. With the constant insurgence of new probes and tracers, PET has allowed a growing capacity of evaluate even deeper the molecular mechanisms underlying the AD development. Recently, there is a renewed interest in track AD using PET new probes sensitive to A-β or neurofibrillary tangles pathology, or both. These new tools are being used to understand how the A-β spreads in the living brain. Although the techniques are still susceptible to sample size, population studied and methods of reconstruction, amyloid PET seems to be useful for detection of early stages of AD [112]. Aiming to elucidate the correlation between the A-β deposition and the astrocytosis, a study combined the multitracer PET imaging, the postmortem autoradiography and the immunohistochemistry analysis of an AD transgenic mouse model (APPswe). The authors found that in early stages of AD, the astrocytosis is noticed even before the appearance of amyloid aggregates. These results highlight the heterogeneous and context-dependent astrocytosis during AD progression, supporting the need of more studies to clarify the functions of different astrocyte populations during the progression of the pathology [118].

According to Hickman and colleagues, AD is one of most difficult clinical challenges of the century. Some of AD biomarkers, risk factors and their implications for the development of new treatments have to be studied in depth. Future works, focusing the earlier stages of AD, are the promising bet to the development of new treatments and the prevention of cognitive decline. Even after extensive study, nowadays, AD remains as a progressive and incurable disease [119].

CONSENT FOR PUBLICATION

Not applicable.

CONFLICT OF INTERESTS

The authors declare no conflict of interests.

ACKNOWLEDGEMENT

Declared none.

REFERENCES

[1]   Weyandt LL. The physiological bases of cognitive and behavioral disorders. Lawrence Erlbaum Associates, Inc. 2006.

[2]   Kipnis J, Filiano AJ. Neuroimmunology in 2017: The central nervous system: privileged by immune connections. Nat Rev Immunol 2018; 18(2): 83-4.
        [http://dx.doi.org/10.1038/nri.2017.152] [PMID: 29279610]

[3]   Keith L Moore, TVN Persaud MGT.. Before we are Born: Essentials of Embriology and Birth Defects. 2016

[4]   Oberman L, Pascual-Leone A. Changes in plasticity across the lifespan: cause of disease and target for intervention. Prog Brain Res 2013; 207: 91-120.
        [http://dx.doi.org/10.1016/B978-0-444-63327-9.00016-3] [PMID: 24309252]

[5]   Petanjek Z, Judaš M, Šimic G, et al. Extraordinary neoteny of synaptic spines in the human prefrontal cortex. Proc Natl Acad Sci USA 2011; 108(32): 13281-6.
        [http://dx.doi.org/10.1073/pnas.1105108108] [PMID: 21788513]

[6]   Blumberg MS, Freeman JH, Robinson SR. Oxford handbook of developmental behavioral neuroscience. Oxford Univ Press 2010; p. 784.

[7]   Kolb B, Mychasiuk R, Gibb R. Brain development, experience, and behavior. Pediatr Blood Cancer

2014; 61(10): 1720-3.
[http://dx.doi.org/10.1002/pbc.24908] [PMID: 24376085]

[8]   Pascual-Leone A, Freitas C, Oberman L, *et al.* Characterizing brain cortical plasticity and network dynamics across the age-span in health and disease with TMS-EEG and TMS-fMRI. Brain Topogr 2011; 24(3-4): 302-15.
[http://dx.doi.org/10.1007/s10548-011-0196-8] [PMID: 21842407]

[9]   Sale A, Berardi N, Maffei L. Environment and brain plasticity: towards an endogenous pharmacotherapy. Physiol Rev 2014; 94(1): 189-234.
[http://dx.doi.org/10.1152/physrev.00036.2012] [PMID: 24382886]

[10]   Tshala-Katumbay D, Mwanza J-C, Rohlman DS, Maestre G, Oriá RB. A global perspective on the influence of environmental exposures on the nervous system. Nature 2015; 527(7578): S187-92.
[http://dx.doi.org/10.1038/nature16034] [PMID: 26580326]

[11]   Berardi N, Sale A, Maffei L. Brain structural and functional development: genetics and experience. Dev Med Child Neurol 2015; 57 (Suppl. 2): 4-9.
[http://dx.doi.org/10.1111/dmcn.12691] [PMID: 25690109]

[12]   Weaver ICGG.. Integrating early life experience, gene expression, brain development, and emergent phenotypes: unraveling the thread of nature *via* nurture. vol. 86C. 2014

[13]   Thirumala P, Hier DB, Patel P. Motor recovery after stroke: lessons from functional brain imaging. Neurol Res 2002; 24(5): 453-8.
[http://dx.doi.org/10.1179/016164102101200320] [PMID: 12117313]

[14]   Dennis M, Spiegler BJ, Simic N, *et al.* Functional plasticity in childhood brain disorders: when, what, how, and whom to assess. Neuropsychol Rev 2014; 24(4): 389-408.
[http://dx.doi.org/10.1007/s11065-014-9261-x] [PMID: 24821533]

[15]   Fine JG, Sung C. Neuroscience of child and adolescent health development. J Couns Psychol 2014; 61(4): 521-7.
[http://dx.doi.org/10.1037/cou0000033] [PMID: 25285711]

[16]   Ohnishi T, Matsuda H, Tabira T, Asada T, Uno M. Changes in brain morphology in Alzheimer disease and normal aging: is Alzheimer disease an exaggerated aging process? AJNR Am J Neuroradiol 2001; 22(9): 1680-5.
[PMID: 11673161]

[17]   Arriagada PV, Marzloff K, Hyman BT. Distribution of Alzheimer-type pathologic changes in nondemented elderly individuals matches the pattern in Alzheimer's disease. Neurology 1992; 42(9): 1681-8.
[http://dx.doi.org/10.1212/WNL.42.9.1681] [PMID: 1307688]

[18]   Brayne C, Calloway P. Normal ageing, impaired cognitive function, and senile dementia of the Alzheimer's type: a continuum? Lancet 1988; 1(8597): 1265-7.
[http://dx.doi.org/10.1016/S0140-6736(88)92081-8] [PMID: 2897526]

[19]   Byun MS, Kim SE, Park J, *et al.* Alzheimer's Disease Neuroimaging Initiative. Heterogeneity of regional brain atrophy patterns associated with distinct progression rates in Alzheimer's disease. PLoS One 2015; 10(11): e0142756.
[http://dx.doi.org/10.1371/journal.pone.0142756] [PMID: 26618360]

[20]   Braak H, Del Tredici K. Neuroanatomy and pathology of sporadic Alzheimer's disease 2015.
[http://dx.doi.org/10.1007/978-3-319-12679-1]

[21]   Arendt T. Alzheimer's disease as a loss of differentiation control in a subset of neurons that retain immature features in the adult brain. Neurobiol Aging 2000; 21(6): 783-96.
[http://dx.doi.org/10.1016/S0197-4580(00)00216-5] [PMID: 11124422]

[22]   Mattson MP, Magnus T. Ageing and neuronal vulnerability. Nat Rev Neurosci 2006; 7(4): 278-94.
[http://dx.doi.org/10.1038/nrn1886] [PMID: 16552414]

[23]   Braak H, Braak E. Frequency of stages of Alzheimer-related lesions in different age categories. Neurobiol Aging 1997; 18(4): 351-7.
[http://dx.doi.org/10.1016/S0197-4580(97)00056-0] [PMID: 9330961]

[24]   Braak H, Del Tredici K, Schultz C, Braak E. Vulnerability of select neuronal types to Alzheimer's disease. Ann N Y Acad Sci 2000; 924: 53-61.
[http://dx.doi.org/10.1111/j.1749-6632.2000.tb05560.x] [PMID: 11193802]

[25]   Morrison BM, Hof PR, Morrison JH. Determinants of neuronal vulnerability in neurodegenerative diseases. Ann Neurol 1998; 44(3) (Suppl. 1): S32-44.
[http://dx.doi.org/10.1002/ana.410440706] [PMID: 9749571]

[26]   Jeffery KJ, Reid IC. Modifiable neuronal connections: an overview for psychiatrists. Am J Psychiatry 1997; 154(2): 156-64.
[http://dx.doi.org/10.1176/ajp.154.2.156] [PMID: 9016262]

[27]   Hasselmo ME. A computational model of the progression of Alzheimer's disease. MD Comput 1997; 14(3): 181-91.
[PMID: 9151508]

[28]   Arendt T, Brückner MK, Bigl V. Maintenance of neuronal plasticity in the reticular core and changes in trophic activity in Alzheimer's disease. Ann N Y Acad Sci 1991; 640: 210-4.
[http://dx.doi.org/10.1111/j.1749-6632.1991.tb00219.x] [PMID: 1776741]

[29]   Arendt T, Brückner MK, Gertz HJ, Marcova L. Cortical distribution of neurofibrillary tangles in Alzheimer's disease matches the pattern of neurons that retain their capacity of plastic remodelling in the adult brain. Neuroscience 1998; 83(4): 991-1002.
[http://dx.doi.org/10.1016/S0306-4522(97)00509-5] [PMID: 9502241]

[30]   Arendt T, Bruckner MK, Bigl V, Marcova L. Dendritic reorganisation in the basal forebrain under degenerative conditions and its defects in Alzheimer's disease. II. Ageing, Korsakoff's disease, Parkinson's disease, and Alzheimer's disease 1995; 222: 198-222.

[31]   Braak H, Braak E. Development of Alzheimer-related neurofibrillary changes in the neocortex inversely recapitulates cortical myelogenesis. Acta Neuropathol 1996; 92(2): 197-201.
[http://dx.doi.org/10.1007/s004010050508] [PMID: 8841666]

[32]   Braak H, Tredici DEL, Schultz C, Braak EVA. Vulnerability of select neuronal types to alzheimer's disease 2000.
[http://dx.doi.org/10.1111/j.1749-6632.2000.tb05560.x]

[33]   Fuster JM. Frontal lobe and cognitive development. J Neurocytol 2002; 31(3-5): 373-85.
[http://dx.doi.org/10.1023/A:1024190429920] [PMID: 12815254]

[34]   Flechsig Of Leipsic P. Developmental (myelogenetic) localisation of the cerebral cortex in the human subject. Lancet 1901; 158: 1027-30.
[http://dx.doi.org/10.1016/S0140-6736(01)01429-5]

[35]   Nagy Z, Esiri MM, Cato AM, Smith AD. Cell cycle markers in the hippocampus in Alzheimer's disease. Acta Neuropathol 1997; 94(1): 6-15.
[http://dx.doi.org/10.1007/s004010050665] [PMID: 9224524]

[36]   Wheal HV, Chen Y, Mitchell J, *et al.* Molecular mechanisms that underlie structural and functional changes at the postsynaptic membrane during synaptic plasticity. Prog Neurobiol 1998; 55(6): 611-40.
[http://dx.doi.org/10.1016/S0301-0082(98)00026-4] [PMID: 9670221]

[37]   Lepelletier F-X, Mann DMA, Robinson AC, Pinteaux E, Boutin H. Early changes in extracellular matrix in Alzheimer's disease. Neuropathol Appl Neurobiol 2015.
[PMID: 26544797]

[38]   Thangavel R, Van Hoesen GW, Zaheer A. The abnormally phosphorylated tau lesion of early Alzheimer's disease. Neurochem Res 2009; 34(1): 118-23.

[http://dx.doi.org/10.1007/s11064-008-9701-1] [PMID: 18437565]

[39] Ferrer I, Soriano E, Tuñón T, Fonseca M, Guionnet N. Parvalbumin immunoreactive neurons in normal human temporal neocortex and in patients with Alzheimer's disease. J Neurol Sci 1991; 106(2): 135-41.
[http://dx.doi.org/10.1016/0022-510X(91)90250-B] [PMID: 1802961]

[40] Chan-Palay VC, Zetzsche T, Höchli M. Parvalbumin neurons in the hippocampus in senile dementia of the alzheimer type, parkinson's disease and multi-infarct dementia. Dement Geriatr Cogn Disord 1991; 2: 297-313.
[http://dx.doi.org/10.1159/000107221]

[41] Fonseca M, Soriano E, Ferrer I, Martinez A, Tuñon T. Chandelier cell axons identified by parvalbumin-immunoreactivity in the normal human temporal cortex and in Alzheimer's disease. Neuroscience 1993; 55(4): 1107-16.
[http://dx.doi.org/10.1016/0306-4522(93)90324-9] [PMID: 8232900]

[42] Bartzokis G. Age-related myelin breakdown: a developmental model of cognitive decline and Alzheimer's disease. Neurobiol Aging 2004; 25(1): 5-18.
[http://dx.doi.org/10.1016/j.neurobiolaging.2003.03.001] [PMID: 14675724]

[43] Noble M. The possible role of myelin destruction as a precipitating event in Alzheimer's disease. Neurobiol Aging 2004; 25(1): 25-31.
[http://dx.doi.org/10.1016/j.neurobiolaging.2003.07.001] [PMID: 14675726]

[44] Peters A, Sethares C. Aging and the myelinated fibers in prefrontal cortex and corpus callosum of the monkey. J Comp Neurol 2002; 442(3): 277-91.
[http://dx.doi.org/10.1002/cne.10099] [PMID: 11774342]

[45] Bartzokis G. Quadratic trajectories of brain myelin content: unifying construct for neuropsychiatric disorders. Neurobiol Aging 2004; 25: 49-62.
[http://dx.doi.org/10.1016/j.neurobiolaging.2003.08.001]

[46] Cai Z, Xiao M. Oligodendrocytes and Alzheimer's disease. Int J Neurosci 2015.
[PMID: 26000818]

[47] Bartzokis G. Alzheimer's disease as homeostatic responses to age-related myelin breakdown. Neurobiol Aging 2011; 32(8): 1341-71.
[http://dx.doi.org/10.1016/j.neurobiolaging.2009.08.007] [PMID: 19775776]

[48] Bartzokis G, Lu PH, Mintz J. Human brain myelination and amyloid beta deposition in Alzheimer's disease. Alzheimers Dement 2007; 3(2): 122-5.
[http://dx.doi.org/10.1016/j.jalz.2007.01.019] [PMID: 18596894]

[49] Ringman JM, O'Neill J, Geschwind D, *et al.* Diffusion tensor imaging in preclinical and presymptomatic carriers of familial Alzheimer's disease mutations. Brain 2007; 130(Pt 7): 1767-76.
[http://dx.doi.org/10.1093/brain/awm102] [PMID: 17522104]

[50] Desai MK, Sudol KL, Janelsins MC, Mastrangelo MA, Frazer ME, Bowers WJ. Triple-transgenic Alzheimer's disease mice exhibit region-specific abnormalities in brain myelination patterns prior to appearance of amyloid and tau pathology. Glia 2009; 57(1): 54-65.
[http://dx.doi.org/10.1002/glia.20734] [PMID: 18661556]

[51] Cai Z, Xiao M. Oligodendrocytes and Alzheimer's disease. Int J Neurosci 2016; 126(2): 97-104.
[http://dx.doi.org/10.3109/00207454.2015.1025778] [PMID: 26000818]

[52] Bartzokis G, Lu PH, Mintz J. Quantifying age-related myelin breakdown with MRI: novel therapeutic targets for preventing cognitive decline and Alzheimer's disease. J Alzheimers Dis 2004; 6(6) (Suppl.): S53-9.
[PMID: 15665415]

[53] Gold BT, Johnson NF, Powell DK. Lifelong bilingualism contributes to cognitive reserve against white matter integrity declines in aging. Neuropsychologia 2013; 51(13): 2841-6.

[http://dx.doi.org/10.1016/j.neuropsychologia.2013.09.037] [PMID: 24103400]

[54]   Stern Y. Cognitive reserve in ageing and Alzheimer's disease. Lancet Neurol 2012; 11(11): 1006-12.
[http://dx.doi.org/10.1016/S1474-4422(12)70191-6] [PMID: 23079557]

[55]   Erickson KI, Weinstein AM, Lopez OL.. Physical activity, brain plasticity, and Alzheimer's disease. Archives of Medical Research 2012; 43(8): 615-21.
[http://dx.doi.org/doi.org/10.1016/j.arcmed.2012.09.008] [PMID: 23085449]

[56]   Serra L, Cercignani M, Petrosini L, *et al.* Neuroanatomical correlates of cognitive reserve in Alzheimer disease. Rejuvenation Res 2011; 14(2): 143-51.
[http://dx.doi.org/10.1089/rej.2010.1103] [PMID: 21204647]

[57]   Stern Y. Cognitive reserve. Neuropsychologia 2009; 47(10): 2015-28.
[http://dx.doi.org/10.1016/j.neuropsychologia.2009.03.004] [PMID: 19467352]

[58]   Braak H, Del Tredici K. Alzheimer's pathogenesis: is there neuron-to-neuron propagation? Acta Neuropathol 2011; 121(5): 589-95.
[http://dx.doi.org/10.1007/s00401-011-0825-z] [PMID: 21516512]

[59]   Shepherd C, McCann H, Halliday GM. Variations in the neuropathology of familial Alzheimer's disease. Acta Neuropathol 2009; 118(1): 37-52.
[http://dx.doi.org/10.1007/s00401-009-0521-4] [PMID: 19306098]

[60]   Abner EL, Kryscio RJ, Schmitt FA, *et al.* "End-stage" neurofibrillary tangle pathology in preclinical Alzheimer's disease: fact or fiction? J Alzheimers Dis 2011; 25(3): 445-53.
[http://dx.doi.org/10.3233/JAD-2011-101980] [PMID: 21471646]

[61]   Braak E, Griffing K, Arai K, Bohl J, Bratzke H, Braak H. Neuropathology of Alzheimer's disease: what is new since A. Alzheimer? Eur Arch Psychiatry Clin Neurosci 1999; 249 (Suppl. 3): 14-22.
[http://dx.doi.org/10.1007/PL00014168] [PMID: 10654095]

[62]   Lepelletier F-X, Mann DMA, Robinson AC, Pinteaux E, Boutin H. Early changes in extracellular matrix in Alzheimer's disease. Neuropathol Appl Neurobiol 2015.
[PMID: 26544797]

[63]   Togo T, Akiyama H, Iseki E, *et al.* Immunohistochemical study of tau accumulation in early stages of Alzheimer-type neurofibrillary lesions. Acta Neuropathol 2004; 107(6): 504-8.
[http://dx.doi.org/10.1007/s00401-004-0842-2] [PMID: 15024583]

[64]   Braak H, Del Tredici K. Alzheimer's disease: pathogenesis and prevention. Alzheimers Dement 2012; 8(3): 227-33.
[http://dx.doi.org/10.1016/j.jalz.2012.01.011] [PMID: 22465174]

[65]   Dugger BN, Hidalgo JA, Chiarolanza G, *et al.* The distribution of phosphorylated tau in spinal cords of Alzheimer's disease and non-demented individuals. J Alzheimers Dis 2013; 34(2): 529-36.
[http://dx.doi.org/10.3233/JAD-121864] [PMID: 23246918]

[66]   Kovács T. The olfactory system in Alzheimer's disease: Pathology, pathophysiology and pathway for therapy. Transl Neurosci 2013; 4: 34-45.
[http://dx.doi.org/10.2478/s13380-013-0108-3]

[67]   Rüb U, Del Tredici K, Schultz C, Büttner-Ennever JA, Braak H. The premotor region essential for rapid vertical eye movements shows early involvement in Alzheimer's disease-related cytoskeletal pathology. Vision Res 2001; 41(16): 2149-56.
[http://dx.doi.org/10.1016/S0042-6989(01)00090-6] [PMID: 11403798]

[68]   Van der Werf YD, Witter MP, Groenewegen HJ. The intralaminar and midline nuclei of the thalamus. Anatomical and functional evidence for participation in processes of arousal and awareness. Brain Res Brain Res Rev 2002; 39(2-3): 107-40.
[http://dx.doi.org/10.1016/S0165-0173(02)00181-9] [PMID: 12423763]

[69]   Mesulam M-M. Cholinergic circuitry of the human nucleus basalis and its fate in Alzheimer's disease.

J Comp Neurol 2013; 521(18): 4124-44.
[http://dx.doi.org/10.1002/cne.23415] [PMID: 23852922]

[70] Rosenberg PB. Nowrangi M a., Lyketsos CG. Neuropsychiatric symptoms in Alzheimer's disease: What might be associated brain circuits? Mol Aspects Med 2015; •••: 1-11.

[71] Lopez OL, Becker JT, Sweet RA, Martin-Sanchez FJ, Hamilton RL. Lewy bodies in the amygdala increase risk for major depression in subjects with Alzheimer disease. Neurology 2006; 67(4): 660-5.
[http://dx.doi.org/10.1212/01.wnl.0000230161.28299.3c] [PMID: 16924019]

[72] Kile SJ, Ellis WG, Olichney JM, Farias S, DeCarli C. Alzheimer abnormalities of the amygdala with Klüver-Bucy syndrome symptoms: an amygdaloid variant of Alzheimer disease. Arch Neurol 2009; 66(1): 125-9.
[http://dx.doi.org/10.1001/archneurol.2008.517] [PMID: 19139311]

[73] Horínek D, Petrovický P, Hort J, *et al.* Amygdalar volume and psychiatric symptoms in Alzheimer's disease: an MRI analysis. Acta Neurol Scand 2006; 113(1): 40-5.
[http://dx.doi.org/10.1111/j.1600-0404.2006.00540.x] [PMID: 16367898]

[74] den Heijer T, Geerlings MI, Hoebeek FE, Hofman A, Koudstaal PJ, Breteler MMB. Use of hippocampal and amygdalar volumes on magnetic resonance imaging to predict dementia in cognitively intact elderly people. Arch Gen Psychiatry 2006; 63(1): 57-62.
[http://dx.doi.org/10.1001/archpsyc.63.1.57] [PMID: 16389197]

[75] Barnes J, Whitwell JL, Frost C, Josephs KAK, Rossor M, Fox NC. Measurements of the amygdala and hippocampus in pathologically confirmed Alzheimer disease and frontotemporal lobar degeneration. Arch Neurol 2006; 63(10): 1434-9.
[http://dx.doi.org/10.1001/archneur.63.10.1434] [PMID: 17030660]

[76] Prestia A, Drago V, Rasser PE, Bonetti M, Thompson PM, Frisoni GB. Cortical changes in incipient Alzheimer's disease. J Alzheimers Dis 2010; 22(4): 1339-49.
[http://dx.doi.org/10.3233/JAD-2010-101191] [PMID: 20930288]

[77] Thal DR, von Arnim C, Griffin WST, *et al.* Pathology of clinical and preclinical Alzheimer's disease. Eur Arch Psychiatry Clin Neurosci 2013; 263 (Suppl. 2): S137-45.
[http://dx.doi.org/10.1007/s00406-013-0449-5] [PMID: 24077890]

[78] Blazquez-Llorca L, Garcia-Marin V, Defelipe J. Pericellular innervation of neurons expressing abnormally hyperphosphorylated tau in the hippocampal formation of Alzheimer's disease patients. Front Neuroanat 2010; 4: 20.
[PMID: 20631843]

[79] Thal DR, Arendt T, Waldmann G, *et al.* Progression of neurofibrillary changes and PHF-τ in end-stage Alzheimer's disease is different from plaque and cortical microglial pathology. Neurobiol Aging 1998; 19(6): 517-25.
[http://dx.doi.org/10.1016/S0197-4580(98)00090-6] [PMID: 10192210]

[80] Braak H, Braak E. Neuropathological stageing of Alzheimer-related changes. Acta Neuropathol 1991; 82(4): 239-59.
[http://dx.doi.org/10.1007/BF00308809] [PMID: 1759558]

[81] Lange I, Kasanova Z, Goossens L, *et al.* The anatomy of fear learning in the cerebellum: A systematic meta-analysis. Neurosci Biobehav Rev 2015; 59: 83-91.
[http://dx.doi.org/10.1016/j.neubiorev.2015.09.019] [PMID: 26441374]

[82] Stoodley CJ. The cerebellum and cognition: evidence from functional imaging studies. Cerebellum 2012; 11(2): 352-65.
[http://dx.doi.org/10.1007/s12311-011-0260-7] [PMID: 21373864]

[83] Wegiel J, Wisniewski HM, Dziewiatkowski J, *et al.* Cerebellar atrophy in Alzheimer's disease — clinicopathological correlations 1999

[84] Sjöbeck M, Dahlén S, Englund E. Neuronal loss in the brainstem and cerebellum-part of the normal

aging process? A morphometric study of the vermis cerebelli and inferior olivary nucleus. J Gerontol A Biol Sci Med Sci 1999; 54(9): B363-8.
[http://dx.doi.org/10.1093/gerona/54.9.B363] [PMID: 10536640]

[85]   Bateman RJ, Aisen PS, De Strooper B, *et al.* Autosomal-dominant Alzheimer's disease: a review and proposal for the prevention of Alzheimer's disease. Alzheimers Res Ther 2011; 3(1): 1.
[http://dx.doi.org/10.1186/alzrt59] [PMID: 21211070]

[86]   Shiino A, Watanabe T, Kitagawa T, *et al.* Different atrophic patterns in early- and late-onset Alzheimer's disease and evaluation of clinical utility of a method of regional z-score analysis using voxel-based morphometry. Dement Geriatr Cogn Disord 2008; 26(2): 175-86.
[http://dx.doi.org/10.1159/000151241] [PMID: 18698140]

[87]   Lista S, O'Bryant SE, Blennow K, *et al.* Biomarkers in Sporadic and Familial Alzheimer's Disease. J Alzheimers Dis 2015; 47(2): 291-317.
[http://dx.doi.org/10.3233/JAD-143006] [PMID: 26401553]

[88]   Chan D, Janssen JC, Whitwell JL, *et al.* Change in rates of cerebral atrophy over time in early-onset Alzheimer's disease: longitudinal MRI study. Lancet 2003; 362(9390): 1121-2.
[http://dx.doi.org/10.1016/S0140-6736(03)14469-8] [PMID: 14550701]

[89]   Ridha BH, Barnes J, Bartlett JW, *et al.* Tracking atrophy progression in familial Alzheimer's disease: a serial MRI study. Lancet Neurol 2006; 5(10): 828-34.
[http://dx.doi.org/10.1016/S1474-4422(06)70550-6] [PMID: 16987729]

[90]   Knight WD, Okello AA, Ryan NS, *et al.* Carbon-11-Pittsburgh compound B positron emission tomography imaging of amyloid deposition in presenilin 1 mutation carriers. Brain 2011; 134(Pt 1): 293-300.
[http://dx.doi.org/10.1093/brain/awq310] [PMID: 21084313]

[91]   Klunk WE, Price JC, Mathis CA, *et al.* Amyloid deposition begins in the striatum of presenilin-1 mutation carriers from two unrelated pedigrees. J Neurosci 2007; 27(23): 6174-84.
[http://dx.doi.org/10.1523/JNEUROSCI.0730-07.2007] [PMID: 17553989]

[92]   Bateman RJ, Xiong C, Benzinger TLS, *et al.* Dominantly Inherited Alzheimer Network. Clinical and biomarker changes in dominantly inherited Alzheimer's disease. N Engl J Med 2012; 367(9): 795-804.
[http://dx.doi.org/10.1056/NEJMoa1202753] [PMID: 22784036]

[93]   Caso F, Agosta F, Mattavelli D, *et al.* White matter degeneration in atypical alzheimer disease. Radiology 2015; 277(1): 162-72.
[http://dx.doi.org/10.1148/radiol.2015142766] [PMID: 26018810]

[94]   Weston PSJ, Nicholas JM, Lehmann M, *et al.* Presymptomatic cortical thinning in familial Alzheimer disease: A longitudinal MRI study. Neurology 2016; 87(19): 2050-7.
[http://dx.doi.org/10.1212/WNL.0000000000003322] [PMID: 27733562]

[95]   Sudo S, Shiozawa M, Cairns NJ, Wada Y. Aberrant accentuation of neurofibrillary degeneration in the hippocampus of Alzheimer's disease with amyloid precursor protein 717 and presenilin-1 gene mutations. J Neurol Sci 2005; 234(1-2): 55-65.
[http://dx.doi.org/10.1016/j.jns.2005.03.043] [PMID: 15946688]

[96]   Thinakaran G, Parent AT. Identification of the role of presenilins beyond Alzheimer's disease. Pharmacol Res 2004; 50(4): 411-8.
[http://dx.doi.org/10.1016/j.phrs.2003.12.026] [PMID: 15304238]

[97]   Singleton AB, Hall R, Ballard CG, *et al.* Pathology of early-onset Alzheimer's disease cases bearing the Thr113-114ins presenilin-1 mutation. Brain 2000; 123(Pt 12): 2467-74.
[http://dx.doi.org/10.1093/brain/123.12.2467] [PMID: 11099448]

[98]   Thordardottir S, Ståhlbom AK, Ferreira D, *et al.* Preclinical cerebrospinal fluid and volumetric magnetic resonance imaging biomarkers in Swedish familial Alzheimer's disease. J Alzheimers Dis 2015; 43(4): 1393-402.

[http://dx.doi.org/10.3233/JAD-140339] [PMID: 25182737]

[99]   Dhikav V, Anand K. Potential predictors of hippocampal atrophy in Alzheimer's disease. Drugs Aging 2011; 28(1): 1-11.
[http://dx.doi.org/10.2165/11586390-000000000-00000] [PMID: 21174483]

[100]   Shi Y, Yamada K, Liddelow SA, *et al.* ApoE4 markedly exacerbates tau-mediated neurodegeneration in a mouse model of tauopathy. Nature 2017; 549(7673): 523-7.
[http://dx.doi.org/10.1038/nature24016] [PMID: 28959956]

[101]   Thaker U, McDonagh AM, Iwatsubo T, Lendon CL, Pickering-Brown SM, Mann DMA. Tau load is associated with apolipoprotein E genotype and the amount of amyloid β protein, Abeta40, in sporadic and familial Alzheimer's disease. Neuropathol Appl Neurobiol 2003; 29(1): 35-44.
[http://dx.doi.org/10.1046/j.1365-2990.2003.00425.x] [PMID: 12581338]

[102]   Fennema-Notestine C, Panizzon MS, Thompson WR, *et al.* Presence of ApoE ε4 allele associated with thinner frontal cortex in middle age. J Alzheimers Dis 2011; 26 (Suppl. 3): 49-60.
[http://dx.doi.org/10.3233/JAD-2011-0002] [PMID: 21971450]

[103]   Manning EN, Barnes J, Cash DM, *et al.* APOE ε4 is associated with disproportionate progressive hippocampal atrophy in AD. PLoS One 2014; 9(5): e97608.
[http://dx.doi.org/10.1371/journal.pone.0097608] [PMID: 24878738]

[104]   Lehtovirta M, Laakso MP, Soininen H, *et al.* Volumes of hippocampus, amygdala and frontal lobe in Alzheimer patients with different apolipoprotein E genotypes. Neuroscience 1995; 67(1): 65-72.
[http://dx.doi.org/10.1016/0306-4522(95)00014-A] [PMID: 7477910]

[105]   Tohgi H, Takahashi S, Kato E, *et al.* Reduced size of right hippocampus in 39- to 80-year-old normal subjects carrying the apolipoprotein E lipoprotein. Neurosci Lett 1997; 236: 21-4.

[106]   Burggren AC, Zeineh MM, Ekstrom AD, *et al.* Reduced cortical thickness in hippocampal subregions among cognitively normal apolipoprotein E e4 carriers. Neuroimage 2008; 41(4): 1177-83.
[http://dx.doi.org/10.1016/j.neuroimage.2008.03.039] [PMID: 18486492]

[107]   Donix M, Burggren AC, Suthana NA, *et al.* Longitudinal changes in medial temporal cortical thickness in normal subjects with the APOE-4 polymorphism. Neuroimage 2010; 53(1): 37-43.
[http://dx.doi.org/10.1016/j.neuroimage.2010.06.009] [PMID: 20541611]

[108]   Okonkwo OC, Xu G, Dowling NM, *et al.* Family history of Alzheimer disease predicts hippocampal atrophy in healthy middle-aged adults. Neurology 2012; 78(22): 1769-76.
[http://dx.doi.org/10.1212/WNL.0b013e3182583047] [PMID: 22592366]

[109]   Suthana NA, Krupa A, Donix M, *et al.* Reduced hippocampal CA2, CA3, and dentate gyrus activity in asymptomatic people at genetic risk for Alzheimer's disease. Neuroimage 2010; 53(3): 1077-84.
[http://dx.doi.org/10.1016/j.neuroimage.2009.12.014] [PMID: 20005961]

[110]   Jack CR Jr, Knopman DS, Jagust WJ, *et al.* Hypothetical model of dynamic biomarkers of the Alzheimer's pathological cascade. Lancet Neurol 2010; 9(1): 119-28.
[http://dx.doi.org/10.1016/S1474-4422(09)70299-6] [PMID: 20083042]

[111]   Weiner MW, Veitch DP, Aisen PS, *et al.* The Alzheimer's Disease Neuroimaging Initiative: a review of papers published since its inception. Alzheimers Dement 2013; 9(5): e111-94.
[http://dx.doi.org/10.1016/j.jalz.2013.05.1769] [PMID: 23932184]

[112]   Ewers M, Frisoni GB, Teipel SJ, *et al.* Staging Alzheimer's disease progression with multimodality neuroimaging. Prog Neurobiol 2011; 95(4): 535-46.
[http://dx.doi.org/10.1016/j.pneurobio.2011.06.004] [PMID: 21718750]

[113]   Sowell ER, Thompson PM, Toga AW. Mapping changes in the human cortex throughout the span of life. Neuroscientist 2004; 10(4): 372-92.
[http://dx.doi.org/10.1177/1073858404263960] [PMID: 15271264]

[114]   Morra JH, Tu Z, Apostolova LG, *et al.* Automated 3D mapping of hippocampal atrophy and its

clinical correlates in 400 subjects with Alzheimer's disease, mild cognitive impairment, and elderly controls. Hum Brain Mapp 2009; 30(9): 2766-88.
[http://dx.doi.org/10.1002/hbm.20708] [PMID: 19172649]

[115] Gogtay N, Thompson PM. Mapping gray matter development: implications for typical development and vulnerability to psychopathology. Brain Cogn 2010; 72(1): 6-15.
[http://dx.doi.org/10.1016/j.bandc.2009.08.009] [PMID: 19796863]

[116] Binnewijzend MAA, Schoonheim MM, Sanz-Arigita E, *et al.* Resting-state fMRI changes in Alzheimer's disease and mild cognitive impairment. Neurobiol Aging 2012; 33(9): 2018-28.
[http://dx.doi.org/10.1016/j.neurobiolaging.2011.07.003] [PMID: 21862179]

[117] Herminghaus S, Frölich L, Gorriz C, *et al.* Brain metabolism in Alzheimer disease and vascular dementia assessed by *in vivo* proton magnetic resonance spectroscopy. Psychiatry Res 2003; 123(3): 183-90.
[http://dx.doi.org/10.1016/S0925-4927(03)00071-4] [PMID: 12928106]

[118] Rodriguez-Vieitez E, Ni R, Gulyás B, *et al.* Astrocytosis precedes amyloid plaque deposition in Alzheimer APPswe transgenic mouse brain: a correlative positron emission tomography and *In vitro* imaging study. Eur J Nucl Med Mol Imaging 2015; 42(7): 1119-32.
[http://dx.doi.org/10.1007/s00259-015-3047-0] [PMID: 25893384]

[119] Hickman RA, Faustin A, Wisniewski T. Alzheimer disease and its growing epidemic: risk factors, biomarkers, and the urgent need for therapeutics. Neurol Clin 2016; 34(4): 941-53.
[http://dx.doi.org/10.1016/j.ncl.2016.06.009] [PMID: 27720002]

[120] Insel PS, Mattsson N, Donohue MC, *et al.* The transitional association between β-amyloid pathology and regional brain atrophy. Alzheimers Dement 2015; 11(10): 1171-9.
[http://dx.doi.org/10.1016/j.jalz.2014.11.002] [PMID: 25499535]

CHAPTER 3

Alterations of Membrane Composition in Alzheimer´s Disease

Manoel Arcisio-Miranda, Rolf Matias Paninka and **Luisa Ribeiro-Silva**[*]

Laboratório de Neurobiologia Estrutural e Funcional (LaNEF), Departamento de Biofísica, Universidade Federal de São Paulo, São Paulo, Brazil

Abstract: Biological membranes are a vital component of all living cells. They consist mainly of lipids and proteins. The proteins are embedded into the lipid structure, whose distribution in an aqueous environment forms a bilayer. The biological membranes have an average thickness of 30Å, determined by the size of the carbon chain of lipids, which range from 14 to 24 carbons. The lipid portion of biological membranes is also fundamental to determine their physicochemical properties such as membrane order, fluidity, and hydrophobicity. As Alzheimer's disease pathology is mainly due to actions of Aβ peptides on the plasma membrane, its modifications are of great importance. In fact, membrane lipids, such as cholesterol, ceramides, gangliosides, and fatty acids, have been implicated in the molecular mechanisms of various stages of Alzheimer's disease pathology. The following chapter describes the main changes in membrane lipid composition in Alzheimer's disease (AD).

Keywords: Ceramide, Cholesterol, Fatty Acids, Glycerophospholipid, Membrane, Sphingolipid, Sphingomyelin.

INTRODUCTION

All living cells and in eukaryotes their intracellular compartments, *e.g.* nucleus, endoplasmatic reticulum, mitochondria and other organelles, are surrounded by biological membranes that separate the cellular content from their environment. The biological membranes are essentially built by lipids and proteins (the ratio of these elements may vary depending on the cell type and organelle – governed by their specific functions) and serve as a highly selective barrier to the transport of substances. Thus, using compartmentalized systems determined by the presence of membranes, cells are able to establish its internal chemical properties and therefore control the myriad of chemical reactions essential for its functioning and survival.

[*] **Corresponding author Luisa Ribeiro-Silva:** LaNEF, Rua Botucatu, 862 – Edifício Ciências Biomédicas - 7° andar, 03262-000, São Paulo, São Paulo, Brazil; Tel: +11 5576-4848 ext. 2337; E-mail: luisars43@gmail.com

Fernando A. Oliveira (Ed.)

The three major lipid components of biological membranes are (Fig. **1**): phospholipids, glycolipids, and sterols. Phospholipids comprise glycerophospholipids and sphingophospholipids. The glycerophospholipids consist of two chains of fatty acids attached to glycerol and a phosphate group. The most abundant glycerophospholipid in biological membranes is phosphatidylcholine, which has a choline molecule attached to the phosphate group. Hydrogen, ethanolamine, serine, glycerol, *myo*-Inositol 4,5-bisphosphate, and phosphatidylglycerol can replace the choline in this position, and these glycerophospholipids are called respectively phosphatidic acid, phosphatidylethanolamine, phosphatidylserine, phosphatidylglycerol, phosphatidylinositol 4,5-bisphosphate, and cardiolipin. Glycolipids can contain either glycerol or sphingosine, and always have a sugar in place of the phosphate group found in phospholipids. In between these two classes of lipids are sphingolipids, which have a chain of fatty acid attached to sphingosine and a phosphate group/choline (sphingophospholipids) or a saccharide (sphingoglycolipids). Sterols form a diverse class of lipids with a quite different structure to that of the phospholipids and glycolipids. An example of a sterol that is commonly found in eukaryotic biological membranes is cholesterol. It consists of a hydroxyl group (hydrophilic head), a tetracyclic core and a short hydrocarbon chain.

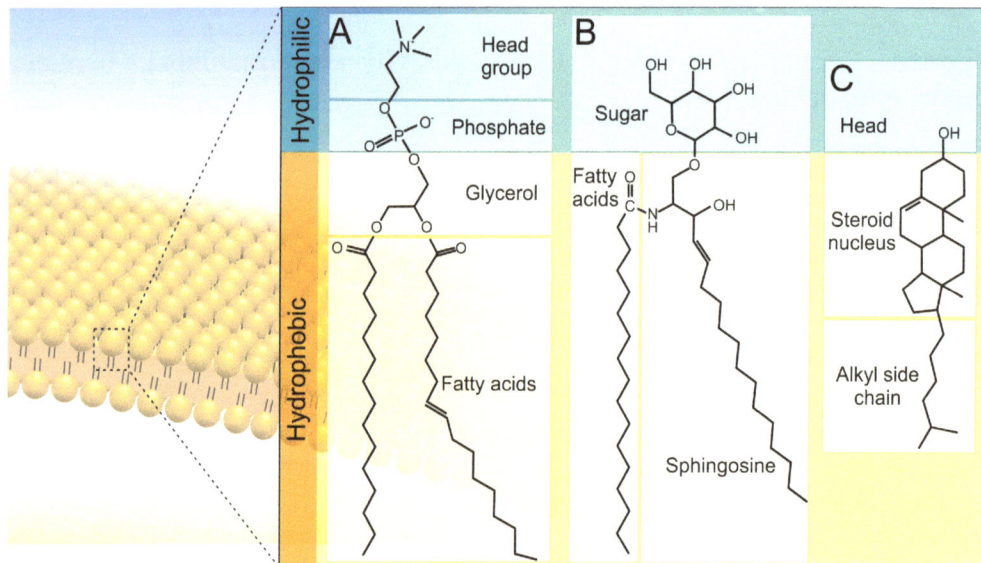

Fig. (1). Schematic representation of the three classes of lipids found in biological membranes. (**A**) Glycerophospholipid, shown here as a phosphatidylcholine. (**B**) Glycosphingolipid. (**C**) Cholesterol.

All the above-described structures determine a common property, all biological membrane lipids have a similar structure consisting of a hydrophilic head (polar) and a hydrophobic tail (nonpolar). Thus, the most favorable environment for the polar head is an aqueous one, whereas for the nonpolar tail is the lipid environment. The amphipathic nature of membrane lipids means that they spontaneously form a bilayer, with the hydrophilic portions facing outward and pointing out to the aqueous environment and the hydrophobic portions facing each other. Interestingly, at first glance, these spontaneous lipid packages in an aqueous environment may be seen as an increase in system's order, in disobedience to the second law of thermodynamics. However, these lipid arrangements are indeed the lowest free energy state for lipids in polar solvents, since it prevents a further ordering of water molecules around the hydrophobic lipid tails (further details about the thermodynamics of the lipid bilayers can be obtained at [1] and [2]).

Membrane proteins play a crucial role in biological membranes; without them, the hydrophobic portion of the membranes would be an "insuperable" barrier to the flux of charged molecules through it. Two classes of proteins assist in transport into or out of cells: (i) peripheral membrane proteins which are temporarily attached or anchored to them *via* covalent bonds and (ii) integral membrane proteins which are fully incorporated into the membrane and traverse its entire length.

In this chapter, we discuss the main alterations of membrane lipid composition in AD.

Alterations in Glycerophospholipid Composition

Phospholipids are the major components of cell membranes making up to approximately 30% of its weight. They are not only structurally important but are also involved in membrane properties and the behavior of membrane proteins such as receptors, ion channels, and enzymes. The composition of phospholipids can alter the membrane physicochemical properties: molecular order, fluidity, thickness, and hydrophobicity.

Membrane phospholipid composition changes in different brain regions. As the brain lipid content is one of the highest in the body, changes in phospholipid levels can lead to pathological processes. Before distinguishing pathological and normal aging processes, elucidating the changes in phospholipid composition occurred during normal aging is needed. In early studies performed using whole brain samples, it was shown that total lipid content increased during the first two decades of age and then began to decrease [3]. A later study analyzing frontal and temporal cortices and white matter of individual from 20 to 100 years of age demonstrated a mild decrease of membrane lipids after the second decade, which became exacerbated after the eighth decade [4]. Specifically, phosphatidylinositol

(PI), phosphatidylethanolamine (PE) and phosphatidylcholine (PC) levels decrease slowly with age, with a loss of less than 10% between 40 to 100 years of age [5]. However, another study showed that in different brain regions the phospholipid content was reduced by 10-20% in individuals between age 89 and 92 compared with 33 to 36-year-old individuals, while in other brain regions, it remained unchanged [6].

The involvement of reduced brain glycerophospholipids levels and its altered brain metabolism in AD pathological process has been suggested in studies from the 1980s and 1990s. Relatively to controls, brain samples from AD individuals have been described as having decreased PI levels [7, 8], and PE levels [7, 9, 10], particularly plasmalogen PE (PPE) is reduced relative to PE [11, 12]. At the same time, alterations in PC levels are contradictory, with reports of unchanged [7, 10], reduction [9, 12] and increase [13]. Moreover, in the frontal cortex, one of the brain regions primarily affected by AD, a reduction of 73% in choline plasmalogen was observed in AD individuals compared to control [14]. As these studies analyzed the phospholipid profile through traditional analytical techniques which requires a substantial amount of sample there is a higher risk of cross-contamination between different regions of the brain and grey and white matter. Using another analytical process, ^{31}P NMR phospholipid profiling, Pettegrew and coauthors found decreased levels of PI, PE and PC in the lipid extracts of combined brain regions from AD individuals compared to age-matched controls, supporting previous findings obtained with the traditional technique [15].

In recent years, the development of mass spectrometry has enabled more sensitive phospholipid profiling using smaller amounts of samples. Taking advantage of this method, Han and coauthors have shown that the levels of PPE change differently in the grey and white matter as AD progress. In the early stage of the disease, PPE levels in the white matter are reduced 40% but remain constant as the disease progresses, while in the grey matter the PPE reduction goes from 10% to 30% during disease progression [16]. It has been suggested that decreases in glycerophospholipid content are due to activation of several phospholipase A$_2$ (PLA$_2$) isoforms, including cytosolic PLA$_2$ (cPLA$_2$), Ca^{++}-independent PLA$_2$ (iPLA$_2$) and secretory PLA$_2$ (sPLA$_2$) [17 - 19].

Phospholipids are also storage depot for lipid mediators such as eicosanoids, platelet activating factors, lysophospholipids, docosanoids, endocannabinoids, and diacylglycerides. These mediators play an important role in various cellular functions, for instance in neuronal homeostasis, immune response, modulation of enzyme activity, mitogenesis, apoptosis, neuroinflammation, and oxidative stress [20]. As most of the glycerophospholipids show a decrease in brains affected with AD, their degradation products are generally found augmented, for example, eicosanoids [21, 22] and cannabinoids [23] are increased while lysophosphatidylcholine is decreased [24]. These degradation products are generally pro-inflammatory and lead to microglial and astrocytic activation, resulting in inflammatory cytokine release, which in turn promotes oxidative stress and neuroinflammation, through diverse mechanisms such as up-regulation of sPLA$_2$ isoforms, cyclooxygenases (COX), and nitric oxide synthase (NOS) [17 - 19, 25].

The cause of augmented PLA$_2$ activity in AD is still not fully understood, though several mechanisms have been proposed. Studies have demonstrated that PLA$_2$ activity can be directly increased by the accumulation of Aβ [26, 27]. Another possibility is that cytokine release, like tumor necrosis factor (TNF-α), interleukin (IL)-1β and IL-6, by activated microglia and astrocytes stimulates cPLA$_2$ activity [28]. Finally, ceramide and ceramide-1-phosphate, metabolites of sphingolipid metabolism that will be discussed in detail later, accumulate in AD brain and also stimulate PLA$_2$ activity [29, 30]. The injury process concerning stimulation of PLA$_2$ is believed to involve sequential activation of each isoform. First, Ca^{++}-independent iPLA$_2$ possibly initiates neural injury by reducing plasmalogens levels, consequently, increasing membrane permeability and Ca^{++} influx. Translocation of cPLA$_2$ to the plasma membrane from the cytosol is facilitated by this Ca^{++} influx, resulting in hydrolysis of membrane PC. As the concentration of Ca^{++} raises and reaches mM levels, sPLA$_2$ may be activated and promote cell injury and death. Therefore, the sequence of stimulation of PLA$_2$ isoform activity is first iPLA$_2$, then cPLA$_2$, and lastly sPLA$_2$. Activation of cPLA$_2$ and iPLA$_2$ generates, respectively, arachidonic acid (AA) and docosahexaenoic acid (DHA), whose involvement in AD pathology is discussed below.

Alterations in Fatty Acids Composition

Membrane fluidity is greatly influenced by the ratio of saturated to unsaturated fatty acids, such that changes in this ratio may implicate in neurological pathologies. Essential fatty acids are those which cannot be synthesized in the body and need to be acquired by food intake. For example, linoleic acid (ω-6 fatty acid) and alpha-linolenic acid (ω-3 fatty acid) are essential polyunsaturated fatty acids (PUFAs) that are required for normal brain function and serve as precursors to the synthesis of other PUFAs, such as DHA and AA. Although DHA can be synthesized by elongation and desaturation of alpha-linolenic acid in the body, only small amounts are indeed endogenously produced and most of DHA is provided by dietary intake, mainly from oily fish. DHA is the most common ω-3 fatty acid in the brain, comprehending approximately 60% of total unsaturated fatty acids present in neuronal membranes. Since it incorporates rapidly into phospholipids of plasma membranes, DHA forms highly disorder domains concentrated in PUFA-containing phospholipids that lack cholesterol, thus, it changes membrane fluidity, which affects neurotransmission, ion channel activity and synaptic plasticity [31].

During the normal aging process, the brain content of PUFAs in specific regions is altered. McGahon and coauthors have found that in the hippocampus of aged rats there is a decrease of AA and DHA [32]. Other studies have also shown a reduction of other PUFAs in an age-dependent manner in the hippocampus, cortex, striatum, and hypothalamus [33, 34]. Furthermore, a progressive decline in saturated fatty acids and consequent increase in monounsaturated fatty acids have been associated with aging. In AD *postmortem* brains, Soderberg and coauthors found decreased levels of DHA in the pons, white matter and, particularly, frontal grey matter and hippocampus [35]. Additionally, not only these changes occur in advanced cases of AD but also in the early stages of the disease [36]. It was suggested that DHA loss occurs due to increased oxidative stress, since DHA is very susceptible to lipid peroxidation, because of its six double bonds, and the observation of augmented peroxidation products of DHA in AD brains [37].

Findings from epidemiological studies show an inverse correlation between elevated fish consumption, consequently DHA intake, and dementia [38]. However, no association between ω-3 fatty acids dietary intake and cognitive decline was found by another study [39]. The protective effect of DHA in AD pathogenesis was further supported by *in vitro* studies and animal models [40, 41]. Overall, it was demonstrated that presence of DHA can reduce Aβ burden [42]. In SH-SY5Y, a neuroblastoma cell line, DHA reduces APP processing by the amyloidogenic pathway by directly inhibiting β- and γ-secretases activity, resulting in a decrease of Aβ levels. At the same time, DHA promotes the non-amyloidogenic pathway by enhancing ADAM17 protein stability [43]. Furthermore, the DHA-mediator NPD1, generated by cPLA$_2$ and 15-lipooxy-genase, has also been shown to elevate the non-amyloidogenic processing of APP and reduce the amyloidogenic pathway, thus diminishing Aβ levels [44]. In addition, NPD1 downregulates inflammatory signaling, apoptosis, and Aβ-induced neurotoxicity acting, thus, as a neuroprotective [45]. Although these results suggest a therapeutic use for DHA in AD, clinical trials with it have not shown promising results.

Alterations in Sphingolipid Composition

Sphingolipids are one of the classes of membrane lipids, which similarly to glycerophospholipids have a polar head and two nonpolar tails, but instead of containing a glycerol backbone they present a sphingosine. This heterogeneous group of lipids, which includes ceramide, sphingomyelin, sphingosine-1 -

phosphate (S1P), and ganglioside, is particular enriched in the central nervous system (CNS), where besides its structural significance, sphingolipid metabolites play a critical role as second messengers to various signaling pathways involved in cell growth and death, proliferation and fusion processes between neuro-transmitter vesicles and the membrane. Therefore, is no surprise that proper sphingolipid metabolism balance is essential to normal brain function, which is evidenced by the fact that some severe brain diseases result from deficiencies in enzymes controlling the sphingolipid metabolism, such as Niemann Pick disease and Tay-Sacks disease. Recently, slight changes in sphingolipids metabolism and levels have been associated with the pathophysiology of neurodegenerative diseases, for example, AD, Amyotrophic Lateral Sclerosis, Parkinson's and HIV-dementia.

During normal aging, it has been observed the occurrence of a progressive increase in ceramides levels in different brain areas [46]. This simple sphingolipid can be created by synthesis *de novo* or by catabolism of sphingomyelin (SM) or glycosphingolipids. In the aged brain, the activity of catabolic enzymes is higher than that of anabolic enzymes [47]. Thus, suggesting that the local catabolism of glycosphingolipids is an important contributor to the increase in ceramide levels observed during aging. At the same time, a study reported augmented levels of SM with aging in the cerebellum, cerebral hemispheres, medulla oblongata and pons [48]. The composition of SM fatty acids is also altered in rat aged brains compared with young brains, with an increase in the monoenoic/saturated ratio in the aged brains. Even though the total ganglioside concentration remains nearly constant between 20 and 70 years of age, there is a slight decrease at more advanced ages [4, 49]. This may be caused by an increase in sialidase activity with age. In addition, there is an increase in the C20- to C18-gangliosides species in the brains of aged humans and rodents [50].

We will address the specific changes in the composition of each subgroup of sphingolipid in AD brains and its importance to AD pathology individually.

Ceramide

There is a consensus in *postmortem* studies that the ceramide levels are elevated in the white and gray matters of AD brains compared to age-matched controls [51, 52]. Even so, one study reported decreased levels of ceramide in the white matter of the middle frontal gyrus [53]. This inconsistency may be related to the stage of the disease in which the samples are collected, as another study has found increased ceramides levels in brain regions of early AD (CDR = 0.5 – very mild dementia, or CDR = 1 – mild dementia) and decreased levels as the disease became more severe (CDR = 2 – moderate dementia, or CDR = 3 – severe dementia) [54].

The very long-chain ceramides (C24:0 and C24:1) are specially altered in AD brains. These ceramides species are enriched in the endosomal and lysosomal compartments, in which APP processing takes place. As differences in ceramide levels occur even at early stages of the disease (CDR of 0.5), it has been proposed to be involved in the promotion of AD. In this context, Katsel and coauthors searched for genetic abnormalities of key enzymes that control sphingolipid metabolism and ceramide synthesis during the progression of AD compared to changes due to normal aging [55]. The study reported an upregulation of enzymes involved in ceramide synthesis, particularly the long –chain ceramides (C22:0 and C24:0), early in the disease progression accompanied by downregulation of glucosylceramide resulting in accumulation of ceramide. Furthermore, brains regions affected early in AD pathogenesis, frontal and temporal cortices, concentrated most of the altered gene expression. In the grey matter of these regions, there was also found an increase in acid sphingomyelinase activity, which metabolizes SM into ceramides [56]. There is a positive correlation between acid sphingomyelinase activity and amyloid β aggregation or phosphorylated tau, implying an involvement of this enzyme in AD neurodegeneration.

Ceramide is a well-known apoptotic inducer and it has neurotoxic properties. In fact, it was shown that Aβ neurotoxicity is dependent on ceramide-induced apoptotic pathways. Lee and coauthors reported that treatment with Aβ in oligodendrocytes induced an increase in neutral sphingomyelinase activity resulting in augmented ceramide levels, and consequently in cell death [57]. This activation has been observed in treatments with $A\beta_{42}$ but not with $A\beta_{40}$ [58]. Even more, ceramide has been shown to alter APP processing and consequently Aβ production [40]. Enhancing ceramide levels, either by direct administration or by increasing neutral sphingomyelinase activity, resulted in augmented Aβ production [59]. This effect is credited to protein stabilization of the β-secretase BACE1 by ceramide, while the γ-secretase is not affected by ceramide levels. Ceramide induces protein stabilization of BACE1 by upregulating the expression of acetyltransferases, ATase1 and ATase2, which acetylates BACE1 and consequently protects the nascent protein from degradation [60]. Taking these results together is clear that ceramide is the driving force in a circulous vitiosus: augmented ceramide levels leads to increased Aβ production, which in turn promotes ceramide accumulation.

Sphingomyelin

Sphingomyelin (SM) is an important component of mammalian cell membranes, comprising about 10-15% of total phospholipid content and even more in the nervous system, as it is especially found in the brain and particularly enriched in myelin sheets [61]. The overall increase in ceramide levels described earlier, suggests an accompanied decrease in SM levels. However, contrary to the *post-mortem* studies on ceramide levels, results of changes in SM level during AD are still inconsistent. A study utilizing an enzymatic assay reported decreased SM levels in soluble fractions from AD brains compared to controls, while in membrane fractions SM levels remained unchanged [56]. This was supported by another study which described reduced SM levels in AD brains, specifically in the middle frontal gyrus, but the same was not seen in the cerebellum [46]. On the other hand, Bandaru and coauthors found increased SM levels in the middle frontal gyrus gray matter of AD brains compared to age-matched controls, while the same brain region white matter did not show any changes [53]. Another study has also described increased SM levels, with differences found in the combined brain regions of AD brains, but not specifically in all regions. While there was an increase in the cerebellum, SM levels remained unchanged in the superior/middle frontal gyrus. This study also observed a positive correlation between SM levels and the number of Aβ plaques, but not with neurofibrillary tangles [15]. In the early stages of the disease, no changes were found in both frontal cortex and cerebellum. In addition, there were no changes across the severity of the disease [54].

Interestingly, neutral sphingomyelinase was found to be upregulated in AD brains, which will consequently result in an increase in SM breakdown. In recent cell culture studies, its activity has been reported to be elevated in presenilin familial AD mutations, thus suggesting an important role for neutral sphingomyelinase in sporadic late onset as well as familial early onset AD pathology [58]. Moreover, SM has been proposed to be involved in neuronal damage through oxidative stress pathways, and inhibition of SM reduced cellular oxidative damage [62]. Importantly, SM itself is described to alter APP processing. Decreased Aβ production was found by increasing SM levels, either by direct administration or by inhibition of neutral sphingomyelinase [58]. Additionally, as discussed earlier $A\beta_{42}$ itself is able to regulate SM metabolism by upregulating neutral sphingomyelinase.

Sphingosine and Sphingosine-1-Phosphate

Sphingosine is a metabolite of ceramide, which like ceramide has pro-apoptotic properties. One study has reported increased levels of sphingosine in brain samples from AD patients, compared to age-matched neurologically normal controls [56]. Two studies found that at least two of the three ceramidases, which converts ceramide to sphingosine, are upregulated in AD brains, which may consequently promote sphingosine accumulation [56, 63]. There are still no studies concerning sphingosine levels at early stages of AD.

Sphingosine-1-phosphate (S1P) is formed by phosphorylation of sphingosine by sphingosine kinases (SK1 or SK2). S1P is considered to be neuroprotective and to have a role in neuronal differentiation. However, a few studies have shown that S1P signaling response is affected by which of the sphingosine kinases are active. Phosphorylation by SK1 creates a ligand that promotes cell growth and proliferation. In turn, phosphorylation by SK2 produces an apoptosis-promoting ligand [64]. One study has found decreased levels of S1P in the frontotemporal grey matter of AD patients, indicating a possible role for S1P in AD pathology [56]. Moreover, it was observed that S1P directly interacts with BACE1 and enhances its proteolytic activity [65]. In addition, S1P accumulation may lead to tau hyperphosphorylation [64]. S1P levels were negatively correlated with amyloid beta and phosphorylated tau levels in the frontotemporal area [56].

Sulfatides

Sulfatides are a sphingolipid subgroup generated from ceramide, which are especially enriched in myelin sheets accounting for 5% of myelin lipids. They are particularly produced by oligodendrocytes and Schwann cells, however, production by neurons and astrocytes at lowers amounts have also been described. Of note, it is known that AD pathology may induce focal demyelination and oligodendrocyte degeneration [66].

These sphingolipids have been described as being the most affected sphingolipid in AD brain, with a remarkable depletion of up to 92% in the gray matter of all regions of AD subjects with a CDR of 0.5 [54]. The same group showed a decrease of up to 51% of sulfatide levels in the white matter. There was no further reduction with the progression of the disease, CDR of 1 to a CDR of 3, which indicates that sulfatide levels are altered early in the disease and remain relatively lower than the control. As sulfatide levels are altered early in AD, possibly these alterations happen at preclinical stages, implying a possible role in AD pathogenesis. These results are partially supported by another study which found decreased sulfatide levels in the middle frontal gyrus white matter of AD patients compared to controls, but they did not confirm the alterations found previously in the gray matter [53]. No differences between AD samples and controls were found in the middle temporal gyrus. Recently, a study using novel techniques of tissue lipidomics has confirmed the decrease of sulfatides in both white and gray matter of pre-frontal cortex in throughout all stages of AD [67].

There is a possible link between sulfatide homeostasis and ApoE trafficking since sulfatide intercellular transport is mediated by APOE-containing lipoproteins in the brain. Among ApoE4 allele carriers, sulfatide levels were higher in the middle frontal gyrus than non-carriers, among AD cases, but not in controls [52]. Thus, the ApoE4 allele may be associated with altered sulfatide levels only in individuals with an underlying neurological disorder. In transgenic mice studies, the highest sulfatide depletion was found in human ApoE4 allele carriers compared to wild-type controls and human ApoE3 allele carriers [68]. Further, APP transgenic mice presented a significant age-related decrease of sulfatide, which was eliminated by ApoE knockout [69]. Sulfatides have also been implicated in ApoE-mediated Aβ clearance. In cell culture studies, treatment with sulfatide promoted a significant decrease in Aβ levels. This has been suggested to be caused by a modification of Aβ clearance by an endocytic pathway [70].

Gangliosides

Gangliosides are a family of glycosphingolipids which contain sialic acid. They are present in the plasma membrane of all vertebrate cells, specifically in the exofacial leaflet, where they are anchored by the ceramide part of their molecule and the oligosaccharide portion project to the extracellular medium. Because of this ubiquitous expression, gangliosides have the most diverse functions, such as serving as antigens, receptors for bacterial toxins, mediating cell adhesion, and mediating and modulating signal transduction. They are most abundant in the nervous system, where its distribution is specific to each cell and regulated by the development, in view of that during cell differentiation changes in gangliosides quantities and species occur. Particularly, in neuronal tissue, gangliosides play an important role in proliferation, differentiation, development, and maintenance of cells.

There are four distinct ganglio-series, in which gangliosides are separated by their number of sialic acid residues: o-series, a-series, b-series, and c-series. In the brain, the a-series (GM1 and GD1a) and the b-series (GD1b and GT1b) are the most common gangliosides. Both of these series have a common precursor, GM3. They are segregated by GD3-synthase (GD3S), which adds a sialic acid to GM3 producing GD3, then, determining the b-series initiation. Thus, GD3S regulates the levels of the major brain gangliosides. The distribution of gangliosides inside the cells is also species specific, for example, GM1 is mostly located in the plasma membrane, but is also present in endocytic organelles, the trans-Golgi network, and the nuclear membrane. In addition, gangliosides are known to not be uniformly distributed in the membrane and to exist in clusters forming microdomains or lipid rafts.

It has been proposed a strong connection between gangliosides metabolism and AD pathology. In fact, early studies on ganglioside metabolism in AD brains suggested an overall decrease in gangliosides levels compared to controls in the majority of brain regions, including cerebral cortex, hippocampus, basal telencephalon, and frontal white matter [71]. According to the age of onset, the pattern and extent of ganglioside alterations are different. In early onset or familial cases, there was a reduction of up to 58-70% of controls concentration in all brain regions gray matter, and a reduction to 81% of that of control in total gangliosides in the frontal white matter [72]. While in late onset cases, the total gangliosides are reduced in a smaller degree and specifically in the frontal white matter, temporal cortex, and hippocampus. Brooksbank and McGovern reported that in the frontal cortex of AD subjects the concentration and composition of total gangliosides remained unchanged compared to age-matched controls, except fractions of GQ1b and GT1L which showed a minor reduction [73]. Moreover, Crino and coauthors found a decrease in total gangliosides in the whole brain from individuals with dementia of Alzheimer's type (DAT) [74]. This reduction affected especially b-series gangliosides in the nucleus basalis of Meyenert, entorhinal, posterior cingulated, visual, and prefrontal cortex. Another study described depletion of the major brain gangliosides (GT1b, GD1b, GD1a, and GM1) in the frontal and temporal cortex, basal telencephalon, and nucleus basalis of Meyenert of AD patients relative to controls [75, 76]. There was also an increase in the levels of simple gangliosides, GM2 and GM3, in the frontal and parietal cortex that may be accompanied with accelerated lysosomal degradation of gangliosides and/or reactive astrogliosis occurring during neuronal loss. These pathological changes have been associated with AD. Such increase of GM3 has been supported by a recent study, which also reported an elevation of glucosylceramide levels, the precursor for ganglioside synthesis [24]. Increase of GM1 and GM2 levels was also observed in lipid rafts fractions from the temporal and frontal cortex of AD brains [77]. The loss of ganglio-series gangliosides is consistent with pathological changes in AD, as these are enriched in neurons and neuronal loss and brain shrinkage are hallmarks of AD pathology.

In summary, ganglioside metabolism is significantly altered during AD progression. While complex gangliosides are depleted, the concentration of simple gangliosides, such as GM1 and GM3, is increased. Since GM3 is the precursor of a-series and b-series gangliosides, its elevation implies modifications in the biosynthesis of these series of gangliosides in a disease-dependent manner. In fact, a strong connection between ganglioside metabolism and APP processing products has been found. APP byproducts have shown the ability to regulate GD3S activity, the key enzyme in segregating the a- and b-series, by two distinct and additive mechanisms. Aβ peptides can directly bind to GM3, reducing substrate availability and thus inhibiting GD3S activity and preventing the conversion of GM3 to GD3 [78]. At the same time, the APP intracellular domain (AICD) can downregulate the gene expression of GD3S, consequently, GD3 levels decrease and GM3 accumulates.

Additionally, GM1 has been associated with various pathomechanisms of AD, such as APP processing, Aβ aggregation, and cytotoxicity. GM1 decreases the production of sAPPα and increases Aβ concentration however it does not alter the levels of sAPPβ [79]. This result suggests that GM1 modulates the activity of α-secretase and γ-secretase, reducing the first and augmenting the second, but does not modify β-secretase activity. GM1 also shifts Aβ production towards the 42-long peptide [80]. Aβ is known to reduce membrane fluidity by binding to GM1. A more rigid membrane is favorable to an amyloidogenic APP processing resulting in increased Aβ production. Thus, Aβ triggers a vicious circle mediated by GM1. Tamboli and coauthors described another link between ganglioside metabolism and APP processing. Reduced Aβ production was observed as a result of inhibition of glucosylceramide-synthase, a key enzyme in ganglioside formation [81]. This effect was proposed to be an outcome of altered APP maturation and transport to cell surface leading to decreased availability of APP to amyloidogenic processing, which occurs in endosomal compartments.

Furthermore, GM1 clusters in the plasma membrane serve as "seeds" for amyloid plaque formation. GM1 interacts directly with Aβ peptide forming GAβ complexes. The β-amyloid peptide has a propensity to aggregate more easily in GAβ complex since the formation of the complex tends to change the secondary structure of Aβ from α-helices to β-sheets [82, 83]. Additional studies showed an enhanced cytotoxicity of accumulation and aggregation of Aβ in cell membranes enriched with GM1 lipid rafts [84]. Even more, it was recently shown that GM1 not only influences these stages of Aβ toxicity but also its ability to form pores [85]. The incidence of GAβ complexes has been reported in both AD brains and aged mice brains. Interestingly, synaptosomes from aged mice presented GM1 clusters, suggesting an increased capability to form GAβ complexes and consequently to initiate Aβ aggregation [86]. Aβ deposition was observed to start primarily in the presynaptic membrane of neuronal cells in AD brains, suggesting an important role for GM1 at early stages of AD pathogenesis [87].

Alterations in Cholesterol Composition

Cholesterol is one of the major components of mammalian cell membranes and a determinant of membrane physicochemical properties, such as fluidity and melting temperature. It also influences multiple membrane functions, for example, it can affect the endocytosis and transport of substrates to proteins embedded in the membrane. The distribution of cholesterol along the membrane is not uniform, as the membrane moves from the ER through the Golgi network to the plasma membrane the cholesterol content increases [88]. In the two leaflets of the lipid bilayer there is also a marked asymmetry, it is enriched in the cytofacial leaflet containing approximately 85% of total cholesterol content [89]. As for the exofacial leaflet, it contains approximately 15% of total cholesterol in the membrane. However, the importance of this asymmetry is not yet fully understood, but alterations in this composition can affect membrane fluidity.

The brain is the most cholesterol-rich organ, accounting for approximately 25% of total free cholesterol content in the organism, even though it only amounts to 2% of total body weight [90]. Cholesterol is majorly present in its free form in the brain. On the contrary of other lipids (*e.g.* fatty acids and SM), cholesterol cannot traverse the blood-brain barrier (BBB), therefore it is exclusively derived from *de novo* biosynthesis from acetyl-coenzyme A catalyzed by the enzyme 3-hydroxy-3-methyl-glutaryl-coenzyme A (HMG-CoA) reductase [91]. Thus, cholesterol levels in the brain are independent of plasma levels of LDL-C. Although both neurons and glial cells are capable of producing cholesterol, the biosynthesis is higher in oligodendrocytes, which are responsible for the myelin sheet; followed by astrocytes whose ability to synthesize is 2 to 3 times greater than that of neurons [92]. During the development, neurons are able to produce most of the cholesterol required for growth and synaptogenesis. However, mature neurons depend on exogenous cholesterol derived out of astrocytes [93]. This demand is met by the astrocytic compartment by secreting ApoE-cholesterol complexes, which are transported to neurons. Astrocytes also play an important role in cholesterol recycling, since they are capable of internalizing and recycling cholesterol released from degenerating nerve terminals [94].

Degradation of cholesterol in the brain is not as simple, as brains cells are not able to do it; cholesterol is exported to the peripheral circulation and disposed of by the liver as bile. This process assists in the maintenance of a steady-state level of cholesterol in the brain. Two independent mechanisms are used to remove cholesterol. The main process of cholesterol clearance is through its conversion by a 24-hydroxylase enzyme to 24S-hydroxycholesterol (24-OH), an oxidized lipophilic metabolite that can freely cross the BBB [95]. The other mechanism is denominated reverse cholesterol transport pathway, which entails the translocation of a portion of brain cholesterol through a membrane transport protein to the blood. This process can be realized by the protein ABCA1. In turn, ABCA1 levels can be partially regulated by oxysterols, including 24-OH [96 - 98].

In the aged brain, there is a decrease in cholesterol levels starting at 20 years of age in the temporal and frontal cortices of human brains [4]. It was also described a slight but significant reduction in the hippocampus and cerebellum total cholesterol concentration [6]. Supporting these results, an age-dependent decrease in cholesterol synthesis in the hippocampus and increase in 24-hydroxylase levels in aged human brain were described [99, 100]. Thus, it may be suggested that the process of aging leads to a reduction in cholesterol synthesis, accompanied by an increase in cholesterol catabolism, resulting in an overall decrease in cholesterol levels. In addition, a study reported that although no significant overall changes were found in the synaptic membranes of aged mice total brain, when the specific levels in the bilayer leaflets were analyzed changes in the asymmetric distribution were found, with a relative enrichment of the exofacial leaflet [101].

The major genetic risk factor for the development of late onset AD is the presence of the allele ε4 of the gene APOE, which encodes a protein involved in cholesterol transport in the brain. APOE as the main risk factor implies an involvement of cholesterol in AD pathology. Several studies have investigated the link between cholesterol and AD, however, there is still no consensus if increased levels of plasma cholesterol raise the risk of developing AD. Kivipelto and coauthors reported a two to three times increased risk of mild dementia and later developing AD in individuals with high levels of total cholesterol [102]. Similarly, low levels of plasma HDL-C were associated with increased risk of AD, while high levels of the same lipoprotein correlated with a larger hippocampal volume and reduced risk of AD [103]. Increased plasma LDL-C and total cholesterol levels were also positively correlated with cognitive impairment [104]. Contrary to these observations, a study has found no association between the concentration of plasma cholesterol and the risk of developing AD [105]. Even so, a few studies associated increased total cholesterol levels in individuals between 70 and 79 years of age with a lower risk of dementia later in life (between 79 and 88 years of age) [104, 106 - 109]. In individuals of 40 to 55 years of age, higher levels of cholesterol have been positively correlated with pathological brain amyloid. These observations were not replicated in older individuals, suggesting an important role for cholesterol in the early or presymptomatic stages of the disease. The different relationship between plasma cholesterol concentration and AD risk has been explained by Shepardson and coauthors, who found that studies finding a negative correlation were done mostly late in the life of patients, while the studies done early in the individual's life reported a positive correlation [110].

In brain samples from AD patients, there is an increase in cholesterol levels compared to controls [111, 112]. The concentration of cholesterol precursors of the mevalonate pathway, farnesylpyrophosphate and geranylpyrophosphate, were also found to be increased. On the other hand, other research groups have reported reduced levels of cholesterol and precursors, lanosterol and lathosterol, in AD brains, accompanied with decreased levels of HMG-CoA reductase [112, 113]. Interestingly, the author points out that the global cholesterol concentration does not reflect the number and distribution of lipid rafts. Moreover, changes in the distribution of cholesterol inside the lipid bilayer were seen in AD brains, with a relative enrichment of the exofacial leaflet from less than 15% to 30% [89].

The role of cholesterol in AD pathology has been extensively studied, however, there are still inconsistent data and conflict between evidence has been described [114 - 116]. Cholesterol is known to affect APP processing and thus Aβ production. The localization of APP and its secretases in the cell membrane is directly affected by the lipid composition of specific regions of the membrane. For example, α-secretase, which activity leads to the non-amyloidogenic cleavage of APP, is mainly located in low-cholesterol nonraft membrane domains [117]. While β- and γ-secretases, responsible for the amyloidogenic processing and production of neurotoxic Aβ peptide, are majorly distributed in lipid rafts regions consisting of high cholesterol, sphingomyelin, and gangliosides [118, 119]. As for APP, it is reported to be present in two separate pools, one located in the lipid rafts domains and the other distributed along the phospholipid-rich regions [120]. Therefore, it is generally accepted that amyloidogenic processing takes place in high-cholesterol lipid rafts regions, whereas non-amyloidogenic processing occurs in phospholipid-rich nonraft domains. Under physiological conditions, most of APP is located in the nonraft pool consequently APP is cleaved predominantly by α-secretase. The normal ratio of production between α-secretase- and β-secretas--generated APP processing products is approximately 90:10 and the amount of neurotoxic Aβ peptides produced are regularly cleared by endogenous pathways. However, in a cholesterol-rich environment, there is an increase in the relative percentage of rafts domains resulting in an augmented contact/activity between APP and β- and γ-secretases leading to an enhanced production of Aβ peptides [114].

Other molecular mechanisms have also been described to explain enhanced Aβ production and plaque deposition with high cholesterol content. Firstly, the presence of cholesterol in cell membrane reduces membrane fluidity which affects the lateral movement of integral membrane proteins, like APP and α-secretase, disfavoring their interaction [121]. Cholesterol also disturbs APP maturation negatively, probably through glycosylation, such that APP does not reach the cell surface and internalizes, reducing the amount of APP available for α-secretase cleavage [122]. Additionally, cholesterol disfavors APP and α-secretase interaction by binding directly to APP at the α-secretase cleavage site [123]. On the other hand, a few studies have reported the contrary effect of cholesterol on Aβ production, with low levels of cholesterol increasing the amount of Aβ peptides [124].

Aggregation of Aβ peptides is a pivotal step in Aβ neurotoxicity and thereupon AD pathogenesis. How cholesterol levels affect this process is still not fully comprehended, with a few contradictory data. A study reported that Aβ oligomers isolated from brain samples of AD individuals interact with lipid raft regions in a cholesterol-dependent manner [125]. At the same time, depleting the cells of cholesterol reduced Aβ aggregation. These results might suggest that reducing the cell cholesterol content have a protective effect against Aβ toxicity, while raising the concentration of cholesterol have a deleterious effect on cell vulnerability to Aβ. However, there are reports of contrary effects of cholesterol on Aβ toxicity [126 - 129]. Cholesterol is believed to modulate Aβ oligomerization and assembly through the conformational modification of other lipid rafts components, like gangliosides. Thereby, the interaction of Aβ with lipid rafts is finely regulated by cholesterol through changes in gangliosides structure and facilitating or hindering the formation of gangliosides clusters. Additionally, Aβ peptides are structurally similar to anti-microbial peptides, by means that both act in the membrane through electrostatic interactions. These are how Aβ recognizes changes in the membrane composition and structure, thus it might be a factor for AD onset [130].

In summary, the relationship between Aβ and cholesterol is not straightforward with modulations on both sides and subtle changes in cholesterol levels and/or distribution across the cell's compartments may alter the final effect on Aβ toxicity.

Role of Oxysterols in AD

Oxysterols are oxidation products of cholesterol metabolism that are created enzymatically or through autoxidation and are closely related to clearance of excess cholesterol from the brain. The main species of oxysterols in the brain are 24S-hydroxycholesterol (24-OH), which is exclusively generated in the CNS and is alternatively denominated cerebrosterol, and 27-hydroxycholesterol (27-OH). The 24-hydroxylase CYP46A1 enzyme that produces 24-OH is exclusively expressed in neuronal cells in the brain and in the retina. Whereas, the enzyme CYP27A1, which generates 27-OH, is ubiquitously expressed in the organism and only a small amount is located in the brain. Being so, most of the 27-OH found in the brain is derived from the peripheral circulation, as 27-OH on the contrary of cholesterol is able to cross the BBB. Inside the brain, 27-OH can be metabolized to 7α-hydroxy-3-oxo-4-cholestenoic acid (7-OH-4-C), which, in turn, crosses the BBB, reaches the peripheral circulation and is then degraded by the liver.

There are a few indications that oxysterols may play an important role in AD pathogenesis. In patients with advanced AD, reduced levels of 24-OH were found in the plasma, whereas 24-OH levels were observed to be increased in CSF samples [131]. On the other hand, no changes in plasma levels of 24-OH in AD patients were reported by another study [132]. As for 27-OH, it was reported to be increased in the CSF of individuals with neurodegeneration [131]. This result was suggested to be caused by an impaired function of the BBB, which would lead to a higher passage of 27-OH from the periphery into the brain. Indeed, a study with brain samples from patients with sporadic AD mutation showed a 50% rise in 27-OH in all brain regions [133, 134]. The same study found a four-fold accumulation of 27-OH in different cortex regions from patients carrying the Swedish APP mutation. The concentration of 24-OH was reported to be reduced in 15-20% that of controls in both forms of Alzheimer's. The increment of 27-OH concentration is believed to be related to a decline in the CYP7B1 enzyme levels found in brain samples from AD patients, resulting in lower conversion of 27-OH into 7-OH-4-C [135]. The expression of the enzymes responsible for oxysterols generation (CYP46A1 and CYP27A1) also showed to be differentially altered in AD brains. CYP27A1, which in the brain is mostly expressed in neurons but in a minor amount is also present in astrocytes and oligodendrocytes, was upregulated in white matter oligodendrocytes [136]. While CYP46A1 showed to be increased in astrocytes and depleted in neurons, selective expression in neuritis around senile plaque was observed.

It was proposed that the balance between 27-OH and 24-OH has a key role in defining amyloidogenesis. This proposition is supported by the increased ratio of 27-OH to 24-OH found in AD brains. However, the mechanisms to oxysterols modulation of APP processing are not clearly elucidated and there are different opinions about their involvement in Aβ production. Accumulation of 24-OH is thought to have an anti-amyloidogenic character since it was described to raise α-secretase activity and the α- to β-secretase activity ratio [137]. This promotion of the non-amyloidogenic processing pathway is probably due to a higher CYP46A1 activity, which by increasing its conversion of cholesterol to 24-OH reduces the total cellular cholesterol concentration and stimulates the α-secretase cleavage of APP. Therefore, the induction of CYP46A1 activity has a beneficial effect on cell viability by preventing Aβ production through modulation of cholesterol metabolism and reduction of cellular cholesterol.

Moreover, 27-OH has also been described as an inhibitor of Aβ generation, but 24-OH is a 1000-fold more potent inhibitor than 27-OH [136]. The effect of 27-OH on Aβ formation is not through direct regulation of α-, β-, or γ-secretases activity, but by upregulation of LXR responsive genes (ABCA1, ABCG1, ApoE) [138]. Contrary to these reports, 27-OH might accelerate neurodegeneration by increasing $A\beta_{42}$ production by upregulating APP and BACE1 and promoting tau hyperphosphorylation [139, 140]. Additionally, oxysterols may participate in augmenting Aβ aggregation and neurotoxicity by interacting and altering specific sites of the peptide [141].

CONCLUDING REMARKS

This chapter has greatly focused on the connection between membrane lipids and

AD pathology. Indeed, several changes in membrane lipid content in AD brains have been reported throughout the years. Cholesterol, sphingolipids, and fatty acids, such as DHA, were found to be directly involved in various steps of AD pathogenesis, *e.g.* APP processing and Aβ production, Aβ aggregation, and cytotoxicity. Therefore, membrane lipids participate in the molecular mechanism of AD pathology through several stages of the disease. However, most of the data is still inconsistent with controversial results reported in different brain regions analyzed. Thus, new studies with a larger cohort and more advanced lipidomic approaches are needed.

SUMMARY OF MAJOR FINDINGS

- This chapter has described various alterations in membrane lipid composition and its relationship with the pathology throughout the development and progressive stages of AD.
- There is an overall decrease in glycerophospholipids in AD brains, result of an increased degradation by PLA2, increasing its byproducts which are pro-inflammatory. Additionally, the presence of these byproducts in the plasma have been suggested as a potential biomarker for AD.
- DHA supplementation is a possible treatment for AD as it diminishes Aβ production and the major PUFAs, DHA and AA, have been found decreased in AD brains.
- Sphingolipids, specially ceramides, sulfatides, and gangliosides, play an important role in the molecular mechanism of AD, as they might be involved in the production, accumulation, aggregation, and cytotoxicity of Aβ peptides.
- Even though there is still no consensus if the levels of plasma cholesterol are a risk factor for AD, there is irrefutable evidence that cholesterol in the brain has a key role in AD pathology.
- Furthermore, oxysterols, oxidations products of cholesterol, make an important contribution to amyloidogenesis.

CONSENT FOR PUBLICATION

Not applicable.

CONFLICT OF INTERESTS

The authors declare no conflict of interests.

ACKNOWLEDGEMENT

This work was supported by The Brazilian Ministry of Education (Coordenação de Aperfeiçoamento de Pessoal de Nível Superior - Capes) and by The National Counsel of Technological and Scientific Development (Grant 142157/2014-7).

REFERENCES

[1]   Nelson DL, Cox MM. Lehninger principles of biochemistry. 5th ed. Book 2008; pp. 1-1294.

[2]   Voet D, Voet JG, Pratt CW. Fundamentals of biochemistry : life at the molecular level. Wiley 2013.

[3]   Rouser G, Yamamoto A. Curvilinear regression course of human brain lipid composition changes with age. Lipids 1968; 3(3): 284-7.
[http://dx.doi.org/10.1007/BF02531202] [PMID: 17805871]

[4]   Svennerholm L, Boström K, Jungbjer B, Olsson L. Membrane lipids of adult human brain: lipid composition of frontal and temporal lobe in subjects of age 20 to 100 years. J Neurochem 1994; 63(5): 1802-11.
[http://dx.doi.org/10.1046/j.1471-4159.1994.63051802.x] [PMID: 7931336]

[5]   Farooqui AA, Liss L, Horrocks LA. Neurochemical aspects of Alzheimer's disease: involvement of membrane phospholipids. Metab Brain Dis 1988; 3(1): 19-35.
[http://dx.doi.org/10.1007/BF01001351] [PMID: 3062351]

[6]   Söderberg M, Edlund C, Kristensson K, Dallner G. Lipid compositions of different regions of the human brain during aging. J Neurochem 1990; 54(2): 415-23.
[http://dx.doi.org/10.1111/j.1471-4159.1990.tb01889.x] [PMID: 2299344]

[7]   Prasad MR, Lovell MA, Yatin M, Dhillon H, Markesbery WR. Regional membrane phospholipid alterations in Alzheimer's disease. Neurochem Res 1998; 23(1): 81-8.
[http://dx.doi.org/10.1023/A:1022457605436] [PMID: 9482271]

[8]   Stokes CE, Hawthorne JN. Reduced phosphoinositide concentrations in anterior temporal cortex of Alzheimer-diseased brains. J Neurochem 1987; 48(4): 1018-21.
[http://dx.doi.org/10.1111/j.1471-4159.1987.tb05619.x] [PMID: 3029323]

[9]   Nitsch RM, Blusztajn JK, Pittas AG, Slack BE, Growdon JH, Wurtman RJ. Evidence for a membrane defect in Alzheimer disease brain. Proc Natl Acad Sci USA 1992; 89(5): 1671-5.
[http://dx.doi.org/10.1073/pnas.89.5.1671] [PMID: 1311847]

[10] Wells K, Farooqui AA, Liss L, Horrocks LA. Neural membrane phospholipids in Alzheimer disease. Neurochem Res 1995; 20(11): 1329-33.
[http://dx.doi.org/10.1007/BF00992508] [PMID: 8786819]

[11] Ginsberg L, Rafique S, Xuereb JH, Rapoport SI, Gershfeld NL. Disease and anatomic specificity of ethanolamine plasmalogen deficiency in Alzheimer's disease brain. Brain Res 1995; 698(1-2): 223-6.
[http://dx.doi.org/10.1016/0006-8993(95)00931-F] [PMID: 8581486]

[12] Guan Z, Wang Y, Cairns NJ, Lantos PL, Dallner G, Sindelar PJ. Decrease and structural modifications of phosphatidylethanolamine plasmalogen in the brain with Alzheimer disease. J Neuropathol Exp Neurol 1999; 58(7): 740-7.
[http://dx.doi.org/10.1097/00005072-199907000-00008] [PMID: 10411344]

[13] Söderberg M, Edlund C, Alafuzoff I, Kristensson K, Dallner G. Lipid composition in different regions of the brain in Alzheimer's disease/senile dementia of Alzheimer's type. J Neurochem 1992; 59(5): 1646-53.
[http://dx.doi.org/10.1111/j.1471-4159.1992.tb10994.x] [PMID: 1402910]

[14] Igarashi M, Ma K, Gao F, Kim H-W, Rapoport SI, Rao JS. Disturbed choline plasmalogen and phospholipid fatty acid concentrations in Alzheimer's disease prefrontal cortex. J Alzheimers Dis 2011; 24(3): 507-17.
[http://dx.doi.org/10.3233/JAD-2011-101608] [PMID: 21297269]

[15]   Pettegrew JW, Panchalingam K, Hamilton RL, McClure RJ. Brain membrane phospholipid alterations in Alzheimer's disease. Neurochem Res 2001; 26(7): 771-82.
[http://dx.doi.org/10.1023/A:1011603916962] [PMID: 11565608]

[16]   Han X, Holtzman DM, McKeel DWJ Jr. Plasmalogen deficiency in early Alzheimer's disease subjects and in animal models: molecular characterization using electrospray ionization mass spectrometry. J Neurochem 2001; 77(4): 1168-80.
[http://dx.doi.org/10.1046/j.1471-4159.2001.00332.x] [PMID: 11359882]

[17]   Farooqui AA, Rapoport SI, Horrocks LA. Membrane phospholipid alterations in Alzheimer's disease: deficiency of ethanolamine plasmalogens. Neurochem Res 1997; 22(4): 523-7.
[http://dx.doi.org/10.1023/A:1027380331807] [PMID: 9130265]

[18]   Stephenson D, Rash K, Smalstig B, *et al.* Cytosolic phospholipase A2 is induced in reactive glia following different forms of neurodegeneration. Glia 1999; 27(2): 110-28.
[http://dx.doi.org/10.1002/(SICI)1098-1136(199908)27:2<110::AID-GLIA2>3.0.CO;2-C]   [PMID: 10417811]

[19]   Farooqui AA, Ong WY, Horrocks LA. Plasmalogens, docosahexaenoic acid and neurological disorders. Adv Exp Med Biol 2003; 544: 335-54.
[http://dx.doi.org/10.1007/978-1-4419-9072-3_45] [PMID: 14713251]

[20]   Farooqui AA, Ong W-Y, Farooqui T. Lipid mediators in the nucleus: Their potential contribution to Alzheimer's disease. Biochim Biophys Acta 2010; 1801(8): 906-16.
[http://dx.doi.org/10.1016/j.bbalip.2010.02.002] [PMID: 20170745]

[21]   Pasinetti GM, Aisen PS. Cyclooxygenase-2 expression is increased in frontal cortex of Alzheimer's disease brain. Neuroscience 1998; 87(2): 319-24.
[http://dx.doi.org/10.1016/S0306-4522(98)00218-8] [PMID: 9740394]

[22]   Qin W, Ho L, Pompl PN, *et al.* Cyclooxygenase (COX)-2 and COX-1 potentiate beta-amyloid peptide generation through mechanisms that involve gamma-secretase activity. J Biol Chem 2003; 278(51): 50970-7.
[http://dx.doi.org/10.1074/jbc.M307699200] [PMID: 14507922]

[23]   Ramírez BG, Blázquez C, Gómez del Pulgar T, Guzmán M, de Ceballos ML. Prevention of Alzheimer's disease pathology by cannabinoids: neuroprotection mediated by blockade of microglial activation. J Neurosci 2005; 25(8): 1904-13.
[http://dx.doi.org/10.1523/JNEUROSCI.4540-04.2005] [PMID: 15728830]

[24]   Chan RB, Oliveira TG, Cortes EP, *et al.* Comparative lipidomic analysis of mouse and human brain with Alzheimer disease. J Biol Chem 2012; 287(4): 2678-88.
[http://dx.doi.org/10.1074/jbc.M111.274142] [PMID: 22134919]

[25]   Frisardi V, Panza F, Seripa D, Farooqui T, Farooqui AA. Glycerophospholipids and glycerophospholipid-derived lipid mediators: a complex meshwork in Alzheimer's disease pathology. Prog Lipid Res 2011; 50(4): 313-30.
[http://dx.doi.org/10.1016/j.plipres.2011.06.001] [PMID: 21703303]

[26]   Kanfer JN, Sorrentino G, Sitar DS. Phospholipases as mediators of amyloid beta peptide neurotoxicity: an early event contributing to neurodegeneration characteristic of Alzheimer's disease. Neurosci Lett 1998; 257(2): 93-6.
[http://dx.doi.org/10.1016/S0304-3940(98)00806-4] [PMID: 9865935]

[27]   Malaplate-Armand C, Florent-Béchard S, Youssef I, *et al.* Soluble oligomers of amyloid-beta peptide induce neuronal apoptosis by activating a cPLA2-dependent sphingomyelinase-ceramide pathway. Neurobiol Dis 2006; 23(1): 178-89.
[http://dx.doi.org/10.1016/j.nbd.2006.02.010] [PMID: 16626961]

[28]   Sun GY, Xu J, Jensen MD, Simonyi A. Phospholipase A2 in the central nervous system: implications for neurodegenerative diseases. J Lipid Res 2004; 45(2): 205-13.

[http://dx.doi.org/10.1194/jlr.R300016-JLR200] [PMID: 14657205]

[29]   Jayadev S, Hayter HL, Andrieu N, *et al.* Phospholipase A2 is necessary for tumor necrosis factor alpha-induced ceramide generation in L929 cells. J Biol Chem 1997; 272(27): 17196-203.
[http://dx.doi.org/10.1074/jbc.272.27.17196] [PMID: 9202042]

[30]   Pettus BJ, Bielawska A, Subramanian P, *et al.* Ceramide 1-phosphate is a direct activator of cytosolic phospholipase A2. J Biol Chem 2004; 279(12): 11320-6.
[http://dx.doi.org/10.1074/jbc.M309262200] [PMID: 14676210]

[31]   Wassall SR, Stillwell W. Polyunsaturated fatty acid-cholesterol interactions: domain formation in membranes. Biochim Biophys Acta 2009; 1788(1): 24-32.
[http://dx.doi.org/10.1016/j.bbamem.2008.10.011] [PMID: 19014904]

[32]   McGahon B, Murray CA, Clements MP, Lynch MA. Analysis of the effect of membrane arachidonic acid concentration on modulation of glutamate release by interleukin-1: an age-related study. Exp Gerontol 1998; 33(4): 343-54.
[http://dx.doi.org/10.1016/S0531-5565(97)00130-7] [PMID: 9639170]

[33]   López GH, Ilincheta de Boschero MG, Castagnet PI, Giusto NM. Age-associated changes in the content and fatty acid composition of brain glycerophospholipids. Comp Biochem Physiol B Biochem Mol Biol 1995; 112(2): 331-43.
[http://dx.doi.org/10.1016/0305-0491(95)00079-8] [PMID: 7584862]

[34]   Ulmann L, Mimouni V, Roux S, Porsolt R, Poisson JP. Brain and hippocampus fatty acid composition in phospholipid classes of aged-relative cognitive deficit rats. Prostaglandins Leukot Essent Fatty Acids 2001; 64(3): 189-95.
[http://dx.doi.org/10.1054/plef.2001.0260] [PMID: 11334555]

[35]   Söderberg M, Edlund C, Kristensson K, Dallner G. Fatty acid composition of brain phospholipids in aging and in Alzheimer's disease. Lipids 1991; 26(6): 421-5.
[http://dx.doi.org/10.1007/BF02536067] [PMID: 1881238]

[36]   Markesbery WR, Kryscio RJ, Lovell MA, Morrow JD. Lipid peroxidation is an early event in the brain in amnestic mild cognitive impairment. Ann Neurol 2005; 58(5): 730-5.
[http://dx.doi.org/10.1002/ana.20629] [PMID: 16240347]

[37]   Montine TJ, Morrow JD. Fatty acid oxidation in the pathogenesis of Alzheimer's disease. Am J Pathol 2005; 166(5): 1283-9.
[http://dx.doi.org/10.1016/S0002-9440(10)62347-4] [PMID: 15855630]

[38]   Kalmijn S, Launer LJ, Ott A, Witteman JC, Hofman A, Breteler MM. Dietary fat intake and the risk of incident dementia in the Rotterdam Study. Ann Neurol 1997; 42(5): 776-82.
[http://dx.doi.org/10.1002/ana.410420514] [PMID: 9392577]

[39]   Engelhart MJ, Geerlings MI, Ruitenberg A, *et al.* Diet and risk of dementia: Does fat matter?: The Rotterdam Study. Neurology 2002; 59(12): 1915-21.
[http://dx.doi.org/10.1212/01.WNL.0000038345.77753.46] [PMID: 12499483]

[40]   Grimm MOW, Zimmer VC, Lehmann J, Grimm HS, Hartmann T. The impact of cholesterol, DHA, and sphingolipids on alzheimer's disease. Biomed Res Int 2013; 2013

[41]   Mohaibes RJ, Fiol-deRoque MA, Torres M, *et al.* The hydroxylated form of docosahexaenoic acid (DHA-H) modifies the brain lipid composition in a model of Alzheimer's disease, improving behavioral motor function and survival. Biochim Biophys Acta - Biomembr 2017; 1859(9 Pt B): 1596-603.

[42]   Green KN, Martinez-Coria H, Khashwji H, *et al.* Dietary docosahexaenoic acid and docosapentaenoic acid ameliorate amyloid-beta and tau pathology *via* a mechanism involving presenilin 1 levels. J Neurosci 2007; 27(16): 4385-95.
[http://dx.doi.org/10.1523/JNEUROSCI.0055-07.2007] [PMID: 17442823]

[43]   Grimm MOW, Kuchenbecker J, Grösgen S, *et al.* Docosahexaenoic acid reduces amyloid beta

production *via* multiple pleiotropic mechanisms. J Biol Chem 2011; 286(16): 14028-39.
[http://dx.doi.org/10.1074/jbc.M110.182329] [PMID: 21324907]

[44]   Zhao Y, Calon F, Julien C, *et al.* Docosahexaenoic acid-derived neuroprotectin D1 induces neuronal
        survival *via* secretase- and PPARγ-mediated mechanisms in Alzheimer's disease models. PLoS One
        2011; 6(1): e15816.
        [http://dx.doi.org/10.1371/journal.pone.0015816] [PMID: 21246057]

[45]   Lukiw WJ, Cui JG, Marcheselli VL, *et al.* A role for docosahexaenoic acid-derived neuroprotectin D1
        in neural cell survival and Alzheimer disease. J Clin Invest 2005; 115(10): 2774-83.
        [http://dx.doi.org/10.1172/JCI25420] [PMID: 16151530]

[46]   Cutler RG, Kelly J, Storie K, *et al.* Involvement of oxidative stress-induced abnormalities in ceramide
        and cholesterol metabolism in brain aging and Alzheimer's disease. Proc Natl Acad Sci USA 2004;
        101(7): 2070-5.
        [http://dx.doi.org/10.1073/pnas.0305799101] [PMID: 14970312]

[47]   Sacket SJ, Chung HY, Okajima F, Im DS. Increase in sphingolipid catabolic enzyme activity during
        aging. Acta Pharmacol Sin 2009; 30(10): 1454-61.
        [http://dx.doi.org/10.1038/aps.2009.136] [PMID: 19749786]

[48]   Giusto NM, Roque ME, Ilincheta de Boschero MG. Effects of aging on the content, composition and
        synthesis of sphingomyelin in the central nervous system. Lipids 1992; 27(11): 835-9.
        [http://dx.doi.org/10.1007/BF02535859] [PMID: 1491598]

[49]   Posse de Chaves EI. Sphingolipids in apoptosis, survival and regeneration in the nervous system.
        Biochim Biophys Acta 2006; 1758(12): 1995-2015.
        [http://dx.doi.org/10.1016/j.bbamem.2006.09.018] [PMID: 17084809]

[50]   Sonnino S, Chigorno V. Ganglioside molecular species containing C18- and C20-sphingosine in
        mammalian nervous tissues and neuronal cell cultures. Biochim Biophys Acta 2000; 1469(2): 63-77.
        [http://dx.doi.org/10.1016/S0005-2736(00)00210-8] [PMID: 10998569]

[51]   Jazvinšćak Jembrek M, Hof PR, Šimić G. Ceramides in alzheimer's disease: key mediators of
        neuronal apoptosis induced by oxidative stress and aβ accumulation. Oxid Med Cell Longev 2015;
        2015: 346783.
        [http://dx.doi.org/10.1155/2015/346783] [PMID: 26090071]

[52]   Mielke MM, Lyketsos CG. Alterations of the sphingolipid pathway in Alzheimer's disease: new
        biomarkers and treatment targets? Neuromolecular Med 2010; 12(4): 331-40.
        [http://dx.doi.org/10.1007/s12017-010-8121-y] [PMID: 20571935]

[53]   Bandaru VV, Troncoso J, Wheeler D, *et al.* ApoE4 disrupts sterol and sphingolipid metabolism in
        Alzheimer's but not normal brain. Neurobiol Aging 2009; 30(4): 591-9.
        [http://dx.doi.org/10.1016/j.neurobiolaging.2007.07.024] [PMID: 17888544]

[54]   Han X, M Holtzman D, McKeel DWJ Jr, Kelley J, Morris JC. Substantial sulfatide deficiency and
        ceramide elevation in very early Alzheimer's disease: potential role in disease pathogenesis. J
        Neurochem 2002; 82(4): 809-18.
        [http://dx.doi.org/10.1046/j.1471-4159.2002.00997.x] [PMID: 12358786]

[55]   Katsel P, Li C, Haroutunian V. Gene expression alterations in the sphingolipid metabolism pathways
        during progression of dementia and Alzheimer's disease: a shift toward ceramide accumulation at the
        earliest recognizable stages of Alzheimer's disease? Neurochem Res 2007; 32(4-5): 845-56.
        [http://dx.doi.org/10.1007/s11064-007-9297-x] [PMID: 17342407]

[56]   He X, Huang Y, Li B, Gong CX, Schuchman EH. Deregulation of sphingolipid metabolism in
        Alzheimer's disease. Neurobiol Aging 2010; 31(3): 398-408.
        [http://dx.doi.org/10.1016/j.neurobiolaging.2008.05.010] [PMID: 18547682]

[57]   Lee JT, Xu J, Lee JM, *et al.* Amyloid-beta peptide induces oligodendrocyte death by activating the
        neutral sphingomyelinase-ceramide pathway. J Cell Biol 2004; 164(1): 123-31.

[http://dx.doi.org/10.1083/jcb.200307017] [PMID: 14709545]

[58]   Grimm MO, Grimm HS, Pätzold AJ, *et al.* Regulation of cholesterol and sphingomyelin metabolism by amyloid-beta and presenilin. Nat Cell Biol 2005; 7(11): 1118-23.
[http://dx.doi.org/10.1038/ncb1313] [PMID: 16227967]

[59]   Puglielli L, Ellis BC, Saunders AJ, Kovacs DM. Ceramide stabilizes beta-site amyloid precursor protein-cleaving enzyme 1 and promotes amyloid beta-peptide biogenesis. J Biol Chem 2003; 278(22): 19777-83.
[http://dx.doi.org/10.1074/jbc.M300466200] [PMID: 12649271]

[60]   Ko MH, Puglielli L. Two endoplasmic reticulum (ER)/ER Golgi intermediate compartment-based lysine acetyltransferases post-translationally regulate BACE1 levels. J Biol Chem 2009; 284(4): 2482-92.
[http://dx.doi.org/10.1074/jbc.M804901200] [PMID: 19011241]

[61]   Ben-David O, Futerman AH. The role of the ceramide acyl chain length in neurodegeneration: involvement of ceramide synthases. Neuromolecular Med 2010; 12(4): 341-50.
[http://dx.doi.org/10.1007/s12017-010-8114-x] [PMID: 20502986]

[62]   Yu ZF, Nikolova-Karakashian M, Zhou D, Cheng G, Schuchman EH, Mattson MP. Pivotal role for acidic sphingomyelinase in cerebral ischemia-induced ceramide and cytokine production, and neuronal apoptosis. J Mol Neurosci 2000; 15(2): 85-97.
[http://dx.doi.org/10.1385/JMN:15:2:85] [PMID: 11220788]

[63]   Huang Y, Tanimukai H, Liu F, Iqbal K, Grundke-Iqbal I, Gong C-X. Elevation of the level and activity of acid ceramidase in Alzheimer's disease brain. Eur J Neurosci 2004; 20(12): 3489-97.
[http://dx.doi.org/10.1111/j.1460-9568.2004.03852.x] [PMID: 15610181]

[64]   Hagen N, Hans M, Hartmann D, Swandulla D, van Echten-Deckert G. Sphingosine-1-phosphate links glycosphingolipid metabolism to neurodegeneration *via* a calpain-mediated mechanism. Cell Death Differ 2011; 18(8): 1356-65.
[http://dx.doi.org/10.1038/cdd.2011.7] [PMID: 21331079]

[65]   Takasugi N, Sasaki T, Suzuki K, *et al.* BACE1 activity is modulated by cell-associated sphingosine--phosphate. J Neurosci 2011; 31(18): 6850-7.
[http://dx.doi.org/10.1523/JNEUROSCI.6467-10.2011] [PMID: 21543615]

[66]   Mitew S, Kirkcaldie MTK, Halliday GM, Shepherd CE, Vickers JC, Dickson TC. Focal demyelination in Alzheimer's disease and transgenic mouse models. Acta Neuropathol 2010; 119(5): 567-77.
[http://dx.doi.org/10.1007/s00401-010-0657-2] [PMID: 20198482]

[67]   Gónzalez de San Román E, Manuel I, Giralt MT, Ferrer I, Rodríguez-Puertas R. Imaging mass spectrometry (IMS) of cortical lipids from preclinical to severe stages of Alzheimer's disease. Biochim Biophys Acta 2017; 1859(9 Pt B): 1604-14.
[http://dx.doi.org/10.1016/j.bbamem.2017.05.009] [PMID: 28527668]

[68]   Han X, Cheng H, Fryer JD, Fagan AM, Holtzman DM. Novel role for apolipoprotein E in the central nervous system. Modulation of sulfatide content. J Biol Chem 2003; 278(10): 8043-51.
[http://dx.doi.org/10.1074/jbc.M212340200] [PMID: 12501252]

[69]   Cheng H, Zhou Y, Holtzman DM, Han X. Apolipoprotein E mediates sulfatide depletion in animal models of Alzheimer's disease. Neurobiol Aging 2010; 31(7): 1188-96.
[http://dx.doi.org/10.1016/j.neurobiolaging.2008.07.020] [PMID: 18762354]

[70]   Zeng Y, Han X. Sulfatides facilitate apolipoprotein E-mediated amyloid-beta peptide clearance through an endocytotic pathway. J Neurochem 2008; 106(3): 1275-86.
[http://dx.doi.org/10.1111/j.1471-4159.2008.05481.x] [PMID: 18485101]

[71]   Ariga T, McDonald MP, Yu RK. Role of ganglioside metabolism in the pathogenesis of Alzheimer's disease--a review. J Lipid Res 2008; 49(6): 1157-75.
[http://dx.doi.org/10.1194/jlr.R800007-JLR200] [PMID: 18334715]

[72]   Svennerholm L, Gottfries CG. Membrane lipids, selectively diminished in Alzheimer brains, suggest synapse loss as a primary event in early-onset form (type I) and demyelination in late-onset form (type II). J Neurochem 1994; 62(3): 1039-47.
[http://dx.doi.org/10.1046/j.1471-4159.1994.62031039.x] [PMID: 8113790]

[73]   Brooksbank BW, McGovern J. Gangliosides in the brain in adult Down's syndrome and Alzheimer's disease. Mol Chem Neuropathol 1989; 11(3): 143-56.
[http://dx.doi.org/10.1007/BF03160048] [PMID: 2534985]

[74]   Crino PB, Ullman MD, Vogt BA, Bird ED, Volicer L. Brain gangliosides in dementia of the Alzheimer type. Arch Neurol 1989; 46(4): 398-401.
[http://dx.doi.org/10.1001/archneur.1989.00520400054019] [PMID: 2705899]

[75]   Kracun I, Kalanj S, Cosovic C, Talan-Hranilovic J. Brain gangliosides in Alzheimer's disease. J Hirnforsch 1990; 31(6): 789-93.
[PMID: 2092064]

[76]   Kracun I, Kalanj S, Talan-Hranilovic J, Cosovic C. Cortical distribution of gangliosides in Alzheimer's disease. Neurochem Int 1992; 20(3): 433-8.
[http://dx.doi.org/10.1016/0197-0186(92)90058-Y] [PMID: 1304338]

[77]   Molander-Melin M, Blennow K, Bogdanovic N, Dellheden B, Månsson J-E, Fredman P. Structural membrane alterations in Alzheimer brains found to be associated with regional disease development; increased density of gangliosides GM1 and GM2 and loss of cholesterol in detergent-resistant membrane domains. J Neurochem 2005; 92(1): 171-82.
[http://dx.doi.org/10.1111/j.1471-4159.2004.02849.x] [PMID: 15606906]

[78]   Grimm MOW, Zinser EG, Grösgen S, *et al.* Amyloid precursor protein (APP) mediated regulation of ganglioside homeostasis linking Alzheimer's disease pathology with ganglioside metabolism. PLoS One 2012; 7(3): e34095.
[http://dx.doi.org/10.1371/journal.pone.0034095] [PMID: 22470521]

[79]   Zha Q, Ruan Y, Hartmann T, Beyreuther K, Zhang D. GM1 ganglioside regulates the proteolysis of amyloid precursor protein. Mol Psychiatry 2004; 9(10): 946-52.
[http://dx.doi.org/10.1038/sj.mp.4001509] [PMID: 15052275]

[80]   Holmes O, Paturi S, Ye W, Wolfe MS, Selkoe DJ. Effects of membrane lipids on the activity and processivity of purified γ-secretase. Biochemistry 2012; 51(17): 3565-75.
[http://dx.doi.org/10.1021/bi300303g] [PMID: 22489600]

[81]   Tamboli IY, Prager K, Barth E, Heneka M, Sandhoff K, Walter J. Inhibition of glycosphingolipid biosynthesis reduces secretion of the beta-amyloid precursor protein and amyloid beta-peptide. J Biol Chem 2005; 280(30): 28110-7.
[http://dx.doi.org/10.1074/jbc.M414525200] [PMID: 15923191]

[82]   Kakio A, Nishimoto S, Yanagisawa K, Kozutsumi Y, Matsuzaki K. Interactions of amyloid beta-protein with various gangliosides in raft-like membranes: importance of GM1 ganglioside-bound form as an endogenous seed for Alzheimer amyloid. Biochemistry 2002; 41(23): 7385-90.
[http://dx.doi.org/10.1021/bi0255874] [PMID: 12044171]

[83]   Utsumi M, Yamaguchi Y, Sasakawa H, Yamamoto N, Yanagisawa K, Kato K. Up-and-down topological mode of amyloid beta-peptide lying on hydrophilic/hydrophobic interface of ganglioside clusters. Glycoconj J 2009; 26(8): 999-1006.
[http://dx.doi.org/10.1007/s10719-008-9216-7] [PMID: 19052862]

[84]   Wakabayashi M, Okada T, Kozutsumi Y, Matsuzaki K. GM1 ganglioside-mediated accumulation of amyloid beta-protein on cell membranes. Biochem Biophys Res Commun 2005; 328(4): 1019-23.
[http://dx.doi.org/10.1016/j.bbrc.2005.01.060] [PMID: 15707979]

[85]   Fernández-Pérez EJ, Sepúlveda FJ, Peoples R, Aguayo LG. Role of membrane GM1 on early neuronal membrane actions of Aβ during onset of Alzheimer's disease. Biochim Biophys Acta 2017; 1863(12):

3105-16.
[http://dx.doi.org/10.1016/j.bbadis.2017.08.013] [PMID: 28844949]

[86] Yamamoto N, Matsubara T, Sato T, Yanagisawa K. Age-dependent high-density clustering of GM1 ganglioside at presynaptic neuritic terminals promotes amyloid beta-protein fibrillogenesis. Biochim Biophys Acta 2008; 1778(12): 2717-26.
[http://dx.doi.org/10.1016/j.bbamem.2008.07.028] [PMID: 18727916]

[87] Bugiani O, Giaccone G, Verga L, *et al.* Alzheimer patients and Down patients: abnormal presynaptic terminals are related to cerebral preamyloid deposits. Neurosci Lett 1990; 119(1): 56-9.
[http://dx.doi.org/10.1016/0304-3940(90)90754-W] [PMID: 1965862]

[88] Schroeder F, Gallegos AM, Atshaves BP, *et al.* Recent advances in membrane microdomains: rafts, caveolae, and intracellular cholesterol trafficking. Exp Biol Med (Maywood) 2001; 226(10): 873-90.
[http://dx.doi.org/10.1177/153537020122601002] [PMID: 11682693]

[89] Hayashi H, Igbavboa U, Hamanaka H, *et al.* Cholesterol is increased in the exofacial leaflet of synaptic plasma membranes of human apolipoprotein E4 knock-in mice. Neuroreport 2002; 13(4): 383-6.
[http://dx.doi.org/10.1097/00001756-200203250-00004] [PMID: 11930145]

[90] Dietschy JM, Turley SD. Cholesterol metabolism in the brain. Curr Opin Lipidol 2001; 12(2): 105-12.
[http://dx.doi.org/10.1097/00041433-200104000-00003] [PMID: 11264981]

[91] Gamba P, Testa G, Sottero B, Gargiulo S, Poli G, Leonarduzzi G. The link between altered cholesterol metabolism and Alzheimer's disease. Ann N Y Acad Sci 2012; 1259(1): 54-64.
[http://dx.doi.org/10.1111/j.1749-6632.2012.06513.x] [PMID: 22758637]

[92] Björkhem I, Meaney S. Brain cholesterol: long secret life behind a barrier. Arterioscler Thromb Vasc Biol 2004; 24(5): 806-15.
[http://dx.doi.org/10.1161/01.ATV.0000120374.59826.1b] [PMID: 14764421]

[93] Pfrieger FW. Cholesterol homeostasis and function in neurons of the central nervous system. Cell Mol Life Sci 2003; 60(6): 1158-71.
[http://dx.doi.org/10.1007/s00018-003-3018-7] [PMID: 12861382]

[94] Jurevics H, Morell P. Cholesterol for synthesis of myelin is made locally, not imported into brain. J Neurochem 1995; 64(2): 895-901.
[http://dx.doi.org/10.1046/j.1471-4159.1995.64020895.x] [PMID: 7830084]

[95] Björkhem I, Lütjohann D, Breuer O, Sakinis A, Wennmalm A. Importance of a novel oxidative mechanism for elimination of brain cholesterol. Turnover of cholesterol and 24(S)-hydroxycholesterol in rat brain as measured with 18O2 techniques *in vivo* and *In vitro*. J Biol Chem 1997; 272(48): 30178-84.
[http://dx.doi.org/10.1074/jbc.272.48.30178] [PMID: 9374499]

[96] Hirsch-Reinshagen V, Maia LF, Burgess BL, *et al.* The absence of ABCA1 decreases soluble ApoE levels but does not diminish amyloid deposition in two murine models of Alzheimer disease. J Biol Chem 2005; 280(52): 43243-56.
[http://dx.doi.org/10.1074/jbc.M508781200] [PMID: 16207707]

[97] Lehmann JM, Kliewer SA, Moore LB, *et al.* Activation of the nuclear receptor LXR by oxysterols defines a new hormone response pathway. J Biol Chem 1997; 272(6): 3137-40.
[http://dx.doi.org/10.1074/jbc.272.6.3137] [PMID: 9013544]

[98] Wang N, Silver DL, Thiele C, Tall AR. ATP-binding cassette transporter A1 (ABCA1) functions as a cholesterol efflux regulatory protein. J Biol Chem 2001; 276(26): 23742-7.
[http://dx.doi.org/10.1074/jbc.M102348200] [PMID: 11309399]

[99] Bjorkhem I, Diczfalusy U. 24(S),25-epoxycholesterol-a potential friend. Arterioscler Thromb Vasc Biol 2004; 24(12): 2209-10.
[http://dx.doi.org/10.1161/01.ATV.0000148704.72481.28] [PMID: 15576644]

[100] Thelen KM, Falkai P, Bayer TA, Lütjohann D. Cholesterol synthesis rate in human hippocampus declines with aging. Neurosci Lett 2006; 403(1-2): 15-9.
[http://dx.doi.org/10.1016/j.neulet.2006.04.034] [PMID: 16701946]

[101] Igbavboa U, Avdulov NA, Schroeder F, Wood WG. Increasing age alters transbilayer fluidity and cholesterol asymmetry in synaptic plasma membranes of mice. J Neurochem 1996; 66(4): 1717-25.
[http://dx.doi.org/10.1046/j.1471-4159.1996.66041717.x] [PMID: 8627330]

[102] Kivipelto M, Helkala EL, Hänninen T, *et al.* Midlife vascular risk factors and late-life mild cognitive impairment: A population-based study. Neurology 2001; 56(12): 1683-9.
[http://dx.doi.org/10.1212/WNL.56.12.1683] [PMID: 11425934]

[103] Wolf H, Grunwald M, Kruggel F, *et al.* Hippocampal volume discriminates between normal cognition; questionable and mild dementia in the elderly. Neurobiol Aging 2001; 22(2): 177-86.
[http://dx.doi.org/10.1016/S0197-4580(00)00238-4] [PMID: 11182467]

[104] Yaffe K, Barrett-Connor E, Lin F, Grady D. Serum lipoprotein levels, statin use, and cognitive function in older women. Arch Neurol 2002; 59(3): 378-84.
[http://dx.doi.org/10.1001/archneur.59.3.378] [PMID: 11890840]

[105] Mielke MM, Lyketsos CG. Lipids and the pathogenesis of Alzheimer's disease: is there a link? Int Rev Psychiatry 2006; 18(2): 173-86.
[http://dx.doi.org/10.1080/09540260600583007] [PMID: 16777671]

[106] Reitz C, Luchsinger J, Tang M-X, Manly J, Mayeux R. Impact of plasma lipids and time on memory performance in healthy elderly without dementia. Neurology 2005; 64(8): 1378-83.
[http://dx.doi.org/10.1212/01.WNL.0000158274.31318.3C] [PMID: 15851727]

[107] Reitz C. Dyslipidemia and dementia: current epidemiology, genetic evidence, and mechanisms behind the associations. J Alzheimers Dis 2012; 30 (Suppl. 2): S127-45.
[http://dx.doi.org/10.3233/JAD-2011-110599] [PMID: 21965313]

[108] Reitz C, Tang M-X, Luchsinger J, Mayeux R. Relation of plasma lipids to Alzheimer disease and vascular dementia. Arch Neurol 2004; 61(5): 705-14.
[http://dx.doi.org/10.1001/archneur.61.5.705] [PMID: 15148148]

[109] Mielke MM, Zandi PP, Sjögren M, *et al.* High total cholesterol levels in late life associated with a reduced risk of dementia. Neurology 2005; 64(10): 1689-95.
[http://dx.doi.org/10.1212/01.WNL.0000161870.78572.A5] [PMID: 15911792]

[110] Shepardson NE, Shankar GM, Selkoe DJ. Cholesterol level and statin use in Alzheimer disease: I. Review of epidemiological and preclinical studies. Arch Neurol 2011; 68(10): 1239-44.
[http://dx.doi.org/10.1001/archneurol.2011.203] [PMID: 21987540]

[111] Hooff GP, Peters I, Wood WG, Müller WE, Eckert GP. Modulation of cholesterol, farnesylpyrophosphate, and geranylgeranylpyrophosphate in neuroblastoma SH-SY5Y-APP695 cells: impact on amyloid beta-protein production. Mol Neurobiol 2010; 41(2-3): 341-50.
[http://dx.doi.org/10.1007/s12035-010-8117-5] [PMID: 20405344]

[112] Kölsch H, Heun R, Jessen F, *et al.* Alterations of cholesterol precursor levels in Alzheimer's disease. Biochim Biophys Acta 2010; 1801(8): 945-50.
[http://dx.doi.org/10.1016/j.bbalip.2010.03.001] [PMID: 20226877]

[113] Leduc V, Jasmin-Bélanger S, Poirier J. APOE and cholesterol homeostasis in Alzheimer's disease. Trends Mol Med 2010; 16(10): 469-77.
[http://dx.doi.org/10.1016/j.molmed.2010.07.008] [PMID: 20817608]

[114] Maulik M, Westaway D, Jhamandas JH, Kar S. Role of cholesterol in APP metabolism and its significance in Alzheimer's disease pathogenesis. Mol Neurobiol 2013; 47(1): 37-63.
[http://dx.doi.org/10.1007/s12035-012-8337-y] [PMID: 22983915]

[115] Luetjohann D, Meichsner S, Pettersson H. Lipids in Alzheimer's disease and their potential for therapy.

Clin Lipidol 2012; 7(1): 65-78.
[http://dx.doi.org/10.2217/clp.11.74]

[116]   Hicks DA, Nalivaeva NN, Turner AJ. Lipid rafts and Alzheimer's disease: protein-lipid interactions and perturbation of signaling. Front Physiol 2012; 3(18): 189.
[PMID: 22737128]

[117]   Kojro E, Gimpl G, Lammich S, Marz W, Fahrenholz F. Low cholesterol stimulates the nonamyloidogenic pathway by its effect on the alpha -secretase ADAM 10. Proc Natl Acad Sci USA 2001; 98(10): 5815-20.
[http://dx.doi.org/10.1073/pnas.081612998] [PMID: 11309494]

[118]   Kalvodova L, Kahya N, Schwille P, *et al.* Lipids as modulators of proteolytic activity of BACE: involvement of cholesterol, glycosphingolipids, and anionic phospholipids *In vitro.* J Biol Chem 2005; 280(44): 36815-23.
[http://dx.doi.org/10.1074/jbc.M504484200] [PMID: 16115865]

[119]   Vetrivel KS, Cheng H, Lin W, *et al.* Association of gamma-secretase with lipid rafts in post-Golgi and endosome membranes. J Biol Chem 2004; 279(43): 44945-54.
[http://dx.doi.org/10.1074/jbc.M407986200] [PMID: 15322084]

[120]   Ehehalt R, Keller P, Haass C, Thiele C, Simons K. Amyloidogenic processing of the Alzheimer beta-amyloid precursor protein depends on lipid rafts. J Cell Biol 2003; 160(1): 113-23.
[http://dx.doi.org/10.1083/jcb.200207113] [PMID: 12515826]

[121]   Chauhan NB. Membrane dynamics, cholesterol homeostasis, and Alzheimer's disease. JLipid Res 2003; 44(0022–2275): 2019-9.

[122]   Vestergaard M, Hamada T, Morita M, Takagi M. Cholesterol, lipids, amyloid Beta, and Alzheimer's. Curr Alzheimer Res 2010; 7(3): 262-70.
[http://dx.doi.org/10.2174/156720510791050821] [PMID: 19715550]

[123]   Yao Z-X, Papadopoulos V. Function of beta-amyloid in cholesterol transport: a lead to neurotoxicity. FASEB J 2002; 16(12): 1677-9.
[http://dx.doi.org/10.1096/fj.02-0285fje] [PMID: 12206998]

[124]   Abad-Rodriguez J, Ledesma MD, Craessaerts K, *et al.* Neuronal membrane cholesterol loss enhances amyloid peptide generation. J Cell Biol 2004; 167(5): 953-60.
[http://dx.doi.org/10.1083/jcb.200404149] [PMID: 15583033]

[125]   Schneider A, Schulz-Schaeffer W, Hartmann T, Schulz JB, Simons M. Cholesterol depletion reduces aggregation of amyloid-beta peptide in hippocampal neurons. Neurobiol Dis 2006; 23(3): 573-7.
[http://dx.doi.org/10.1016/j.nbd.2006.04.015] [PMID: 16777421]

[126]   Arispe N, Doh M. Plasma membrane cholesterol controls the cytotoxicity of Alzheimer's disease AbetaP (1-40) and (1-42) peptides. FASEB J 2002; 16(12): 1526-36.
[http://dx.doi.org/10.1096/fj.02-0829com] [PMID: 12374775]

[127]   Sponne I, Fifre A, Koziel V, Oster T, Olivier J-L, Pillot T. Membrane cholesterol interferes with neuronal apoptosis induced by soluble oligomers but not fibrils of amyloid-beta peptide. FASEB J 2004; 18(7): 836-8.
[http://dx.doi.org/10.1096/fj.03-0372fje] [PMID: 15001562]

[128]   Yip CM, Elton EA, Darabie AA, Morrison MR, McLaurin J. Cholesterol, a modulator of membrane-associated Abeta-fibrillogenesis and neurotoxicity. J Mol Biol 2001; 311(4): 723-34.
[http://dx.doi.org/10.1006/jmbi.2001.4881] [PMID: 11518526]

[129]   Zhou Y, Richardson JS. Cholesterol protects PC12 cells from beta-amyloid induced calcium disordering and cytotoxicity. Neuroreport 1996; 7(15-17): 2487-90.
[http://dx.doi.org/10.1097/00001756-199611040-00017] [PMID: 8981409]

[130]   Drolle E, Negoda A, Hammond K, Pavlov E, Leonenko Z. Changes in lipid membranes may trigger amyloid toxicity in Alzheimer's disease. PLoS One 2017; 12(8): e0182194.

[http://dx.doi.org/10.1371/journal.pone.0182194] [PMID: 28767712]

[131] Leoni V, Masterman T, Mousavi FS, *et al.* Diagnostic use of cerebral and extracerebral oxysterols. Clin Chem Lab Med 2004; 42(2): 186-91.
[http://dx.doi.org/10.1515/CCLM.2004.034] [PMID: 15061359]

[132] Papassotiropoulos A, Lütjohann D, Bagli M, *et al.* 24S-hydroxycholesterol in cerebrospinal fluid is elevated in early stages of dementia. J Psychiatr Res 2002; 36(1): 27-32.
[http://dx.doi.org/10.1016/S0022-3956(01)00050-4] [PMID: 11755458]

[133] Heverin M, Bogdanovic N, Lütjohann D, *et al.* Changes in the levels of cerebral and extracerebral sterols in the brain of patients with Alzheimer's disease. J Lipid Res 2004; 45(1): 186-93.
[http://dx.doi.org/10.1194/jlr.M300320-JLR200] [PMID: 14523054]

[134] Shafaati M, Marutle A, Pettersson H, *et al.* Marked accumulation of 27-hydroxycholesterol in the brains of Alzheimer's patients with the Swedish APP 670/671 mutation. J Lipid Res 2011; 52(5): 1004-10.
[http://dx.doi.org/10.1194/jlr.M014548] [PMID: 21335619]

[135] Yau JL, Rasmuson S, Andrew R, *et al.* Dehydroepiandrosterone 7-hydroxylase CYP7B: predominant expression in primate hippocampus and reduced expression in Alzheimer's disease. Neuroscience 2003; 121(2): 307-14.
[http://dx.doi.org/10.1016/S0306-4522(03)00438-X] [PMID: 14521990]

[136] Brown J III, Theisler C, Silberman S, *et al.* Differential expression of cholesterol hydroxylases in Alzheimer's disease. J Biol Chem 2004; 279(33): 34674-81.
[http://dx.doi.org/10.1074/jbc.M402324200] [PMID: 15148325]

[137] Gamba P, Testa G, Gargiulo S, Staurenghi E, Poli G, Leonarduzzi G. Oxidized cholesterol as the driving force behind the development of Alzheimer's disease. Front Aging Neurosci 2015; 7: 119.
[http://dx.doi.org/10.3389/fnagi.2015.00119] [PMID: 26150787]

[138] Kim WS, Chan SL, Hill AF, Guillemin GJ, Garner B. Impact of 27-hydroxycholesterol on amyloid-beta peptide production and ATP-binding cassette transporter expression in primary human neurons. J Alzheimers Dis 2009; 16(1): 121-31.
[http://dx.doi.org/10.3233/JAD-2009-0944] [PMID: 19158428]

[139] Marwarha G, Dasari B, Prasanthi JRP, Schommer J, Ghribi O. Leptin reduces the accumulation of Abeta and phosphorylated tau induced by 27-hydroxycholesterol in rabbit organotypic slices. J Alzheimers Dis 2010; 19(3): 1007-19.
[http://dx.doi.org/10.3233/JAD-2010-1298] [PMID: 20157255]

[140] Prasanthi JR, Huls A, Thomasson S, Thompson A, Schommer E, Ghribi O. Differential effects of 24-hydroxycholesterol and 27-hydroxycholesterol on beta-amyloid precursor protein levels and processing in human neuroblastoma SH-SY5Y cells. Mol Neurodegener 2009; 4: 1.
[http://dx.doi.org/10.1186/1750-1326-4-1] [PMID: 19126211]

[141] Usui K, Hulleman JD, Paulsson JF, Siegel SJ, Powers ET, Kelly JW. Site-specific modification of Alzheimer's peptides by cholesterol oxidation products enhances aggregation energetics and neurotoxicity. Proc Natl Acad Sci USA 2009; 106(44): 18563-8.
[http://dx.doi.org/10.1073/pnas.0804758106] [PMID: 19841277]

CHAPTER 4

Amyloidogenic Peptide Structure, Aggregation, And Membrane Interaction

Manoel Arcisio-Miranda and **Laíz da Costa Silva-Gonçalves**[*]

Laboratório de Neurobiologia Estrutural e Funcional (LaNEF), Departamento de Biofísica, Universidade Federal de São Paulo, São Paulo, Brazil

Abstract: It is estimated that 44 millions of people have Alzheimer's disease (AD) or related dementia around the world. The AD is an irreversible progressive brain disorder that destroys the memory and thinking and causes the loss of cognitive functions. The development of AD is strongly correlated with the development of plaques and tangles in the brain. Beta-amyloid (Aβ) peptides are the main compound in the brain plaques however, their neurotoxic effects remain unclear. These peptides are generated from Amyloid Precursor Protein (APP) and the APP processing may be modulated by many factors, such as lipid rafts. Aβ coexists in different forms in the brain and the exact neurotoxic effect of each one is not understood. The majority of the studies about Aβ neurotoxicity suggests that the fibrillar form is the most neurotoxic and for this reason, much effort has been employed to understand mechanisms that modulate or inhibit the fibrillation process. Other studies suggest that the main neurotoxic form is the oligomer, which forms channels in the lipid membrane and induces cell death. In this chapter, we explore the mechanism of Aβ's production and fibrillation, and the factors that can modulate it.

Keywords: Aggregation, Amyloidogenesis, Amyloid Fibrils, Amyloid Inhibitors, APP, β-Amyloid Peptides, Membrane.

INTRODUCTION

Alzheimer's Disease (AD) is the most common cause of dementia in elderly people [1] and is considered a global epidemic [2, 3]. The chances of developing AD double every 5 years after the age 65 years, and it is estimated that 11% of the population over this age are already affected with AD [2, 3]. Many hypotheses have been proposed to explain the development of AD since your causes remain unknown. Among these hypotheses are the altered mitochondrial activity, neuroinflammation, the altered metabolism of cholesterol or insulin [4 - 8], and the dendritic hypotheses [9, 10]. Beyond these hypotheses are the amyloid

[*] **Corresponding author Laíz da Costa Silva-Gonçalves:** LaNEF, Rua Botucatu, 862 – Edifício Ciências Biomédicas - 7° andar, 03262-000, São Paulo, São Paulo, Brazil; Tel: +11 5576-4848 ext. 2337; E-mail: laiz.lcs@gmail.com

Fernando A. Oliveira (Ed.)

cascade and phosphorylated tau protein hypotheses. One of the hallmarks of the amyloid cascade hypotheses is the increased production of the considered a more neurotoxic form of the β-amyloid (Aβ) peptide, *i.e.* the $A\beta_{42}$, and its accumulation in the form of senile plaques within the central nervous system (CNS) [1, 11]. Several studies suggest that these factors determine the main phenotypes of the AD, which are increased inflammatory response and oxidative stress, changes in the homeostasis of CNS, and synaptic dysfunction. As a result of these changes, there is a progressive increase in cell death when compared with healthy individuals [12, 13].

As we will see in this chapter, Aβ peptides may exist in the CNS in different configurations, from monomers to fibrils. Although there is no consensus in the literature regarding the most neurotoxic between them, many studies point to intracellular calcium dysregulation signaling as the main factor that triggers cell death, independent of the causing configuration. The main mechanism by which Aβ peptides can alter cellular Ca^{2+} homeostasis involves changes in membrane Ca^{2+} permeability; however, the precise mechanism remains to be determined. Three major mechanisms are proposed: (i) interactions with endogenous Ca^{2+}-permeable channels, disruption of lipid membrane integrity, and formation of Ca^{2+}-permeable channels by Aβ peptides (for a review of these mechanisms, please see [14]).

Several groups have been testing the cytotoxicity effects of the two main forms of Aβ peptides, the $A\beta_{40}$ and $A\beta_{42}$. The results generated by these groups were obtained in different experimental conditions, such as the number of cells, incubation time, aggregation state, and the method used to quantify the effects on cell viability. The cytotoxicity data collected in different cell lines are summarized in Table **1**.

Table 1. Cytotoxic effect of $A\beta_{40}$ and $A\beta_{42}$ in different cell lines.

Cell Line	$[A\beta_{40}]$ (μMol L^{-1})	$[A\beta_{42}]$ (μMol L^{-1})	Ref.
Rat Primary Astrocyte	0,1-10	-	[15, 16]
Oligodendrocytes	0,2-20	-	[17]
Rat Primary Cortical Neurons	5-25	1-25	[18 - 22]
HeLa	0,023 - 5	-	[23, 24]
Rat Brain Endothelial cell	10	0,1 - 30	[25, 26]
B12	10	-	[27]
PC-12	0,05 - 2,5	0,05 - 20	[28 - 32]
Primary Human Neurons	$10^{-3} - 10^{-6}$	$10^{-3} - 10^{-6}$	[33]
SH-SY5Y	10	1 - 20	[34 - 37]

(Table 1) cont.....

Cell Line	$[A\beta_{40}]$ (μMol L^{-1})	$[A\beta_{42}]$ (μMol L^{-1})	Ref.
Mice/Rat Primary Hippocampal Neurons	-	0,1 - 20	[11, 26, 38 - 41]
HT22	-	1-10	[42]
NT2	-	0,04-5	[43]
EcR293	-	0,04-5	[43]
Huvec	-	50	[44]
B12	-	10	[27]

Amyloid Precursor Protein and Amyloid β Peptide Processing Pathways

Aβ peptides are produced by serial cleavage pathways, through the action of secretases α, β or γ, which occur in the N-terminal and/or transmembrane portions of the Amyloid Precursor Protein (APP).

The APP is a transmembrane glycoprotein with MW between 110 and 135 kDa [45]. Its physiological function is not well established; but an action as vesicular receptor for the motor protein kinesin-I has been hypothesized [46 - 50]. Other functions attributed to the APP are the regulation of neuronal survival, protection against toxic external stimuli, synaptic plasticity and cellular adhesion [9]. This protein has a large extracellular domain (88% of the protein length), a single membrane-spanning domain and a short cytoplasmatic domain (47 amino acids) [51 - 53]. The N-terminal and the C-terminal are directed to the extracellular and to the cytoplasmatic compartments, respectively. The heterogeneous MW arises mainly because the full-length human APP has three isoforms - APP$_{695}$, APP$_{751,}$ and APP$_{770}$ – derived from alternative splicing of exon 7, which encodes a Kunitz-type protease inhibitor (KPI) domain and exon 8, which encodes an OX-2 homology sequence [49, 54 - 57]. APP$_{695}$ lacks KPI and OX-2, APP$_{751}$ contains KPI, and APP$_{770}$ contains KPI and OX-2 [58, 59]. APP$_{751}$ and APP$_{770}$ are widely expressed in neuronal and non-neuronal cells and found in large quantities in the brain of AD patients [49, 60, 61]. APP$_{695}$ is expressed more highly in neurons and in very small quantities in other cells.

The APP is initially cleaved by α- or β-secretases, which directly compete for it [62 - 64]. The enzyme α-secretase is a zinc metalloproteinase whereas the β-secretase is an integral membrane aspartyl protease encoded by the β-site APP-cleaving enzyme 1 gene (BACE1) [45]. The cleavage by α-secretase is defined as nonamyloidogenic pathway (Fig. 1) and occurs at the position 83 amino acids from the C terminal, generating two fragments: APPsα, which is secreted in the extracellular medium and α-Carboxy Terminal Fragment (α-CTF), which remains anchored in the membrane [52, 58, 62, 65]. Subsequently, the α-CTF fragment is cleaved by γ-secretase, a membrane-bound complex of at least four components including the presenilins, nicastrin, and the genes APH-1 and PEN-2 [45], releasing the p53 peptide in the extracellular space and the APP Intracellular Domain (AICD) in the cytoplasm [46, 48, 66].

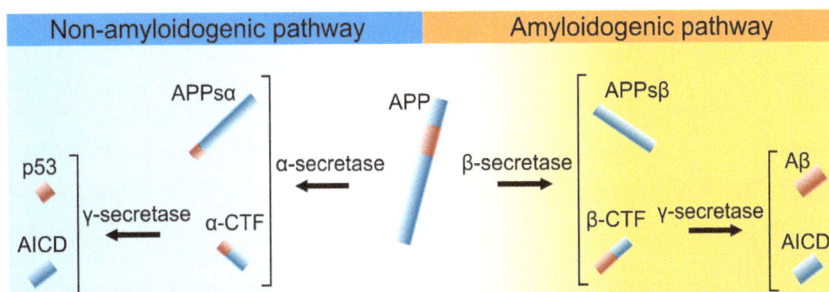

Fig. (1). Processing pathways of APP to produce Aβ and others peptides. APP can be processed in two different pathways: In a non-amyloidogenic pathway, the full-length APP is initially cleaved by α-secretase, yielding APPsα (which is released to extracellular space) and α-CTF (which remains anchored in the lipid membrane). Next, α-CTF is cleaved by γ-secretase releasing p53 peptide in the extracellular space and the APP Intracellular Domain (AICD) in the cytoplasm. The amyloidogenic pathway begins with the cleavage of the full-length APP by β-secretase, yielding APPsβ (which is released to extracellular space) and β-CTF (which remains anchored in the lipid membrane). β-CTF is than cleaved by γ-secretase releasing Aβ peptide in the extracellular space and the APP Intracellular Domain (AICD) in the cytoplasm.

In the amyloidogenic pathway, APP is cleaved by β-secretase at the position located 99 amino acids from the C terminal, generating two fragments: APPsβ and β-CTF. After the cleavage by γ-secretase, β-CTF is converted in AICD and in Aβ peptide which is released in the cytoplasm and in the extracellular space, respectively [46, 49, 52, 67]. The γ-secretase cleavage is heterogeneous generating peptides with various lengths (39 to 43 amino acids) [68]. Most of the Aβ peptides produced have 40 amino acids ($A\beta_{40}$), but a little fraction has 42 amino acids ($A\beta_{42}$) [69] (Fig. **2**). The addition of two hydrophobic amino acids in $A\beta_{42}$ favors the oligomeric and fibrillar forms, being considered the most neurotoxic form of Aβ peptides [48, 70]. The 43 amino acids species ($A\beta_{43}$) is a rarer isoform of Aβ peptide and is more harmful than $A\beta_{42}$ [71].

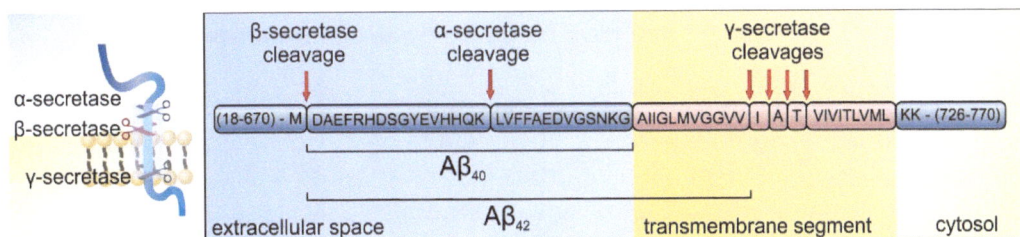

Fig. (2). APP Cleavage Sites. There are distinct cleavage sites of APP protein by secretases. APP can be cleaved by β-secretase in a position before the Aβ sequence and the resulting fragments are cleaved by γ-secretase in different positions within the transmembrane segment, generating different Aβ peptides isoforms. APP also can cleave by α-secretase, within the Aβ sequence.

Major Factors that Modulate the Production of Aβ Peptides

Inhibition of β-Secretase Activity

This line of evidence comes mainly from genetic studies, which demonstrate that the inhibition of β-secretase activity can ameliorate several phenotypes of AD disease. Devi & Ohno (2010) demonstrated that BACE1 -/- homozygous knockout mice fail to produce Aβ peptides and do not develop amyloid plaques, reducing the impairment of conditioned memory of AD-prone mice [72]. Already, Jonsson *et al.* [73], who searched for coding variants in APP gene in a set of whole-genome sequence data from 1,795 Icelanders, found that a single coding mutation (A673T) in the APP gene protects against the Alzheimer's disease and cognitive decline in the elderly people (without AD), supporting the hypothesis that reducing the β-cleavage of APP may protect against the disease.

Pharmacological inhibition of β-secretase is also possible and has been considered a promising strategy for clinical usage in AD patients. In this sense, several drugs, such as CTS-21166, LY2886721, E2609, HPP854, and RG7129, have been evaluated in terms of efficiency in different clinical trial stages. However, clinical development of such inhibitors has suffered three major difficulties: (i) potential β-secretase inhibitors must also be able to penetrate both the plasma and endosomal membranes to access to the intracellular compartments where endogenous β-secretase is located; (ii) potential side effects have also been grown. It is now accepted that β-secretase may modulate the activity of numerous other proteins, including proteins involved in myelination and sodium homeostasis and in normal cell metabolism [73 - 75], which suggests a risk of morbidity with long-term β-secretase inhibition; and (iii) liver toxicity.

Activation of α-Secretase Activity

This seems to be an obvious therapeutic strategy. As described above, in the non-amyloidogenic pathway, APP is first cleaved by α-secretase along the Aβ peptide region, precluding its formation [67, 76, 77]. The stimulation of this enzyme has been shown to have a protective role in AD patients [78 - 80]. However, the ongoing uncertain over potential side effects of upregulation of the α-secretase has been limited the development of direct activators of it. However, several studies have demonstrated that a number of drugs currently use as a part of the treatment of AD patients, such as Selegiline® and Atorvastatin®, increase the activity of α-secretase [77, 81 - 86].

Inhibition of γ-Secretase Complex Activity

As we have seen above, the last step in the amyloidogenic pathway is the cleavage of β-CTF by γ-secretase complex. In this sense, the inhibition of its activity has also been considered promising to reduce the production of Aβ and thus, used in the treatment of AD patients [87]. However, the γ-secretase complex activity can generate a wide range of substrates with diverse physiological functions. One of these substrates is Notch, a cell surface signaling receptor that is essential for many aspects of cell development and differentiation [88 - 92]. It may also play a role in tumor suppression [93]. For these reasons, potential side effects with toxicity in γ-secretase inhibition can be predicted to occur.

Moreover, clinical trials of inhibiting γ-secretase activity demonstrate adverse effects on cognitive recovery ability in AD patients [94]. Thus, the future of this strategy as an AD treatment may depend on the successful development of γ-secretase complex-selective compounds, *i.e.*, with no effects on the activity of other substrates [95, 96]. For this purpose, various γ-secretase modulators (GSMs) was tested. These inhibitors block the action of the γ-secretase enzyme but maintain their action in others processing pathways [97].

Effects of Biological Membrane Composition in the Synthesis of Aβ Peptides

Once the APP and the processing enzymes are membrane proteins, several studies suggest that changes in the physical properties of biological membranes by changes in lipid composition can influence the processing and generation of Aβ peptides. In this sense, the model of membrane compartmentalization has been proposed. This model suggests that APP would be located in two separate regions of the membrane, with different physicochemical properties; a region associated with cholesterol lipid clusters where Aβ is generated and a second region that is not related to lipid clusters, where the α-secretase acts, determining the non-amyloidogenic pathway [98 - 100]. Using neuroblastoma N2a cells, Ehehalt *et al.* (2003) demonstrated that depletion of cholesterol, by treating the cells with Lovastatin (which inhibits cholesterol synthesis) or Methyl-β-cyclodextrin (which removes cholesterol from the membranes), inhibits the production of Aβ peptides [62]. Enrichment of cells with cholesterol promotes opposite effect. Other studies show a direct relationship between the membrane cholesterol levels and activity of β-secretase, while Lovastatin increases the activity of α-secretase [101, 102].

The compartmentalization model then suggests that alterations in the fluidity of biological membranes modify the processability of Aβ peptides. Interestingly, Kojro *et al.* (2001) demonstrated that alterations in membrane fluidity, by modulating the cholesterol content, reduce the production of Aβ by preventing the interaction of the substrate with its proteases. The substitution of cholesterol for cholestane, which induces little or no alteration in membrane fluidity, reduces the production of Aβ by α-secretase; conversely, substitution for lanosterol, which increases membrane fluidity, increases the production of Aβ by α-secretase [99].

Another factor that can alter the activity of processing enzymes of Aβ peptides is the presence of fatty acids as constituents of biological membranes. Studies in rats show that diets enriched with polyunsaturated fatty acids can reduce AD-like pathology [103]. For example, long-term supplementation with docosahexaenoic acid (DHA, 20:5) improved spatial memory, decreased cerebral deposition of Aβ and slightly increased the cerebral blood volume, indicating that DHA enriched diets can reduce AD-like pathology. Similar to that observed with the reduction in cholesterol content, the increase of polyunsaturated fatty acids can increase the fluidity of biological membranes, stimulating the activity of α-secretase. However, the relationship between the degree of unsaturation of fatty acids and changes in the α-secretase activity is still controversial. Yang *et al.* (2011) showed that human neuroblastoma cells SH-SY5Y treated with arachidonic acid (AA, 20:4), eicosapentaenoic acid (EPA, 20:5), and DHA for 24h showed increased membrane fluidity and Aβ produced by alpha-secretase. Similar effects were not observed when cells were treated with the fatty acids stearic (18:0), oleic (18:1), linoleic (18:2) and α-linolenic (18:3), suggesting that only fatty acids with four or more double bonds are able to increase the fluidity of the membrane and lead to an increase in the production of Aβ by α-secretase [104]. However, another study shows that PSwt-1 cells treated with oleic and linoleic acids increase the activity of α-secretase and the production of Aβ [105].

The Aβ Peptides and the Fiber Formation Process

The two main amyloidogenic peptides produced by the cleavage of APP proteins are $A\beta_{40}$ and $A\beta_{42}$ [45, 67, 106]. These peptides are highly homologous to each other; but the addition of two hydrophobic amino acids at the C-terminus of $A\beta_{42}$ makes it more neurotoxic and more prone to aggregate than the $A\beta_{40}$ form, which means that the $A\beta_{42}$ peptide is more related with the AD [107 - 110]. In solution, Aβ monomer can be structured in two conformations: (i) as a random coil [111] or (ii) as two regions of α-helix, at residues 8-25 and 28-38, separated by a flexible hinge [112]. At pH 7.4, these peptides have a net charge of +3 and can form β-sheet structures during the dimerization process [1]. The Aβ dimmers can assemble into higher order aggregates such as oligomers and fibrils. The conversion rate of these peptides into oligomers is not similar. $A\beta_{42}$ have greater tendency to fibrillation and is more toxic than $A\beta_{40}$ [45, 69, 108, 109, 113, 114].

Interestingly, these two peptides are not only pathological forms, *i.e.*, they are also present in the brain and in cerebrospinal fluid of healthy individuals. In this condition, $A\beta_{40}$ and $A\beta_{42}$ coexist in a molar ratio of 9:1 [69, 113]. However, in the brain AD patients, there is a shift to a higher level of $A\beta_{42}$, determining a ratio of

3:7 [113]. Importantly, some studies have demonstrated that this difference in ratio between the $A\beta_{40}$ and $A\beta_{42}$ may interfere with the stability, neurotoxic potential, and kinetics of aggregation of each other [113]. It has been shown that $A\beta_{40}$ decreases $A\beta_{42}$ aggregation, while $A\beta_{42}$ induces $A\beta_{40}$ aggregation. *In vivo* studies confirm this observation and have shown that higher levels of $A\beta_{40}$ might protect the brain [113].

The extracellular deposition of $A\beta$ peptides in the form of senile plaques is a typical phenotype of the AD [45, 62, 63, 113, 115 - 117]. This process is associated by many researchers with the neurotoxic action of $A\beta$ peptides, but the exact mechanism of neurotoxicity is still unknown and under debate. Some studies suggest the fibril form as the most neurotoxic form [118], while others support the oligomeric and protofibril forms [1, 107, 119 - 124]. However, albeit the molecular events that determine amyloid fibrillation are not still well understood, the cell surface has been considered as the site for the formation of amyloid fibers [125 - 130]; in this scenario, the membrane acts as a platform to enhance the local concentration of $A\beta$ or to promote the formation of specific structures that facilitate the fibrillar elongation [127 - 130]. *In vitro* studies show that the $A\beta$ can adopt different morphologies depending on the experimental conditions; thereby affecting the morphology of the fibers. This can influence the toxicity of aggregates and support the idea that this process can occur *via* multiple mechanisms [113, 131 - 133].

The amyloid aggregates and fibers are insoluble in an aqueous medium. The process by which the soluble $A\beta$ peptides are converted into insoluble aggregates or fibers is known as amyloidogenesis [134 - 136]. The most accepted theory that describes the amyloid fibril formation is based on the nucleation-dependent model (Fig. **3a**) [137, 138]. In this model, the amyloidogenesis occurs in two distinct phases, named nucleation and elongation [137]. The monomeric form of $A\beta$ peptide can adopt α-helical and/or unordered structures [111, 112]. During the nucleation phase, the monomers suffer conformational changes and self-associate to form oligomeric nuclei [137, 139]. This process is thermodynamically unfavorable and occurs after prolonged incubation periods [138]. Once the nucleus is formed, monomeric peptides are added to the template. This gives rise to the abruptly accelerated fibrillar growth phase, *i.e.* the elongation phase [137, 140 - 142]. As monomeric peptides are consumed, the elongation phase is decelerated to a stationary phase, where no additional fibrillar growth occurs [138]. As a result, the kinetics of β-amyloid fibril formation is well represented by a sigmoidal curve (Fig. **3b**) with a nucleation/lag phase followed by a rapid elongation phase, followed by a saturation phase [137, 143, 144]. The nucleation phase is the rate-limiting step for the entire fibrillation process [138]. This phase can be shortened by the addition of preformed nuclei to an incubation mixture of amyloidogenic proteins, abolishing the nucleation phase [138].

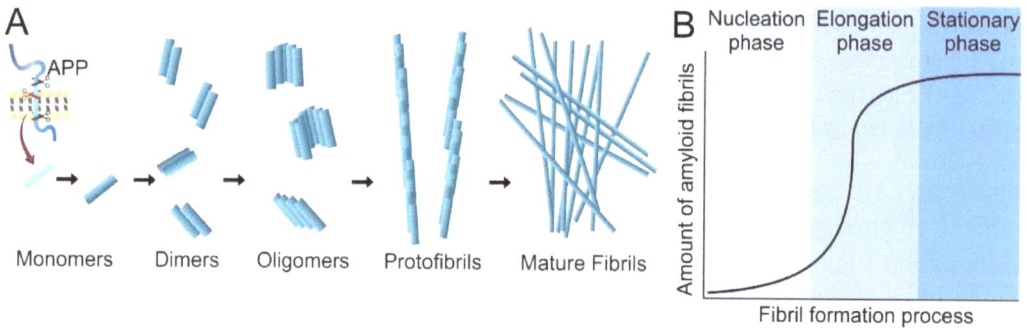

Fig. (3). Nucleation-dependent model and kinetics curve of fibril formation. (a) Amyloid fibrillation process occurs in two distinct phases: in the nucleation phase, Aβ monomers undergo a conformational change to form the oligomeric nucleus. In sequence, monomeric proteins are rapidly accreted to the nucleus and form larger protofibrils until the saturation. The final phase consists of a reduction in the addition of monomers, and the process reaches a stationary phase. (b) The amyloid formation is well represented by a sigmoidal curve in with a lag phase followed by an elongation phase and a stationary phase.

Major Factors that Modulate the Aggregation of Aβ Peptides

Several studies have shown that aggregation of Aβ can be modulated by various compounds. However, different data are obtained depending on the experimental conditions and there is no consensus on the action of several of these compounds in different forms Aβ single peptide, oligomer, and fibril.

Effects of Membrane Lipid Composition

As described in the previous chapter, biological membranes are composed of a number of lipids with amphipathic characteristics. These lipids can influence the formation of amyloid fibrils (*i.e.,* fibrinogenesis process) by mechanisms whose molecular events are still unknown. Our current knowledge about the relationship between lipid components of biological membranes and their influence on fibrinogenesis come mainly from studies of model systems that include the amyloidogenic peptides and lipid vesicles of different compositions. All these studies led to the following conclusion: the influence of the membrane on fibrinogenesis is highly dependent on the chemical nature of the lipid constituting the membrane and the mode of interaction of the protein with the membrane. Thus, it has been attributed to various classes of membrane lipids ability to promote fibrillation of β-amyloids.

Anionic lipids are a major component of biological membranes induced increase in Aβ-amyloid fibrillation process. Chauhan *et al.* (2000) demonstrated that acidic phospholipids such as phosphatidic acid, phosphatidylserine, phosphatidylinositol (PI), phosphatidylinositol 4-phosphate, phosphatidylinositol 4,5-P2, and cardiolipin can increase Aβ fibrillation, while neutral lipids (diacylglycerol, cholesterol, and cerebrosides) and zwitterionic lipids (phosphatidylcholine, phosphatidylethanolamine, and sphingomyelin) do not affect Aβ fibrillation [145]. It has been shown that the fibrillation $A\beta_{42}$ by PI results from the interaction of the peptide with the phosphate group and the inositol ring of PI molecule. However, other studies have provided evidence that the acceleration of the Aβ fibrillation may also be induced by the presence of gangliosides, mixtures of zwitterionic lipids (PC and PE) with ganglioside and cholesterol, and lipid agglomerates containing sphingolipids and cholesterol [146, 147].

Effects of Metallic Ions

High concentrations of Metallic Ions (MI) such as Cu^{2+}, Fe^{3+}, Zn^{2+}, Al^{3+}, and others can induce the Aβ aggregation [1]. MI can inhibit or enhance the fibril formation depending on the fibrillar conditions [1]; these ions also enhance the AD toxicity in model animals [1, 148]. The main MI studied are Cu^{2+} and Zn^{2+} because of their presence as free ions within synaptic vesicles. They are released into the synaptic cleft during neurotransmission [149 - 151]. The affinity between Aβ peptides and Cu^{2+} is higher than with Aβ peptides and Zn^{2+} [148]. Cu^{2+} as well as Zn^{2+} causes Aβ aggregation and may enhance the fibril formation *in vitro*, however, the extent of aggregation caused by Cu^{2+} is smaller and more slowly than the aggregation caused by Zn^{2+} [148]. The formation of Aβ: Cu^{2+} complex leads to the generation of ROS that can cause oxidative stress and neurotoxicity [152, 153]. Fe^{2+} and Fe^{3+} are described to promote Aβ aggregation, but with different rate constants [1]. In physiological conditions, Al^{3+} strongly promote Aβ aggregation but in a distinct rate and extent of the aggregation caused by Zn^{2+} [1]. The Aβ:Al^{3+} complex is more cytotoxic than the complexes formed between Aβ and Cu^{2+}, Zn^{2+} and Fe^{3+} [154, 155]. The effect of metallic ions on Aβ aggregation has been correlated with oxidative stress [156, 157].

Effects of Metal Chelators

The cell treatment with metal chelators results in the dissolution of aggregated Aβ from the AD brain extracts [1]. One of the several Cu/Zn chelators is the clioquinol (CQ) which are able to inhibit and reverse Zn/Cu-induced aggregation of $A\beta_{40}$ and $A\beta_{42}$*in vitro* and to decrease the Aβ amyloid deposits in animal models of the AD [158 - 160]. The administration of CQ to AD patients reduce progression of cognitive decline and coincide with the decrease of $A\beta_{42}$ plasma levels [161]. Other metal ligands that reduce Aβ levels include 8-hydroxy-quinoline (8-HQ), phenanthroline derivatives and pyrrolidine dithiocarbamate (PDTC) [162]. A third-generation clioquinol, PBT2, reduced the toxic oligomers, reversed the Aβ-induced loss of neurotransmission and improved cognition in a mouse model of the AD [162].

Effects of Sulfonated Dyes

The main representative of this amyloidogenesis inhibitors family is the congo red (CR). It was reported that CR can inhibit the fibrillation and the neurotoxicity of Aβ peptides [163, 164]. For $A\beta_{40}$, CR blocks the fibril formation by binding to preformed fibrils and reducing their toxicity [163]. For $A\beta_{42}$, CR also blocks the toxicity of fibrils but did not prevent their formation [163]. However, this dye cannot cross the blood-brain barrier and is carcinogenic if orally administrated [165].

Effects of Polyphenols

This group of synthetic or natural small molecules is composed of one or more aromatic phenolic rings [166]. Many kinds of natural polyphenols have been shown to have anti-amyloidogenic effects [167]. Some of the polyphenols cause destabilization of Aβ fibrils *in vitro* in a dose-dependent manner and can inhibit the fibril formation of both $A\beta_{40}$ and $A\beta_{42}$ [168, 169].

Epigallocatechin-3-gallate (EGCG) is the main polyphenol of green tea and have been shown to be an Aβ anti-aggregating compound [170]. EECG promotes the formation of unstructured and nontoxic Aβ aggregates and is able to remodel mature Aβ fibrils and toxic oligomers into smaller non-toxic aggregates [170].

Resveratrol (3, 5, 4′-trihydroxystilbene) is a nonflavonoid polyphenol found in red wines and other plants. This polyphenol has many biological effects and directly interfere with Aβ aggregation, reducing the Aβ processing through the inhibition of BACE-1 activity [170] or by converting the toxic oligomers in nontoxic species through a direct binding [170], attenuating the Aβ toxicity [170, 171] and lowering the extracellular accumulation of Aβ [170].

One of the polyphenols most studies is curcumin, a natural polyphenol that has been shown to have a variety of pharmacological activities including antidiabetic, antihypertensive, anticancer, anti-inflammatory, antimicrobial properties, and only minimal adverse effects have been reported. Also, it has been shown that curcumin inhibits the formation and the extension of $A\beta_{40}$ and $A\beta_{42}$ fibrils and destabilizes Aβ preformed fibrils in a dose-dependent manner [109, 169, 172 - 174]. Curcumin also decreases the levels of insoluble and soluble Aβ and the plaque in many affected brain regions [174], decreases the neurotoxicity of the Aβ aggregates, reduces the Aβ fibril conversion and changes or accelerates the conversion of toxic oligomers in nontoxic Aβ forms [170]. These characteristics make the curcumin an efficient β-sheet breaker. Some studies suggest that the neuroprotective capabilities of curcumin result from their ability to alter the kinetics of Aβ fibrillation [162]. This compound also binds to Cu^{2+} and Fe^{2+} ions, which inhibit the Aβ aggregation [170].

Flavonoids

The flavonoids are considered another class of compounds that directly affect the processing of Aβ. They exhibit neuroprotective effects in AD by multiple mechanisms. The two most promise flavonoids are Myricetin and Quercetin. Myricetin prevents the conformational change of Aβ from a random coil to a β-sheet rich structure and inhibits the Aβ aggregation [170]. Quercetin inhibits the Aβ fibril formation and protects the neuronal cells against Aβ-induced toxicity [170].

Effects of Other Compounds

Many other compounds have been tested as potential drugs in AD treatment but the majority of the studies are still *in vitro* test phase. Melatonin, a pineal hormone secreted during the dark phase of the circadian cycle, is reduced in AD patients. However, melatonin has a demonstrated capacity in inhibiting the amyloid fibril formation [175 - 180]. Other compounds reduced in AD patients and used in the treatment of dementia are the vitamins [181 - 189]. Some of these compounds inhibit the formation of Aβ fibrils *in vitro* in a dose-dependent manner [190]. Tetracyclines interfere with the accumulation of Aβ, in the development of Aβ fibrils, and cause destabilization of Aβ fibrils [168, 191 - 194]. Nicotine protects neurons against Aβ toxicity, inhibiting $A\beta_{40}$ and $A\beta_{42}$ fibril formation and destabilizing preformed fibrils. Also, it has been shown that the chronic treatment with nicotine reduces Aβ deposits in the brain of AD mice [195 - 198].

Recent Findings in AD Treatments

The latest decades were characterized by many efforts to develop therapeutic strategies against the AD. In the beginning, the main strategy was the inhibition of the β- and γ-secretases, but as previously discussed in this chapter, these strategies have encountered many challenges. Thus, other strategies have been formulated and tested to inhibit the formation of aggregates or to increase the clearance of existing aggregates. These strategies are briefly discussed below.

β-sheet Breakers Peptides

β-sheet breakers peptides are a class of compounds that inhibit and reverse Aβ misfolding and aggregation [199]. The action of these peptides is driven by your capacity of recognition and binding to Aβ motif (17-20). This process depends on the number of H-bonds, hydrophobic interaction and the planar structure of β-sheet. The breaking effect is modulated by the reduction of H-bonds and introduction of a breaker element [200].

One of the first tested peptides was the peptide iAβ5 (LPFFD) that showed to be able to prevent neuronal death induced by the oligomeric Aβ structures [199, 201]. β-sheet breakers are susceptible to peptidases degradation and exhibit very short half-lives *in vivo* [199]. An attempt to reduce this effect in iAβ5 was the acetylation of the N-terminal and amidation of the C-terminal [199], which increases the stability of this peptide.

Other effective peptides tested were the rGffLKGr-1,5-diaminopentane, H102 (HKQLPFFEED), NH2-D-TRP-AIb-OH and NF11 (NAVRWSLMRPF) that possess proven anti- or disaggregating effect in amyloid fibrillation process [201].

Active Immunotherapy

In recent years, some of the treatments developed against AD include immunotherapy techniques. The advantage of active immunotherapy is the long-term antibody production from short-term drug administration at limited cost [202]. The first trial with active immunization has halted because 6% of the participants develop T cell-mediated meningoencephalitis [2, 202]. Others vaccines (ACC-001 and CAD106) have been tested after this episode, and have sought to generate antibodies restricted to the N-terminus. CAD106 is the only one that advanced to the phase 3 trials [202].

Passive Immunotherapy

One of the mechanisms studied in the treatment of the AD is the administration of exogenous antibodies. This technique is based on the peripheral sink phenomenon, where administered antibodies can bind and circulating soluble Aβ species, leading to changes in Aβ concentration ratio between CNS and plasma [203]. The advantage of passive immunization is the consistent antibody titers and the possibility of stopping the treatment if side effects were observed [202]. On the other hand, the drawbacks of monoclonal antibodies (mAbs) are the need for repeated administrations and the cost of production [202]. In the last years, some mAbs were engineered against Aβ. These immunotherapeutics and your main characteristics are summarized in Table **2** [2, 202 - 204]. No mAb targeting Aβ has demonstrated significant efficacy so far, however, the safety and tolerability profile of these antibodies has been acceptable [202].

Table 2. Characteristics of monoclonal antibodies used in the AD treatment researchers.

Antibody	Origin	Subclass	Antibody Target	Mechanism
Bapineuzumab	Humanized	IgG1	N terminus ($A\beta_{1-5}$)	Clears both fibrillar and soluble $A\beta$
Solanezumab	Humanized	IgG1	Mid-domain ($A\beta_{16-24}$)	Increases clearance of monomers
Poneuzumab	Humanized	IgG2	C-terminal amino acids ($A\beta_{1-40}$)	Induce immune effector function
Gantenerumab	Human	IgG1	Fibrillar $A\beta$ ($A\beta_{3-12;18-27}$)	Binds a conformational epitope expressed on $A\beta$ fibrils
Crenezumab	Humanized	IgG4	Mid-domain ($A\beta_{13-24}$)	Binds a conformational epitope expressed on $A\beta$ fibrils
BAN2401	Humanized	IgG1	Protofibrils	Binds and clears soluble $A\beta$ protofibrils
Aducanumab	Human	IgG1	Soluble $A\beta$ oligomers, insoluble fibrils	Reacts with $A\beta$ aggregates, including soluble oligomers and insoluble fibrils

Main Techniques for Monitoring the Fibril Formation

To understand the molecular mechanism of amyloid aggregation in the AD and identify drug candidates to modulate the fibrillation process is necessary to understand the molecular mechanism of protein aggregation. For this purpose, various techniques have been applied to monitor the fibril formation *in vitro*.

X-Ray Crystallography: this technique is used to examine the atomic structure of crystals using diffraction patterns of X-ray radiation directed at homogeneous single crystals in which molecules exist in highly ordered repetitive units [205]. The diffraction signals are collected and converted into 3D density maps which are used to deduce the positions of the atom nuclei. With these data and complementary chemical information, 3D models of molecules or macromolecular assemblies in the crystal are obtained [205]. This technique has been used to determine the structures of amyloidogenic proteins that natively form a stable fold, *i.e.*, in their nonamyloidogenic form because the degree of order of fibrils formed by amyloidogenic peptides is not high enough to produce high-resolution diffraction patterns [205]. The critical step for X-ray crystallography is obtaining a crystal with high diffraction quality. On the other hand, X-ray diffraction methods do not require single crystals and have been applied for the determination of secondary structures of amyloid fibril [205].

Nuclear Magnetic Resonance (NMR): With this technique is possible to determine the structure of the protein through the magnetic properties of the nuclei in the atoms [205]. NMR occurs when nuclei with nonzero spin quantum numbers are placed in a magnetic field and subject to radiofrequency irradiation

[205]. In biological samples, there are some nuclei, 1H, 13C, 15N, 19F and 31P, with the magnetic spin of 1/2 which are the most informative. The resonance signals and their characteristics, *i.e.* chemical shift, linewidth, J-coupling, cross-peaks and nuclear Overhauser effect (NOE) are correlated to the nuclear environment and can be used for determining 3D structures [205]. Solid-state NMR is available for obtaining high-resolution structural information of amyloid fibrils [205]

Solution-State Nuclear Magnetic Resonance (NMR) is a method for study 3D structures of soluble samples. Resonances of the nuclei 1H, 13C and 15N and interactions among them often can resolve all or most of the individual amino acids in small proteins [205]. Changes in spectroscopic features such as chemical shift, linewidth, cross-peaks and NOE can be used to monitor the transition from monomer to oligomer [206, 207]. This technique is used to study amyloidogenic proteins in monomeric form but is not useful when the monomers aggregate in oligomers due to the eventual extinction of the signal [206]. Despite the advantage of using soluble samples, the heterogeneous nature of amyloidogenic oligomers and the high concentrations need for NMR experiments make the study of these proteins very difficult [208].

Solid-state NMR can also be used in studies of insoluble and non-crystalline solid-state nuclear system that are not suitable for solution-state NMR or X-Ray crystallography [205].

Circular Dichroism Spectroscopy (CD): CD measures the differential absorption of circularly polarized light by a chiral center as a function of wavelength [205]. This is a common method used for qualitative determination of the secondary structure of proteins. During the amyloidogenesis, this method can be used to monitor the formation of β-sheet structures, resulting from the aggregation of amyloidogenic peptides into protofibrils and fibrils [205, 209]. Each stage of aggregation has a characteristic secondary structure; monomers and small oligomers consist of mainly unordered/α-helical structures and intermediate fibrillar oligomers, protofibrils, and mature fibrils consist of β-sheet structures [210 - 213]. Details such as regions with different structures into a single protein and the orientation of monomers into a β-sheet (parallel or antiparallel) cannot be determined [205]. Quantitative assessment of secondary structures can be achieved by deconvolution of experimental spectra using algorithms that use libraries of existing know structures [109, 214, 215]. However, caution should be taken in interpreting CD spectra of fibrillar protein because the majority of these libraries does not include amyloidogenic and random coil proteins into the reference sets [209]. An advantage of CD is its tolerance of a wide range of pH and temperature [205].

Fourier Transform Infrared Spectroscopy (FTIR): FTIR analyzes molecular bond vibration frequencies and as well as CD Spectroscopy is useful to monitor the secondary structure of protein aggregates in solution [209]. A strong absorption band at ~1600–1700cm^{-1} in Infrared (IR) spectra of proteins has been assigned to the vibration of C=O bonds in the polypeptide main chain. This spectral feature is particularly sensitive to and therefore serves as an informative proxy for, secondary structural elements [205]. Then the deconvolution of this band gives the secondary structure content through the relationship between peak position and the type of secondary structures [205]. The main bands for the detection of fibrils are at 1626 and 1632cm^{-1} for parallel β-sheet structure and at 1690cm^{-1} for antiparallel ones [205]. An advantage of this technique is the possibility of obtaining good resolution of secondary structures within the β-sheet group (parallel and anti-parallel β-sheets) [205].

Thioflavin T (ThT) Assay: ThT and your derivatives are the most used method to monitor aggregation of amyloidogenic proteins *in vitro* and *in vivo*, respectively [209]. This small molecule dye that forms micelles in aqueous solutions and binds to beta-sheet structures result in intensified fluorescence signals relative to unbound ThT [216]. Tht also can be used as a staining agent for fluorescence microscopy, confocal microscopy, and total-internal-reflection fluorescence microscopy (TIRFM) of amyloidogenic proteins [217, 218]. Tht is excited at 342 nm and the emission occurs at 430 nm, however, after binding to amyloid proteins, the excitation and emission of ThT undergo a shift to 444 nm and 482 nm, respectively [219]. Tht binding is initiated and increased in proportion to the content of β-sheet in the system. The aggregation profile monitored by ThT is typically a sigmoidal curve consisting of three different regions that correspond to the phases of fibril formation [220 - 225]. Tht cannot detect the prefibrillar oligomers that lack the β-sheet structures [226, 227].

Congo Red (CR): CR is a small molecule probe used to identify amyloid fibrils both in brain tissue and *in vitro* [228 - 231]. This molecule binds to β-sheet structures in amyloid fibrils and as a consequence shifts their maximum absorbance from 490 to 540 nm and green birefringence with crossed polarized light [209]. However, as well as ThT, CR does not shift their maximum absorbance after binding to prefibrillar oligomers [209]; for this reason, CR could be used to characterize protofibrils and fibrillar oligomers. CR is not employed to characterize prefibrillar oligomers that do not have defined stacked beta-sheet structure [209]. The exact mechanism o CR binding to amyloid fibrils is not understood.

Fluorescence Reporter Fusion to C-Terminus of a Target Aβ Protein:
Fluorescent proteins such as green fluorescent protein (GFP) and variants can be

fused to a target protein to visualize their expression inside the cells [209]. This approach can monitor the extent of target protein misfolding and aggregation through the measurement of fluorescence intensity [109, 232, 233]. In these experiments, the fluorescence intensity is directly proportional to how correctly the target protein has folded. An increase in the misfolding and aggregation of target proteins causes a reduction in the solubility of these proteins which causes a decrease in the cellular fluorescence intensity [232].

Transmission Electron Microscopy (TEM), Scanning Transmission Electron Microscopy (STEM) and Atomic Force Microscopy (AFM): These techniques are used to visualize the morphology of β-amyloid aggregates [210, 221 - 223, 225, 229, 234 - 238] and provide qualitative and quantitative information about the quaternary structures at the nanometer level. With these techniques are possible to monitor the length, width, curvature and surface features of protein aggregates [228, 239 - 244].

In TEM a cathode ray source is used to emit and accelerate a high-voltage electron beam, which is focused by electrostatic and electromagnetic lenses. When the electrons pass through a thin and electron-transparent specimen an image containing information about the structure of the specimen is formed [205]. This technique is used to monitor the formation, inhibition, and disaggregation of larger protofibrils/fibrils, but not for monitor small prefibrillar conformers, limited by your degree of resolution, which should be higher than 20 nm [226, 245, 246].

In the STEM, a field emission gun delivers a subnanometer beam of -100 kV onto a specimen. The electron beam scans the specimen and the scattered electrons are collected by various detectors located behind the specimen. The image of the specimen is generated as the focused beam moves step by step over them; the image intensity is directly proportional to the mass of irradiated region [205]. STEM provides images of isolated and unstained specimens allowing for accurate quantitative mass determination of individual molecules [247]. STEM is used to characterize the homogeneity and structural properties of transient quaternary structure intermediates in the fibril-formation pathway of β-amyloid proteins [248].

AFM provides three-dimensional resolution of protein sample characteristics and is then well-suited for studying smaller prefibrillar aggregates with low expected error [249]. A laser beam detects the extent of bending and the deflection of the laser is translated to force units by a photodetector. The force is maintained constant while scanning across the surface and the vertical movement of the tip generates the surface contour, which is recorded as the topography map of the sample [205]. AFM has been used to investigate the assembly dynamics of several amyloidogenic proteins. One advantage of AFM over TEM is the continuous monitoring of the growth of oligomers and fibrils in solution [225]. However, the sample preparation for AFM often takes longer and involves more steps, limiting your use [242].

CONCLUDING REMARKS

In this chapter, we explore the mechanisms of Aβ peptide processing and aggregation and the forms to modulate each of these steps. The APP processing can be modulated by the inhibition or enhancement of the secretases involved in the APP cleavage as well as by the membrane composition. The lipid membrane can act as a site to enhance the local concentration of Aβ or to promote the formation of specific structures that facilitate the fibril formation. This hypothesis can be related to the alterations in the lipid composition of the cell membranes during the AD development. Many conditions can modulate the Aβ morphologies *in vitro*, which are correlated with the toxicity of these fibrils. Other compounds such as metallic ions and polyphenols are described as modulators of β-amyloid aggregation. To monitor fibril formation and their characteristics many techniques are described. The main topics discussed in this chapter and the main conclusions of each one are pointed in the Box **1**. Despite all efforts to elucidate the amyloidogenesis many factors remain unclear and need further study.

Box 1. Major conclusions on the subjects discussed in each topic of this chapter.

Processing of Amyloid Precursor Protein (APP)	APP can be processed in two distinct pathways. In the amyloidogenic pathway, one of the products of the processing is the Aβ peptide, which is pointed as a critical factor in the development of the Alzheimer Disease (AD).
Major factors that modulate the Aβ peptides production	The APP processing involves at least three distinct enzymes (α, β, and γ-secretases) whose activation or inhibition has been considered as a potential therapeutic target in AD treatment.
Effects of Biological membranes in Aβ peptides synthesis	Many studies suggest that APP processing may be influenced by the physical properties of biological membranes, as the fluidity, and by the presence of fatty acids.
Fibril formation process	One of the hallmarks of the AD is the deposition of senile plaques that are formed by the aggregation of Aβ peptides. This process involves two distinct phases named nucleation and elongation.
Modulation of Aβ peptides aggregation	Several substances as metallic ions and sulfonated dyes have been tested as an anti-aggregating agent; however, some of them are cytotoxic to the cells. One alternative to the use of these substances is the natural compounds as flavonoids or polyphenols, which attenuates the Aβ cytotoxic and aggregating.
Therapeutic Strategies against Aβ aggregation	Alternative strategies for the inhibition of β or γ-secretases are the use of Beta-sheet breakers peptides or immunotherapy techniques to inhibit the formation of Aβ fibrils or increase the clearance of the aggregates.

CONSENT FOR PUBLICATION

Not applicable.

CONFLICT OF INTEREST

The authors declare no conflict of interest.

ACKNOWLEDGEMENT

This work was supported by The National Counsel of Technological and Scientific Development (Grant 142066/2014-1) and, by Fundação de Amparo à Pesquisa do Estado de São Paulo (Grant 2012/02065-0).

REFERENCES

[1]   Hamley IW. The amyloid beta peptide: a chemist's perspective. Role in Alzheimer's and fibrillization. Chem Rev 2012; 112(10): 5147-92.
[http://dx.doi.org/10.1021/cr3000994] [PMID: 22813427]

[2]   Wang Y, Yan T, Lu H, Yin W, Lin B, Fan W, *et al.* Lessons from Anti-Amyloid-β Immunotherapies in Alzheimer Disease: Aiming at a Moving Target. Neurodegener Dis 2017; 17(6): 242-50.

[3]   Alzheimer's Disease Facts and Figures Includes a Special Report on the Personal Financial Impact of Alzheimer's on Families , 2016 [cited 2018 May 1]; Available from: https://www.alz.org/documents_custom/2016-facts-and-figures.pdf

[4]   Castello MA, Soriano S. On the origin of Alzheimer's disease. Trials and tribulations of the amyloid hypothesis. Ageing Res Rev 2014; 13: 10-2.

[5]   Drachman DA. The amyloid hypothesis, time to move on: Amyloid is the downstream result, not cause, of Alzheimer's disease. Alzheimer's Dement 2014; 10(3): 372-80.

[6]   Ferreira ST, Clarke JR, Bomfim TR, De Felice FG. Inflammation, defective insulin signaling, and neuronal dysfunction in Alzheimer's disease. Alzheimer's Dement 2014; 10(1): S76-83.
[http://dx.doi.org/10.1016/j.jalz.2013.12.010]

[7]   De Felice FG. Alzheimer's disease and insulin resistance: translating basic science into clinical applications. J Clin Invest 2013; 123(2): 531-9.

[8]   De Felice FG, Ferreira ST. Inflammation, defective insulin signaling, and mitochondrial dysfunction as common molecular denominators connecting type 2 diabetes to alzheimer disease. Diabetes 2014; 63(7): 2262-72.

[9]   Folch J, Ettcheto M, Petrov D, *et al.* Review of the advances in treatment for Alzheimer disease: Strategies for combating β-amyloid protein. Neurología. 2018;33(1):47–58.

[10]   Cochran JN, Hall AM, Roberson ED. The dendritic hypothesis for Alzheimer's disease pathophysiology. Brain Res Bull. 2014; 103: 18–28.
[http://dx.doi.org/10.1016/j.brainresbull.2013.12.004]

[11]   Hoppe JB, Frozza RL, Pires EN, Meneghetti AB, Salbego C. The curry spice curcumin attenuates beta-amyloid-induced toxicity through beta-catenin and PI3K signaling in rat organotypic hippocampal slice culture. Neurol Res. 2013; 35(8): 857–66.

[12]   Verdile G, Fuller S, Atwood CS, Laws SM, Gandy SE, Martins RN. The role of beta amyloid in Alzheimer's disease: still a cause of everything or the only one who got caught? Pharmacol Res. 2004 Oct;50(4):397–409. Available from: http://www. ncbi.nlm.nih.gov/pubmed/15304237

[13]   Tanzi RE, Bertram L. Twenty years of the Alzheimer's disease amyloid hypothesis: a genetic perspective. Cell. 2005 Feb 25;120(4):545–55. Available from: http://www.ncbi.nlm.nih.gov/pubmed/15734686 [http://dx.doi.org/10.1016/j.cell.2005.02.008]

[14]   Demuro A, Parker I, Stutzmann GE. 2010. Stutzmann GE. Calcium signaling and amyloid toxicity in Alzheimer disease. J Biol Chem. 2010 Apr 23 [cited 2016 Oct 17];285(17):12463–8. Available from: http://www.ncbi.nlm.nih.gov/pubmed/20212036

[15]   Brera B, Serrano A, de Ceballos ML. β-amyloid peptides are cytotoxic to astrocytes in culture: a role for oxidative stress. Neurobiol Dis 2000; 7(4): 395-405. [http://dx.doi.org/10.1006/nbdi.2000.0313] [PMID: 10964610]

[16]   de Ceballos ML, Brera B, Fernández-Tomé MP. β-Amyloid-induced cytotoxicity, peroxide generation and blockade of glutamate uptake in cultured astrocytes. Clin Chem Lab Med 2001; 39(4): 317-8. [http://dx.doi.org/10.1515/CCLM.2001.049] [PMID: 11388655]

[17]   Xu J, Chen S, Ahmed SH, Chen H, Ku G, Goldberg MP, *et al.* Amyloid-B Peptides Are Cytotoxic to Oligodendrocytes. J Neurosci 2001; 21: 1-5. [http://dx.doi.org/10.1523/JNEUROSCI.21-01-j0001.2001]

[18]   Dai X, Sun Y, Gao Z, Jiang Z. Copper enhances amyloid-β peptide neurotoxicity and non β-aggregation: a series of experiments conducted upon copper-bound and copper-free amyloid-β peptide. J Mol Neurosci 2010; 41(1): 66-73. [http://dx.doi.org/10.1007/s12031-009-9282-8] [PMID: 19685013]

[19]   Aguirre-Rueda D, Guerra-Ojeda S, Aldasoro M, *et al.* WIN 55,212-2, agonist of cannabinoid receptors, prevents amyloid β1-42 effects on astrocytes in primary culture. PLoS One 2015; 10(4): e0122843. [http://dx.doi.org/10.1371/journal.pone.0122843] [PMID: 25874692]

[20]   Kumar J, Namsechi R, Sim VL. Structure-based peptide design to modulate amyloid beta aggregation and reduce cytotoxicity. PLoS One 2015; 10(6): e0129087. [http://dx.doi.org/10.1371/journal.pone.0129087] [PMID: 26070139]

[21]   Suwanna N, Thangnipon W, Soi-Ampornkul R. Neuroprotective effects of diarylpropionitrile against β-amyloid peptide-induced neurotoxicity in rat cultured cortical neurons. Neurosci Lett 2014; 578: 44-9. [Internet]. [http://dx.doi.org/10.1016/j.neulet.2014.06.029] [PMID: 24960633]

[22]   Ditaranto K, Tekirian TL, Yang AJ. Lysosomal membrane damage in soluble Abeta-mediated cell death in Alzheimer's disease. Neurobiol Dis 2001; 8(1): 19-31. [http://dx.doi.org/10.1006/nbdi.2000.0364] [PMID: 11162237]

[23]   Nishimura S, Murasugi T, Kubo T, *et al.* RS-4252 inhibits amyloid beta-induced cytotoxicity in HeLa cells. Pharmacol Toxicol 2003; 93(1): 29-32. [http://dx.doi.org/10.1034/j.1600-0773.2003.930104.x] [PMID: 12828571]

[24]   Catto M, Arnesano F, Palazzo G, *et al.* Investigation on the influence of (Z) -3- (2- (3-chlorophenyl) hydrazono) - and toxicity. Arch Biochem Biophys Elsevier Inc 2014; 560: 73-82. [http://dx.doi.org/10.1016/j.abb.2014.07.015]

[25]   Paris D, Parker TA, Town T, *et al.* Role of peroxynitrite in the vasoactive and cytotoxic effects of Alzheimer's beta-amyloid1-40 peptide. Exp Neurol 1998; 152(1): 116-22. [http://dx.doi.org/10.1006/exnr.1998.6828] [PMID: 9682018]

[26]   Veszelka S, Tóth AE, Walter FR, *et al.* Docosahexaenoic acid reduces amyloid-β induced toxicity in cells of the neurovascular unit. J Alzheimers Dis 2013; 36(3): 487-501. [http://dx.doi.org/10.3233/JAD-120163] [PMID: 23645098]

[27]   Liu Y, Schubert D. Cytotoxic amyloid peptides inhibit cellular bromide (MTT) reduction by enhancing MTT formazan exocytosis. J Neurochem 1997; 69(6): 2285-93. [http://dx.doi.org/10.1046/j.1471-4159.1997.69062285.x] [PMID: 9375659]

[28] Irie Y, Keung WM. Rhizoma acori graminei and its active principles protect PC-12 cells from the toxic effect of amyloid-beta peptide. Brain Res 2003; 963(1-2): 282-9.
[http://dx.doi.org/10.1016/S0006-8993(02)04050-7] [PMID: 12560134]

[29] Bansal S, Maurya IK, Yadav N, *et al.* C-terminal fragment, aβ32-37 analogues protect against aβ aggregation-induced toxicity. ACS Chem Neurosci 2016; 7(5): 615-23.
[http://dx.doi.org/10.1021/acschemneuro.6b00006] [PMID: 26835536]

[30] Takai E, Uda K, Yoshida T, Zako T, Maeda M, Shiraki K. Cysteine inhibits the fibrillisation and cytotoxicity of amyloid-β 40 and 42: implications for the contribution of the thiophilic interaction. Phys Chem Chem Phys 2014; 16(8): 3566-72.
[http://dx.doi.org/10.1039/c3cp54245a] [PMID: 24413447]

[31] Arispe N, Doh M. Plasma membrane cholesterol controls the cytotoxicity of Alzheimer's disease AbetaP (1-40) and (1-42) peptides. FASEB J 2002; 16(12): 1526-36.
[http://dx.doi.org/10.1096/fj.02-0829com] [PMID: 12374775]

[32] Zeng GF, Zong SH, Zhang ZY, *et al.* the role of 6-gingerol on inhibiting amyloid β protein-induced apoptosis in pc12 cells. Rejuvenation Res 2015; 18(5): 413-21.
[http://dx.doi.org/10.1089/rej.2014.1657] [PMID: 25811848]

[33] Zhang Y, McLaughlin R, Goodyer C, LeBlanc A. Selective cytotoxicity of intracellular amyloid beta peptide1-42 through p53 and Bax in cultured primary human neurons. J Cell Biol 2002; 156(3): 519-29.
[http://dx.doi.org/10.1083/jcb.200110119] [PMID: 11815632]

[34] Meng P, Yoshida H, Tanji K, *et al.* Carnosic acid attenuates apoptosis induced by amyloid-β 1-42 or 1-43 in SH-SY5Y human neuroblastoma cells. Neurosci Res 2015; 94: 1-9. [Internet].
[http://dx.doi.org/10.1016/j.neures.2014.12.003] [PMID: 25510380]

[35] Fernàndez-Busquets X, Ponce J, Bravo R, *et al.* Modulation of amyloid β peptide(1-42) cytotoxicity and aggregation *in vitro* by glucose and chondroitin sulfate. Curr Alzheimer Res 2010; 7(5): 428-38.
[http://dx.doi.org/10.2174/156720510791383787] [PMID: 20043808]

[36] Lv X, Li W, Luo Y, *et al.* Exploring the differences between mouse mAβ(1-42) and human hAβ(1-42) for Alzheimer's disease related properties and neuronal cytotoxicity. Chem Commun (Camb) 2013; 49(52): 5865-7.
[http://dx.doi.org/10.1039/c3cc40779a] [PMID: 23700581]

[37] Wang Y, Liu L, Hu W, Li G. Mechanism of soluble beta-amyloid 25-35 neurotoxicity in primary cultured rat cortical neurons. Neurosci Lett 2016; 618: 72-6. [Internet].
[http://dx.doi.org/10.1016/j.neulet.2016.02.050] [PMID: 26940239]

[38] Alhebshi AH, Gotoh M, Suzuki I. Biochemical and Biophysical Research Comm unications Thymoquinone protects cultured rat primary neurons against amyloid β -induced neurotoxicity. Biochem Biophys Res Commun Elsevier Inc 2013; 433(4): 362-7.

[39] Zeng X, Wang T, Jiang L, *et al.* Diazoxide and cyclosporin A protect primary cholinergic neurons against β-amyloid (1-42)-induced cytotoxicity. Neurol Res 2013; 35(5): 529-36.
[http://dx.doi.org/10.1179/1743132813Y.0000000202] [PMID: 23595141]

[40] Jiang F, Mao Y, Liu H, *et al.* magnesium lithospermate b protects neurons against amyloid β (1-42--induced neurotoxicity through the nf-κB pathway. Neurochem Res 2015; 40(9): 1954-65.
[http://dx.doi.org/10.1007/s11064-015-1691-1] [PMID: 26285901]

[41] Majd S, Zarifkar A, Rastegar K, Takhshid MA. Different fibrillar Abeta 1-42 concentrations induce adult hippocampal neurons to reenter various phases of the cell cycle. Brain Res 2008; 1218: 224-9.
[http://dx.doi.org/10.1016/j.brainres.2008.04.050] [PMID: 18533137]

[42] Wu M, Jia J, Lei C, *et al.* Cannabinoid receptor CB1 is involved in nicotine-induced protection against Aβ1-42 neurotoxicity in HT22 cells. J Mol Neurosci 2015; 55(3): 778-87.
[http://dx.doi.org/10.1007/s12031-014-0422-4] [PMID: 25262246]

[43]   Liu ML, Hong ST. Early phase of amyloid β42-induced cytotoxicity in neuronal cells is associated with vacuole formation and enhancement of exocytosis. Exp Mol Med 2005; 37(6): 559-66. [http://dx.doi.org/10.1038/emm.2005.69] [PMID: 16391517]

[44]   Suhara T, Magrané J, Rosen K, *et al.* Abeta42 generation is toxic to endothelial cells and inhibits eNOS function through an Akt/GSK-3β signaling-dependent mechanism. Neurobiol Aging 2003; 24(3): 437-51. [http://dx.doi.org/10.1016/S0197-4580(02)00135-5] [PMID: 12600720]

[45]   Selkoe DJ. Alzheimer's disease: genes, proteins, and therapy. Physiol Rev. 2001 Apr;81(2):741–66. Available from: http://www.ncbi.nlm.nih.gov/pubmed/11274343 [http://dx.doi.org/10.1152/physrev.2001.81.2.741]

[46]   Wilquet V, De Strooper B. Amyloid-beta precursor protein processing in neurodegeneration. Curr Opin Neurobiol 2004; 14(5): 582-8. [http://dx.doi.org/10.1016/j.conb.2004.08.001] [PMID: 15464891]

[47]   Wilkins HM, Swerdlow RH. Amyloid precursor protein processing and bioenergetics Brain Res Bull. Elsevier Inc. 2016. Internet Available from: http://dx.doi.org/10.1016/j.brainresbull.2016.08.009

[48]   Arbor SC, LaFontaine M, Cumbay M. Amyloid-beta Alzheimer targets - protein processing, lipid rafts, and amyloid-beta pores. Yale J Biol Med 2016; 89(1): 5-21. [PMID: 27505013]

[49]   Iversen LL, Mortishire-Smith RJ, Pollack SJ, Shearman MS. The toxicity *in vitro* of beta-amyloid protein. Biochem J 1995; 311(Pt 1): 1-16. [http://dx.doi.org/10.1042/bj3110001] [PMID: 7575439]

[50]   Kang J, Lemaire HG, Unterbeck A, *et al.* The precursor of Alzheimer's disease amyloid A4 protein resembles a cell-surface receptor. Nature. 1987;325(6106):733–6. Available from: http://www.ncbi.nlm.nih.gov/pubmed/2881207 [http://dx.doi.org/10.1038/325733a0]

[51]   O'Brien RJ, Wong PC. Amyloid precursor protein processing and Alzheimer's disease. Annu Rev Neurosci. 2011;34:185–204. Available from: http://www.ncbi. nlm.nih.gov/pubmed/21456963 [http://dx.doi.org/10.1146/annurev-neuro-061010-113613]

[52]   Montoliu-Gaya L, Villegas S. Protein structures in Alzheimer's disease: The basis for rationale therapeutic design. Arch Biochem Biophys Elsevier Ltd 2015; 588: 1-14.

[53]   Schreiber A, Fischer S, Lang T. The amyloid precursor protein forms plasmalemmal clusters *via* its pathogenic amyloid-β domain. Biophys J The Biophysical Society 2012; 102(6): 1411-7. [http://dx.doi.org/10.1016/j.bpj.2012.02.031]

[54]   Zhang Y, Thompson R, Zhang H, Xu H. APP processing in Alzheimer's disease Mol Brain 2011; 4(3) [http://dx.doi.org/10.1186/1756-6606-4-3]

[55]   Hu Y, Wen Q, Liang W, *et al.* Osthole reverses beta-amyloid peptide cytotoxicity on neural cells by enhancing cyclic AMP response element-binding protein phosphorylation. Biol Pharm Bull 2013; 36(12): 1950-8. [http://dx.doi.org/10.1248/bpb.b13-00561] [PMID: 24432380]

[56]   Kang J, Müller-Hill B. Differential splicing of Alzheimer's disease amyloid A4 precursor RNA in rat tissues: PreA4(695) mRNA is predominantly produced in rat and human brain. Biochem Biophys Res Commun. 1990; 166(3): 1192–200.

[57]   Rohan de Silva HA, Jen A, Wickenden C, Jen LS, Wilkinson SL, Patel AJ. Cell-specific expression of beta-amyloid precursor protein isoform mRNAs and proteins in neurons and astrocytes. Brain Res Mol Brain Res. 1997; 47(1–2): 147–56. Available from: http://www.ncbi.nlm.nih.gov/pubmed/9221912

[58]   Cappai R. Making sense of the amyloid precursor protein: its tail tells an interesting tale. J Neurochem 2014; 130(3): 325-7.

[http://dx.doi.org/10.1111/jnc.12707] [PMID: 24673147]

[59] Zhang H, Ma Q, Zhang Y, Xu H. 2012. Proteolytic processing of Alzheimer's β-amyloid precursor protein. J Neurochem. 2012;9–21.

[60] Menéndez-González M, Pérez-Pinera P, Martínez-Rivera M, Calatayud MT, Blázquez Menes B. APP processing and the APP-KPI domain involvement in the amyloid cascade. Neurodegener Dis. 2005;2(6):277–83. Available from: http://www.ncbi. nlm.nih.gov/pubmed/16909010 [http://dx.doi.org/10.1159/000092315]

[61] Bordji K, Becerril-Ortega J, Nicole O, Buisson A. 2010. Activation of extrasynaptic, but not synaptic, NMDA receptors modifies amyloid precursor protein expression pattern and increases amyloid-ß production. J Neurosci. 2010;30(47):15927–42. Available from: http://www.ncbi.nlm.nih.gov/pubmed/21106831

[62] Ehehalt R, Keller P, Haass C, Thiele C, Simons K. Amyloidogenic processing of the Alzheimer β-amyloid precursor protein depends on lipid rafts. J Cell Biol 2003; 160(1): 113-23. [http://dx.doi.org/10.1083/jcb.200207113] [PMID: 12515826]

[63] Karran E, Mercken M, De Strooper B. The amyloid cascade hypothesis for Alzheimer's disease: an appraisal for the development of therapeutics. Nat Rev Drug Discov. 2011;10(9):698–712. Available from: http://www.ncbi.nlm.nih.gov/pubmed/21852788 [http://dx.doi.org/10.1038/nrd3505]

[64] Jankowsky JL, Fadale DJ, Anderson J, Xu GM, Gonzales V, Jenkins NA, *et al.* 2004. Mutant presenilins specifically elevate the levels of the 42 residue beta-amyloid peptide *in vivo*: evidence for augmentation of a 42-specific gamma secretase. Hum Mol Genet. 2004;13(2):159–70. Available from: http://www.ncbi.nlm.nih.gov/pubmed/14645205

[65] Kojro E, Fahrenholz F. The non-amyloidogenic pathway: structure and function of alpha-secretases. Subcell Biochem. 2005;38:105–27. Available from: http://www.ncbi. nlm.nih.gov/pubmed/15709475 [http://dx.doi.org/10.1007/0-387-23226-5_5]

[66] Haass C, Hung AY, Schlossmacher MG, Teplow DB, Selkoe DJ. 1993. beta-Amyloid peptide and a 3-kDa fragment are derived by distinct cellular mechanisms. J Biol Chem. American Society for Biochemistry and Molecular Biology; 1993;268(5):3021–4. Available from: http://www.ncbi.nlm.nih.gov/pubmed/8428976

[67] Haass C, Selkoe DJ. Cellular processing of beta-amyloid precursor protein and the genesis of amyloid beta-peptide. Cell. 1993;75(6):1039–42. Available from: http://www.ncbi.nlm.nih.gov/pubmed/8261505

[68] LaFerla FM, Green KN, Oddo S. Intracellular amyloid-beta in Alzheimer's disease. Nat Rev Neurosci. 2007;8(7):499–509. Available from: http://www.ncbi.nlm. nih.gov/pubmed/17551515

[69] Jarrett JT, Berger EP, Lansbury PT. The carboxy terminus of the beta amyloid protein is critical for the seeding of amyloid formation: implications for the pathogenesis of Alzheimer's disease. Biochemistry. 1993;32(18):4693–7. Available from: http://www.ncbi.nlm. nih.gov/pubmed/8490014 [http://dx.doi.org/10.1021/bi00069a001]

[70] Marr RA, Hafez DM. Amyloid-beta and Alzheimer's disease: the role of neprilysin-2 in amyloid-beta clearance. Front Aging Neurosci 2014; 6(187): 187. [PMID: 25165447]

[71] Saito T, Suemoto T, Brouwers N, Sleegers K, Funamoto S, Mihira N, *et al.* Potent amyloidogenicity and pathogenicity of Aβ43. Nat Neurosci. 2011;14(8):1023–32. Available from: http://www.ncbi.nlm.nih.gov/pubmed/21725313 [http://dx.doi.org/10.1038/nn.2858]

[72] Devi L, Ohno M. Genetic reductions of beta-site amyloid precursor protein-cleaving enzyme 1 and amyloid-beta ameliorate impairment of conditioned taste aversion memory in 5XFAD Alzheimer's disease model mice. Eur J Neurosci. NIH Public Access; 2010;31(1):110–8. Available from:

http://www.ncbi.nlm.nih.gov/pubmed/20092558

[73]   Jonsson T, Atwal JK, Steinberg S, Snaedal J, Jonsson PV, Bjornsson S, *et al.* 2012. A mutation in APP protects against Alzheimer's disease and age-related cognitive decline. Nature. Nature Research; 2012;488(7409):96–9. Available from: http://www.nature.com/doifinder/10.1038/nature11283 [http://dx.doi.org/10.1038/nature11283]

[74]   Haass C, Schlossmacher MG, Hung AY, Vigo-Pelfrey C, Mellon A, Ostaszewski BL, *et al.* Amyloid beta-peptide is produced by cultured cells during normal metabolism. Nature. 1992;359(6393):322–5. Available from: http://www.ncbi.nlm.nih.gov/pubmed/1383826

[75]   Hu X, Hicks CW, He W, Wong P, Macklin WB, Trapp BD, *et al.* Bace1 modulates myelination in the central and peripheral nervous system. Nat Neurosci. 2006;9(12):1520–5. Available from: http://www.ncbi.nlm.nih.gov/pubmed/17099708 [http://dx.doi.org/10.1038/nn1797]

[76]   Kuhn P-H, Wang H, Dislich B, Colombo A, Zeitschel U, Ellwart JW, *et al.* ADAM10 is the physiologically relevant, constitutive alpha-secretase of the amyloid precursor protein in primary neurons. EMBO J. 2010;29(17):3020–32. Available from: http://www.ncbi.nlm.nih.gov/pubmed/20676056

[77]   De Strooper B, Vassar R, Golde T. The secretases: enzymes with therapeutic potential in Alzheimer disease. Nat Rev Neurol 2010; 6(2): 99-107. [http://dx.doi.org/10.1038/nrneurol.2009.218] [PMID: 20139999]

[78]   Furukawa K, Sopher BL, Rydel RE, Begley JG, Pham DG, Martin GM, *et al.* Increased activity-regulating and neuroprotective efficacy of alpha-secretase-derived secreted amyloid precursor protein conferred by a C-terminal heparin-binding domain. J Neurochem. 1996;67(5):1882–96. Available from: http://www.ncbi.nlm.nih.gov/pubmed/8863493

[79]   Lichtenthaler SF. α-secretase in Alzheimer's disease: molecular identity, regulation and therapeutic potential. J Neurochem. 2011;116(1):10–21. Available from: http://www.ncbi.nlm.nih.gov/pubmed/21044078

[80]   Ring S, Weyer SW, Kilian SB, Waldron E, Pietrzik CU, Filippov MA, *et al.* The secreted beta-amyloid precursor protein ectodomain APPs alpha is sufficient to rescue the anatomical, behavioral, and electrophysiological abnormalities of APP-deficient mice. J Neurosci. 2007;27(29):7817–26. Available from: http://www.ncbi.nlm.nih.gov/pubmed/17634375

[81]   Bandyopadhyay S, Goldstein LE, Lahiri DK, Rogers JT. Role of the APP non-amyloidogenic signaling pathway and targeting alpha-secretase as an alternative drug target for treatment of Alzheimer's disease. Curr Med Chem. 2007;14(27):2848–64. Available from: http://www.ncbi.nlm.nih.gov/pubmed/18045131

[82]   Yang H-Q, Sun Z-K, Ba M-W, Xu J, Xing Y. Involvement of protein trafficking in deprenyl-induced alpha-secretase activity regulation in PC12 cells. Eur J Pharmacol. 2009;610(1–3):37–41. Available from: http://www.ncbi.nlm.nih.gov/pubmed/19324034

[83]   Hong-Qi Y, Zhi-Kun S, Sheng-Di C. Hong-Qi Y, Zhi-Kun S, Sheng-Di C. Current advances in the treatment of Alzheimer's disease: focused on considerations targeting Aβ and tau. Transl Neurodegener. Available from: http://www.ncbi.nlm.nih.gov/pubmed/23210837 [http://dx.doi.org/10.1186/2047-9158-1-21]

[84]   Filip V, Kolibás E. Selegiline in the treatment of Alzheimer's disease: a long-term randomized placebo-controlled trial. Czech and Slovak Senile Dementia of Alzheimer Type Study Group. J Psychiatry Neurosci. 1999;24(3):234–43. Available from: http://www.ncbi.nlm.nih.gov/pubmed/10354658

[85]   Zamrini E, McGwin G, Roseman JM. Association between statin use and Alzheimer's disease. Neuroepidemiology.;23(1–2):94–8. Available from: http://www.ncbi. nlm.nih.gov/pubmed/14739574 [http://dx.doi.org/10.1159/000073981]

[86]   Parvathy S, Ehrlich M, Pedrini S, Diaz N, Refolo L, Buxbaum JD, *et al.* Atorvastatin-induced activation of Alzheimer's alpha secretase is resistant to standard inhibitors of protein phosphorylation-regulated ectodomain shedding. J Neurochem. Blackwell Science Ltd; 2004;90(4):1005–10. Available from: http://doi.wiley.com/10.1111/j.1471-4159.2004.02521.x

[87]   Macleod R, Hillert E-K, Cameron RT, Baillie GS. The role and therapeutic targeting of α - , β - and γ - secretase in Alzheimer's disease. Futur Sci. 2015;1(3):1–16. Available from: http://www.future-science.com/doi/pdf/10.4155/fso.15.9

[88]   De Strooper B, Annaert W, Cupers P, Saftig P, Craessaerts K, Mumm JS, *et al.* A presenilin--dependent gamma-secretase-like protease mediates release of Notch intracellular domain. Nature. 1999;398(6727):518–22. Available from: http://www.ncbi.nlm.nih.gov/pubmed/10206645

[89]   Lleó A, Berezovska O, Ramdya P, Fukumoto H, Raju S, Shah T, *et al.* Notch1 competes with the amyloid precursor protein for gamma-secretase and down-regulates presenilin-1 gene expression. J Biol Chem. 2003;278(48):47370–5. Available from: http://www.ncbi.nlm.nih.gov/pubmed/12960155

[90]   Sorensen EB, Conner SD. γ-secretase-dependent cleavage initiates notch signaling from the plasma membrane. Traffic. 2010;11(9):1234–45. Available from: http://www.ncbi.nlm.nih.gov/pubmed/20573067

[91]   Androutsellis-Theotokis A, Leker RR, Soldner F, Hoeppner DJ, Ravin R, Poser SW, *et al.* Notch signalling regulates stem cell numbers *in vitro* and *in vivo*. Nature. 2006;442(7104):823–6. Available from: http://www.ncbi.nlm.nih.gov/pubmed/16799564 [http://dx.doi.org/10.1038/nature04940]

[92]   Artavanis-Tsakonas S, Rand MD, Lake RJ. Notch signaling: cell fate control and signal integration in development. Science. 1999;284(5415):770–6. Available from: http://www.ncbi.nlm.nih.gov/pubmed/10221902 [http://dx.doi.org/10.1126/science.284.5415.770]

[93]   Reichrath J, Reichrath S. Notch-signaling and nonmelanoma skin cancer: an ancient friend, revisited. Adv Exp Med Biol. 2012;727:265–71. Available from: http://www.ncbi.nlm.nih.gov/pubmed/22399354 [http://dx.doi.org/10.1007/978-1-4614-0899-4_20]

[94]   Golde TE, Koo EH, Felsenstein KM, Osborne BA, Miele L. γ-Secretase inhibitors and modulators. Biochim Biophys Acta. 2013;1828(12):2898–907. Available from: http://www.ncbi.nlm.nih.gov/pubmed/23791707

[95]   Augelli-Szafran CE, Wei H-X, Lu D, Zhang J, Gu Y, Yang T, *et al.* Discovery of notch-sparing gamma-secretase inhibitors. Curr Alzheimer Res. 2010;7(3):207–9. Available from: http://www.ncbi.nlm.nih.gov/pubmed/20088802

[96]   Crump CJ, Johnson DS, Li Y-M. Development and mechanism of γ-secretase modulators for Alzheimer's disease. Biochemistry. 2013;52(19):3197–216. Available from: http://www.ncbi.nlm.nih.gov/pubmed/23614767 [http://dx.doi.org/10.1021/bi400377p]

[97]   Wolfe MS. γ-Secretase as a Target for Alzheimer's Disease. In: Advances in pharmacology . 2012. p. 127–53. Available from: http://www.ncbi.nlm.nih.gov/pubmed/22840746

[98]   Tun H, Marlow L, Pinnix I, Kinsey R, Sambamurti K. Lipid rafts play an important role in A beta biogenesis by regulating the beta-secretase pathway. J Mol Neurosci. 2002;19(1–2):31–5. Available from: http://www.ncbi.nlm.nih.gov/pubmed/12212790

[99]   Kojro E, Gimpl G, Lammich S, Marz W, Fahrenholz F. Low cholesterol stimulates the nonamyloidogenic pathway by its effect on the alpha -secretase ADAM 10. Proc Natl Acad Sci USA 2001; 98(10): 5815-20. [http://dx.doi.org/10.1073/pnas.081612998] [PMID: 11309494]

[100] Vetrivel KS, Cheng H, Lin W, Sakurai T, Li T, Nukina N, *et al.* Association of gamma-secretase with

lipid rafts in post-Golgi and endosome membranes. J Biol Chem. 2004;279(43):44945–54. Available from: http://www.ncbi.nlm.nih.gov/pubmed/15322084

[101] Xiu J, Nordberg A, Qi X, Guan Z-Z. Influence of cholesterol and lovastatin on alpha-form of secreted amyloid precursor protein and expression of alpha7 nicotinic receptor on astrocytes. Neurochem Int. 2006;49(5):459–65. Available from: http://www.ncbi.nlm. nih.gov/pubmed/16675062

[102] Liu WW, Todd S, Coulson DTR, Irvine GB, Passmore AP, McGuinness B, *et al.* A novel reciprocal and biphasic relationship between membrane cholesterol and beta-secretase activity in SH-SY5Y cells and in human platelets. J Neurochem. 2009;108(2):341–9. Available from: http://www.ncbi.nlm.nih.gov/pubmed/19094065

[103] Hooijmans CR, Van der Zee CEEM, Dederen PJ, Brouwer KM, Reijmer YD, van Groen T, *et al.* 2009. DHA and cholesterol containing diets influence Alzheimer-like pathology, cognition and cerebral vasculature in APPswe/PS1dE9 mice. Neurobiol Dis. 2009;33(3):482–98. Available from: http://www.ncbi.nlm.nih.gov/pubmed/19130883

[104] Yang X, Sheng W, Sun GY, Lee JC-M. Effects of fatty acid unsaturation numbers on membrane fluidity and α-secretase-dependent amyloid precursor protein processing 2011. Neurochem Int. 2011 Feb;58(3):321–9. Available from: http://www.ncbi.nlm. nih.gov/pubmed/21184792 [http://dx.doi.org/10.1016/j.neuint.2010.12.004]

[105] Liu Y, Yang L, Conde-Knape K, Beher D, Shearman MS, Shachter NS. 2004. Fatty acids increase presenilin-1 levels and [gamma]-secretase activity in PSwt-1 cells. J Lipid Res. 2004;45(12):2368–76. Available from: http://www.ncbi.nlm.nih.gov/pubmed/15375184

[106] Morley JE, Farr SA. The role of amyloid-beta in the regulation of memory 2014. Biochem Pharmacol. 2014 Apr 15;88(4):479–85. Available from: http://www.ncbi.nlm. nih.gov/pubmed/24398426 [http://dx.doi.org/10.1016/j.bcp.2013.12.018]

[107] Sasahara K, Morigaki K, Mori Y. Uptake of raft components into amyloid β-peptide aggregates and membrane damage 2015. Anal Biochem. 2015 Jul 15;481:18–26. Available from: http://www.ncbi.nlm.nih.gov/pubmed/25908557 [http://dx.doi.org/10.1016/j.ab.2015.04.014]

[108] Iwatsubo T, Odaka A, Suzuki N, Mizusawa H, Nukina N, Ihara Y. Visualization of A beta 42(43) and A beta 40 in senile plaques with end-specific A beta monoclonals: evidence that an initially deposited species is A beta 42(43). Neuron. 1994;13(1):45–53. Available from: http://www.ncbi.nlm.nih.gov/pubmed/8043280

[109] Kim W, Hecht MH. Sequence determinants of enhanced amyloidogenicity of Alzheimer Aβ42 peptide relative to Aβ40. J Biol Chem. 2005;280(41):35069–76. Available from: http://www.ncbi.nlm.nih.gov/pubmed/16079141

[110] Tran L, Ha-Duong T. Exploring the Alzheimer amyloid-β peptide conformational ensemble: A review of molecular dynamics approaches Peptides. 2015 Jul;69:86–91. Available from: http://www.ncbi.nlm.nih.gov/pubmed/25908410 [http://dx.doi.org/10.1016/j.peptides.2015.04.009]

[111] Singh SK, Singh A, Prakash V. Structure modeling and dynamics driven mutation and phosphorylation analysis of Beta-amyloid peptides. Bioinformation. 2014;10(9):569–74. http://www.ncbi.nlm.nih.gov/pubmed/25352724

[112] Urbanc B, Cruz L, Ding F, *et al.* Molecular dynamics simulation of amyloid beta dimer formation Biophys J. 2004;87(4):2310–21. Available from: http://www.ncbi.nlm.nih.gov/pubmed/15454432

[113] Korsak M, Kozyreva T. Beta Amyloid Hallmarks: From Intrinsically Disordered Proteins to Alzheimer's Disease. Adv Exp Med Biol. 2015;870:401–21. Available from: http://www.ncbi.nlm.nih.gov/pubmed/26387111

[114] Lansbury PT, Lashuel HA. A century-old debate on protein aggregation and neurodegeneration enters the clinic Nature. 2006;443(7113):774–9. Available from:

http://www.ncbi.nlm.nih.gov/pubmed/17051203
[http://dx.doi.org/10.1038/nature05290]

[115]   Avdulov NA, Chochina SV, Igbavboa U, *et al.* Amyloid beta-peptides increase annular and bulk fluidity and induce lipid peroxidation in brain synaptic plasma membranes. J Neurochem. 1997;68(5):2086–91. Available from: http://www.ncbi.nlm.nih.gov/pubmed/9109536

[116]   Eckert GP, Wood WG, Müller WE. Membrane disordering effects of beta-amyloid peptides Subcell Biochem. 2005;38:319–37. Available from:http://www.ncbi.nlm.nih.gov/pubmed/15709486

[117]   Hardy J, Selkoe DJ. The amyloid hypothesis of Alzheimer's disease: progress and problems on the road to therapeutics Science. 2002;297(5580):353–6. Available from: http://www.ncbi.nlm.nih.gov/pubmed/12130773
[http://dx.doi.org/10.1126/science.1072994]

[118]   Lorenzo A, Yankner BA. Amyloid fibril toxicity in Alzheimer's disease and diabetes Ann N Y Acad Sci. 1996;777:89–95. Available from: http://www.ncbi.nlm. nih.gov/pubmed/8624132

[119]   Glabe CG, Kayed R. Common structure and toxic function of amyloid oligomers implies a common mechanism of pathogenesis Neurology. 2006;66(2 Suppl 1):S74-8. Available from: http://www.ncbi.nlm.nih.gov/pubmed/16432151
[http://dx.doi.org/10.1212/01.wnl.0000192103.24796.42]

[120]   Haass C, Selkoe DJ. Soluble protein oligomers in neurodegeneration: lessons from the Alzheimer's amyloid beta-peptide Nat Rev Mol Cell Biol. 2007;8(2):101–12. Available from: http://www.ncbi.nlm.nih.gov/pubmed/17245412
[http://dx.doi.org/10.1038/nrm2101]

[121]   Knowles TPJ, Vendruscolo M, Dobson CM. The amyloid state and its association with protein misfolding diseases Nat Rev Mol Cell Biol. Nature Research; 2014;15(6):384–96. Available from: http://www.nature.com/doifinder/10.1038/nrm3810
[http://dx.doi.org/10.1038/nrm3810]

[122]   Jang H, Connelly L, Arce FT, *et al.* Alzheimer's disease: which type of amyloid-preventing drug agents to employ? Phys Chem Chem Phys. 2013;15(23):8868–77. Available from: http://www.ncbi.nlm.nih.gov/pubmed/23450150
[http://dx.doi.org/10.1039/c3cp00017f]

[123]   Zhao LN, Long H, Mu Y, Chew LY. The toxicity of amyloid β oligomers Int J Mol Sci. 2012;13(6):7303–27. Available from: http://www.ncbi.nlm. nih.gov/pubmed/ 22837695

[124]   Garai K, Sahoo B, Kaushalya SK, Desai R, Maiti S. Zinc lowers amyloid-beta toxicity by selectively precipitating aggregation intermediates Biochemistry. 2007;46(37):10655–63. http://www.ncbi.nlm.nih.gov/pubmed/17718543

[125]   Delgado DA, Doherty K, Cheng Q, *et al.* Distinct Membrane Disruption Pathways Are Induced by 40-Residue β-Amyloid Peptides. J Biol Chem. 2016;291(23):12233–44. Available from:http://www.jbc.org/lookup/doi/10.1074/jbc.M116. 720656

[126]   Engel MFM, Khemtémourian L, Kleijer CC, *et al.* Membrane damage by human islet amyloid polypeptide through fibril growth at the membrane Proc Natl Acad Sci USA. National Academy of Sciences; 2008;105(16):6033–8. Available from: http://www.ncbi.nlm.nih.gov/pubmed/18408164
[http://dx.doi.org/10.1073/pnas.0708354105]

[127]   Matsuzaki K. Physicochemical interactions of amyloid β-peptide with lipid bilayers. Biochim Biophys Acta - Biomembr 2007; 1768(8): 1935-42.
[http://dx.doi.org/10.1016/j.bbamem.2007.02.009]

[128]   Yang X, Askarova S, Lee JC-M. Membrane biophysics and mechanics in Alzheimer's disease Mol Neurobiol. 2010;41(2–3):138–48. Available from: http://www.ncbi.nlm.nih.gov/pubmed/20437210
[http://dx.doi.org/10.1007/s12035-010-8121-9]

[129]   Williams TL, Serpell LC. Membrane and surface interactions of Alzheimer's Aβ peptide--insights into

the mechanism of cytotoxicity. FEBS J. 2011;278(20):3905–17. Available from: http://www.ncbi.nlm.nih.gov/pubmed/21722314

[130] Kotler SA, Walsh P, Brender JR, Ramamoorthy A. Differences between amyloid-β aggregation in solution and on the membrane: insights into elucidation of the mechanistic details of Alzheimer's disease. Chem Soc Rev 2014; 43(19): 6692-700. Available from: http://www.ncbi.nlm.nih.gov/pubmed/24464312 [http://dx.doi.org/10.1039/C3CS60431D]

[131] Lu J-X, Qiang W, Yau W-M, Schwieters CD, Meredith SC, Tycko R. Molecular structure of β-amyloid fibrils in Alzheimer's disease brain tissue 2013. Cell. 2013;154(6):1257–68. Available from: http://www.ncbi.nlm.nih.gov/pubmed/24034249 [http://dx.doi.org/10.1016/j.cell.2013.08.035]

[132] Paravastu AK, Qahwash I, Leapman RD, Meredith SC, Tycko R. Seeded growth of beta-amyloid fibrils from Alzheimer's brain-derived fibrils produces a distinct fibril structure Proc Natl Acad Sci USA. 2009;106(18):7443–8. Available from: http://www. ncbi.nlm.nih.gov/pubmed/19376973

[133] Petkova AT, Leapman RD, Guo Z, Yau W-M, Mattson MP, Tycko R. Self-propagating, molecular-level polymorphism in Alzheimer's beta-amyloid fibrils Science. 2005;307(5707):262–5. Available from: http://www.ncbi.nlm.nih.gov/pubmed/15653506

[134] Merlini G, Bellotti V. Molecular mechanisms of amyloidosis. N Engl J Med. 2003;349(6):583–96. Available from: http://www.ncbi.nlm.nih.gov/pubmed/12904524

[135] Thirumalai D, Klimov DK, Dima RI. Emerging ideas on the molecular basis of protein and peptide aggregation Curr Opin Struct Biol. 2003;13(2):146–59. Available from: http://www.ncbi.nlm.nih.gov/pubmed/12727507 [http://dx.doi.org/10.1016/S0959-440X(03)00032-0]

[136] Dobson CM. Protein misfolding, evolution and disease Trends Biochem Sci. 1999;24(9):329–32. Available from: http://www.ncbi.nlm.nih.gov/pubmed/10470028 [http://dx.doi.org/10.1016/S0968-0004(99)01445-0]

[137] Arosio P, Knowles TPJ, Linse S. On the lag phase in amyloid fibril formation Phys Chem Chem Phys. 2015;17(12):7606–18. Available from: http://www.ncbi. nlm.nih.gov/pubmed/25719972 [http://dx.doi.org/10.1039/C4CP05563B]

[138] Bhak G, Choe Y-J, Paik SR. Mechanism of amyloidogenesis: nucleation-dependent fibrillation *versus* double-concerted fibrillation. BMB Rep 2009; 42(9): 541-51. [http://dx.doi.org/10.5483/BMBRep.2009.42.9.541] [PMID: 19788854]

[139] Taneja V, Verma M, Vats A. Toxic species in amyloid disorders: Oligomers or mature fibrils. Ann Indian Acad Neurol. 2015;18(2):138. Available from: http://www.annalsofian.org/text.asp?2015/18/2/138/144284

[140] Campioni S, Mannini B, López-Alonso JP, *et al*. Salt anions promote the conversion of HypF-N into amyloid-like oligomers and modulate the structure of the oligomers and the monomeric precursor state. J Mol Biol. 2012;424(3–4):132–49. http://www.ncbi.nlm.nih.gov/pubmed/23041425

[141] Marek PJ, Patsalo V, Green DF, Raleigh DP. Ionic strength effects on amyloid formation by amylin are a complicated interplay among Debye screening, ion selectivity, and Hofmeister effects Biochemistry. 2012;51(43):8478–90. Available from: http://www.ncbi.nlm.nih.gov/pubmed/23016872 [http://dx.doi.org/10.1021/bi300574r]

[142] Klement K, Wieligmann K, Meinhardt J, Hortschansky P, Richter W, Fändrich M. Effect of different salt ions on the propensity of aggregation and on the structure of Alzheimer's abeta(1-40) amyloid fibrils. J Mol Biol. 2007;373(5):1321–33. Available from: http://www.ncbi.nlm.nih.gov/pubmed/17905305

[143] Naiki H, Gejyo F. Kinetic analysis of amyloid fibril formation Methods Enzymol. 1999;309:305–18. Available from: http://www.ncbi.nlm.nih.gov/pubmed/10507032

[http://dx.doi.org/10.1016/S0076-6879(99)09022-9]

[144] Ferrone F. Analysis of protein aggregation kinetics Methods Enzymol. 1999;309:256–74. Available from: http://www.ncbi.nlm.nih.gov/pubmed/10507029 [http://dx.doi.org/10.1016/S0076-6879(99)09019-9]

[145] Chauhan A, Ray I, Chauhan VP. Interaction of amyloid beta-protein with anionic phospholipids: possible involvement of Lys28 and C-terminus aliphatic amino acids. Neurochem Res. 2000;25(3):423–9. Available from: http://www.ncbi.nlm.nih.gov/pubmed/ 10761989

[146] Matsuzaki K, Kato K, Yanagisawa K. Abeta polymerization through interaction with membrane gangliosides Biochim Biophys Acta. 2010;1801(8):868–77. Available from: http://www.ncbi.nlm.nih.gov/pubmed/20117237

[147] Gorbenko GP, Kinnunen PKJ. The role of lipid-protein interactions in amyloid-type protein fibril formation Chem Phys Lipids. 2006;141(1–2):72–82. Available from: http://www.ncbi.nlm.nih.gov/pubmed/16569401 [http://dx.doi.org/10.1016/j.chemphyslip.2006.02.006]

[148] Tõugu V, Tiiman A, Palumaa P. Interactions of Zn(II) and Cu(II) ions with Alzheimer's amyloid-beta peptide. Metal ion binding, contribution to fibrillization and toxicity. Metallomics. 2011;3(3):250–61. Available from: http://www.ncbi.nlm.nih.gov/pubmed/21359283

[149] Hung YH, Bush AI, Cherny RA. Copper in the brain and Alzheimer's disease. J Biol Inorg Chem. 2010;15(1):61–76. Available from: http://www.ncbi.nlm.nih.gov/ pubmed/19862561

[150] Barnham KJ, Bush AI. Metals in Alzheimer's and Parkinson's diseases ;12(2):222–8. Available from: http://www.ncbi.nlm.nih.gov/pubmed/18342639 [http://dx.doi.org/10.1016/j.cbpa.2008.02.019]

[151] Schlief ML. NMDA receptor activation mediates copper homeostasis in hippocampal neurons. J Neurosci. 2005;25(1):239–46. Available from: http://www.jneurosci.org/cgi/doi/10.1523/JNEUROSCI.3699-04.2005

[152] Huang X, Cuajungco MP, Atwood CS, *et al.* Cu(II) potentiation of alzheimer abeta neurotoxicity. Correlation with cell-free hydrogen peroxide production and metal reduction. J Biol Chem. 1999;274 (52):37111–6. Available from: http://www.ncbi.nlm.nih.gov/pubmed/10601271

[153] Smith DG, Cappai R, Barnham KJ. The redox chemistry of the Alzheimer's disease amyloid beta peptide Biochim Biophys Acta. 2007;1768(8):1976–90. Available from: http://www.ncbi.nlm.nih.gov/pubmed/17433250

[154] Drago D, Bettella M, Bolognin S, *et al.* Potential pathogenic role of beta-amyloid(1-42)-aluminum complex in Alzheimer's disease. Int J Biochem Cell Biol. 2008;40(4):731–46. Available from: http://www.ncbi.nlm.nih.gov/ pubmed/18060826

[155] Ricchelli F, Drago D, Filippi B, Tognon G, Zatta P. Aluminum-triggered structural modifications and aggregation of beta-amyloids 2005. Cell Mol Life Sci. 2005;62(15):1724–33. Available from: http://www.ncbi.nlm.nih.gov/pubmed/15990957

[156] Sayre LM, Perry G, Smith MA. Redox metals and neurodegenerative disease. Curr Opin Chem Biol. Elsevier Current Trends 1999; 3(2): 220-5. [PMID: 10226049]

[157] Rottkamp CA, Raina AK, Zhu X, *et al.* Redox-active iron mediates amyloid-beta toxicity Free Radic Biol Med. 2001;30(4):447–50. Available from: http://www.ncbi.nlm.nih.gov/pubmed/11182300

[158] Cherny RA, Atwood CS, Xilinas ME, *et al.* Treatment with a copper-zinc chelator markedly and rapidly inhibits beta-amyloid accumulation in Alzheimer's disease transgenic mice Neuron. 2001;30(3):665–76. Available from: http://www.ncbi.nlm.nih.gov/pubmed/11430801

[159] Bush AI, Pettingell WH, Multhaup G. Rapid induction of Alzheimer A beta amyloid formation by zinc. Science. 1994;265(5177):1464–7. Available from: http://www.ncbi.nlm.nih.gov/pubmed/8073293

[160] Atwood CS, Moir RD, Huang X, Scarpa RC, Bacarra NM, Romano DM, *et al.* Dramatic aggregation of Alzheimer abeta by Cu(II) is induced by conditions representing physiological acidosis. J Biol Chem. 1998;273(21):12817–26. Available from: http://www.ncbi.nlm.nih.gov/pubmed/9582309

[161] Ritchie CW, Bush AI, Mackinnon A, Macfarlane S, Mastwyk M, MacGregor L, *et al.* Metal-protein attenuation with iodochlorhydroxyquin (clioquinol) targeting Abeta amyloid deposition and toxicity in Alzheimer disease: a pilot phase 2 clinical trial. Arch Neurol. 2003;60(12):1685–91. Available from: http://www.ncbi.nlm.nih.gov/pubmed/14676042

[162] Hawkes CA, Ng V, McLaurin J. Small molecule inhibitors of Aβ-aggregation and neurotoxicity. Drug Dev Res 2009; 70(2): 111-24.
[http://dx.doi.org/10.1002/ddr.20290]

[163] Lorenzo A, Yankner BA. Beta-amyloid neurotoxicity requires fibril formation and is inhibited by congo   red   Proc   Natl   Acad   Sci   USA.   1994;91(25):12243–7.   Available   from: http://www.ncbi.nlm.nih.gov/pubmed/7991613
[http://dx.doi.org/10.1073/pnas.91.25.12243]

[164] Fraser PE, Nguyen JT, Chin DT, Kirschner DA. Effects of sulfate ions on Alzheimer beta/A4 peptide assemblies: implications   for   amyloid   fibril-proteoglycan   interactions.   J   Neurochem. 1992;59(4):1531–40. Available from: http://www.ncbi.nlm.nih.gov/pubmed/ 1402902

[165] Frid P, Anisimov SV, Popovic N. Congo red and protein aggregation in neurodegenerative diseases Brain Res Rev. 2007;53(1):135–60. Available from: http://www.ncbi.nlm.nih.gov/pubmed/16959325
[http://dx.doi.org/10.1016/j.brainresrev.2006.08.001]

[166] Ramassamy C. Emerging role of polyphenolic compounds in the treatment of neurodegenerative diseases: a review of their intracellular targets Eur J Pharmacol. 2006;545(1):51–64. Available from: http://www.ncbi.nlm.nih.gov/pubmed/16904103
[http://dx.doi.org/10.1016/j.ejphar.2006.06.025]

[167] Hamaguchi T, Ono K, Yamada M. Anti-amyloidogenic therapies: strategies for prevention and treatment of Alzheimer's disease. Cell Mol Life Sci 2006; 63(13): 1538-52.
[http://dx.doi.org/10.1007/s00018-005-5599-9] [PMID: 16804637]

[168] Ono K, Yoshiike Y, Takashima A, Hasegawa K, Naiki H, Yamada M. Potent anti-amyloidogenic and fibril-destabilizing effects of polyphenols *in vitro*: implications for the prevention and therapeutics of Alzheimer's   disease.   J   Neurochem.   2003;87(1):172–81.   Available   from: http://www.ncbi.nlm.nih.gov/pubmed/12969264

[169] Ono K, Hasegawa K, Naiki H, Yamada M. Anti-amyloidogenic activity of tannic acid and its activity to destabilize Alzheimer's beta-amyloid fibrils in vitro Biochim Biophys Acta. 2004;1690(3):193–202. Available from: http://www.ncbi.nlm.nih.gov/pubmed/ 15511626

[170] Bu X-L, Rao PPN, Wang Y-J. Anti-amyloid aggregation activity of natural compounds: implications for alzheimer's drug discovery. Mol Neurobiol. 2016;53(6):3565–75. Available from: http://www.ncbi.nlm.nih.gov/pubmed/26099310

[171] Huang T-C, Lu K-T, Wo Y-YP, Wu Y-J, Yang Y-L. Resveratrol protects rats from aβ-induced neurotoxicity by the reduction of iNOS expression and lipid peroxidation. PLoS One. 2011;6(12):e29102. Available from: http://www.ncbi.nlm.nih.gov/ pubmed/22220203

[172] Park S-Y, Kim DSHL. Discovery of natural products from *Curcuma longa* that protect cells from beta-amyloid insult: a drug discovery effort against Alzheimer's disease. J Nat Prod. 2002;65(9):1227–31. Available from: http://www.ncbi.nlm.nih.gov/pubmed/12350137

[173] Yang SF, Wu ZJ, Yang ZQ, *et al.* Protective effect of ecdysterone on PC12 cells cytotoxicity induced by beta-amyloid25-35. Chin J Integr Med 2005; 11(4): 293-6.
[http://dx.doi.org/10.1007/BF02835792] [PMID: 16417781]

[174] Lim GP, Chu T, Yang F, Beech W, Frautschy SA, Cole GM. The curry spice curcumin reduces oxidative   damage   and   amyloid   pathology   in   an   Alzheimer   transgenic   mouse.   J   Neurosci.

2001;21(21):8370–7. Available from: http://www.ncbi.nlm.nih.gov/ pubmed/11606625

[175]   Reiter RJ. The ageing pineal gland and its physiological consequences Bioessays. 1992;14(3):169–75. Available from: http://www.ncbi.nlm.nih.gov/pubmed/1586370
[http://dx.doi.org/10.1002/bies.950140307]

[176]   Souêtre E, Salvati E, Krebs B, Belugou JL, Darcourt G. Abnormal melatonin response to 5-methoxypsoralen in dementia. Am J Psychiatry. 1989;146(8):1037–40. Available from: http://www.ncbi.nlm.nih.gov/pubmed/2750976

[177]   Mishima K, Okawa M, Hishikawa Y, Hozumi S, Hori H, Takahashi K. Morning bright light therapy for sleep and behavior disorders in elderly patients with dementia Acta Psychiatr Scand. 1994;89(1):1–7. Available from: http://www.ncbi.nlm.nih.gov/ pubmed/8140901
[http://dx.doi.org/10.1111/j.1600-0447.1994.tb01477.x]

[178]   Liu RY, Zhou JN, van Heerikhuize J, Hofman MA, Swaab DF. Decreased melatonin levels in postmortem cerebrospinal fluid in relation to aging, Alzheimer's disease, and apolipoprotein E-epsilon4/4 genotype. J Clin Endocrinol Metab. 1999;84(1):323–7. Available from: http://www.ncbi.nlm.nih.gov/pubmed/9920102

[179]   Pappolla M, Bozner P, Soto C, *et al.* Inhibition of Alzheimer beta-fibrillogenesis by melatonin. J Biol Chem. 1998;273(13):7185–8. Available from: http://www.ncbi.nlm.nih.gov/pubmed/9516407

[180]   Poeggeler B, Miravalle L, Zagorski MG, *et al.* Melatonin reverses the profibrillogenic activity of apolipoprotein E4 on the Alzheimer amyloid Abeta peptide Biochemistry. 2001;40(49):14995–5001. Available from: http://www.ncbi.nlm.nih.gov/pubmed/11732920

[181]   Jama JW, Launer LJ, Witteman JC, *et al.* Dietary antioxidants and cognitive function in a population-based sample of older persons The Rotterdam Study. Am J Epidemiol. 1996;144(3):275–80. Available from: http://www.ncbi.nlm.nih.gov/pubmed/8686696
[http://dx.doi.org/10.1093/oxfordjournals.aje.a008922]

[182]   Zaman Z, Roche S, Fielden P, Frost PG, Niriella DC, Cayley AC. Plasma concentrations of vitamins A and E and carotenoids in Alzheimer's disease. Age Ageing. 1992;21(2):91–4. Available from: http://www.ncbi.nlm.nih.gov/pubmed/1575097

[183]   Jiménez-Jiménez FJ, de Bustos F, Molina JA, *et al.* Cerebrospinal fluid levels of alpha-tocopherol (vitamin E) in Alzheimer's disease. J Neural Transm. 1997;104(6–7):703–10. Available from: http://www.ncbi.nlm.nih.gov/ pubmed/9444569

[184]   Rivière S, Birlouez-Aragon I, Nourhashémi F, Vellas B. Low plasma vitamin C in Alzheimer patients despite an adequate diet Int J Geriatr Psychiatry. 1998;13(11):749–54. Available from: http://www.ncbi.nlm.nih.gov/pubmed/9850871

[185]   Jiménez-Jiménez FJ, Molina JA, de Bustos F, *et al.* Serum levels of beta-carotene, alpha-carotene and vitamin A in patients with Alzheimer's disease Eur J Neurol. 1999;6(4):495–7. Available from: http://www.ncbi.nlm.nih.gov/ pubmed/10362906
[http://dx.doi.org/10.1046/j.1468-1331.1999.640495.x]

[186]   Sano M, Ernesto C, Thomas RG, *et al.* A controlled trial of selegiline, alpha-tocopherol, or both as treatment for Alzheimer's disease The Alzheimer's Disease Cooperative Study. N Engl J Med. 1997;336(17):1216–22. Available from: http://www.ncbi.nlm.nih.gov/pubmed/9110909
[http://dx.doi.org/10.1056/NEJM199704243361704]

[187]   Morris MC, Beckett LA, Scherr PA, *et al.* Vitamin E and vitamin C supplement use and risk of incident Alzheimer disease. Alzheimer Dis Assoc Disord. 1998;12(3):121–6. Available from: http://www.ncbi.nlm.nih.gov/pubmed/9772012

[188]   Paleologos M, Cumming RG, Lazarus R. Cohort study of vitamin C intake and cognitive impairment Am J Epidemiol. 1998;148(1):45–50. Available from: http://www.ncbi.nlm.nih.gov/pubmed/9663403
[http://dx.doi.org/10.1093/oxfordjournals.aje.a009559]

[189]   Morris MC, Evans DA, Bienias JL, Tangney CC, Wilson RS. Vitamin E and cognitive decline in older

persons. Arch Neurol. 2002;59(7):1125–32. Available from: http://www.ncbi.nlm.nih.gov/pubmed/12117360

[190] Ono K, Yoshiike Y, Takashima A, Hasegawa K, Naiki H, Yamada M. Vitamin A exhibits potent antiamyloidogenic and fibril-destabilizing effects in vitro Exp Neurol. 2004;189(2):380–92. Available from: http://www.ncbi.nlm.nih.gov/pubmed/15380488 [http://dx.doi.org/10.1016/j.expneurol.2004.05.035]

[191] Tomiyama T, Asano S, Suwa Y, *et al*. Rifampicin prevents the aggregation and neurotoxicity of amyloid beta protein in vitro Biochem Biophys Res Commun. 1994;204(1):76–83. Available from: http://www.ncbi.nlm.nih.gov/pubmed/7945395

[192] Tomiyama T, Shoji A, Kataoka K, *et al*. Inhibition of amyloid beta protein aggregation and neurotoxicity by rifampicin J Biol Chem. 1996;271(12):6839–44. Available from: http://www.ncbi.nlm.nih.gov/pubmed/8636108

[193] Naiki H, Hasegawa K, Yamaguchi I, Nakamura H, Gejyo F, Nakakuki K. Apolipoprotein E and antioxidants have different mechanisms of inhibiting Alzheimer's beta-amyloid fibril formation *in vitro*. Biochemistry. 1998;37(51):17882–9. Available from: http://www.ncbi.nlm.nih.gov/pubmed/9922155

[194] Forloni G, Colombo L, Girola L, Tagliavini F, Salmona M. Anti-amyloidogenic activity of tetracyclines: studies in vitro FEBS Lett. 2001;487(3):404–7. Available from: http://www.ncbi.nlm.nih.gov/pubmed/11163366 [http://dx.doi.org/10.1016/S0014-5793(00)02380-2]

[195] Zamani MR, Allen YS, Owen GP, Gray JA. Nicotine modulates the neurotoxic effect of β☐amyloid protei… : NeuroReport. Neuropharmacol Neurotoxicology. 1997;8(2):513–7. Available from: http://journals.lww.com/neuroreport/Abstract/1997/01200/Nicotine_modulates_the_neurotoxic_effect_of.27.aspx

[196] Salomon AR, Marcinowski KJ, Friedland RP, Zagorski MG. Nicotine inhibits amyloid formation by the beta-peptide Biochemistry. 1996;35(42):13568–78. Available from: http://www.ncbi.nlm.nih.gov/pubmed/8885836

[197] Ono K, Hasegawa K, Yamada M, Naiki H. Nicotine breaks down preformed Alzheimer's beta-amyloid fibrils in vitro Biol Psychiatry. 2002;52(9):880–6. Available from: http://www.ncbi.nlm.nih.gov/pubmed/12399141

[198] Nordberg A, Hellström-Lindahl E, Lee M, *et al*. Chronic nicotine treatment reduces beta-amyloidosis in the brain of a mouse model of Alzheimer's disease (APPsw). J Neurochem. 2002;81(3):655–8. Available from: http://www.ncbi.nlm.nih.gov/pubmed/12065674

[199] Bieler S, Soto C. Beta-sheet breakers for Alzheimer's disease therapy Curr Drug Targets. 2004;5(6):553–8. Available from: http://www.ncbi.nlm.nih.gov/ pubmed/15270201

[200] Paul A, Kumar S, Kalita S, Ghosh AK, Mondal AC, Mandal B. A Peptide Based Pro-drug Disrupts Alzheimer's Amyloid into Non-toxic Species and Reduces Aβ Induced Toxicity in vitro Int J Pept Res Ther. Springer Netherlands; 2018;24(1):201–11. Available from: http://link.springer.com/10.1007/s10989-017-9602-8 [http://dx.doi.org/10.1007/s10989-017-9602-8]

[201] Ghosh A, Pradhan N, Bera S, *et al*. Inhibition and Degradation of Amyloid Beta (Aβ40) Fibrillation by Designed Small Peptide: A Combined Spectroscopy, Microscopy, and Cell Toxicity Study. ACS Chem Neurosci. 2017;8(4):718–22. Available from: http://www.ncbi.nlm.nih.gov/pubmed/28061031

[202] van Dyck CH. Anti-Amyloid-β monoclonal antibodies for alzheimer's disease: pitfalls and promise. Biol Psychiatry. 2018;83(4):311–9. Available from: http://www.ncbi.nlm.nih.gov/pubmed/28967385

[203] Cehlar O, Skrabana R, Revajova V, Novak M. Structural aspects of Alzheimer's disease immunotherapy targeted against amyloid-beta peptide Bratislava Med J. 2018;119(04):201–4. Available from: http://www.ncbi.nlm.nih.gov/pubmed/29663816

[http://dx.doi.org/10.4149/BLL_2018_037]

[204] Penninkilampi R, Brothers HM, Eslick GD. Safety and efficacy of anti-amyloid-β immunotherapy in alzheimer's disease: a systematic review and meta-analysis. J Neuroimmune Pharmacol. 2017;12(1):194–203. Available from: http://www.ncbi.nlm.nih.gov/ pubmed/28025724

[205] Li H, Rahimi F, Sinha S, Maiti P, Bitan G. Amyloids and protein aggregation – analytical methods. Encycl Anal Chem 2009; pp. 1-32.

[206] Zeeb M, Balbach J. Protein folding studied by real-time NMR spectroscopy Methods. 2004;34(1):65–74. Available from: http://www.ncbi.nlm.nih.gov/pubmed/15283916 [http://dx.doi.org/10.1016/j.ymeth.2004.03.014]

[207] Dyson HJ, Wright PE. Unfolded proteins and protein folding studied by NMR Chem Rev. 2004;104(8):3607–22. Available from: http://www.ncbi.nlm.nih.gov/ pubmed/15303830

[208] Mandal PK, Pettegrew JW, McKeag DW, Mandal R. Alzheimer's disease: halothane induces aβ peptide to oligomeric form—solution NMR studies. Neurochem Res. Springer US; 2006;31(7):883–90. Available from: http://link.springer.com/10.1007/ s11064-006-9092-0

[209] Gregoire S, Irwin J, Kwon I. Techniques for monitoring protein misfolding and aggregation *in vitro* and in living cells. Korean J Chem Eng 2012; 29(6): 693-702. [http://dx.doi.org/10.1007/s11814-012-0060-x] [PMID: 23565019]

[210] Wu JW, Breydo L, Isas JM, *et al.* Fibrillar oligomers nucleate the oligomerization of monomeric amyloid beta but do not seed fibril formation. J Biol Chem. 2010;285(9):6071–9. Available from: http://www.ncbi.nlm.nih.gov/ pubmed/20018889

[211] Kayed R, Pensalfini A, Margol L, *et al.* Annular protofibrils are a structurally and functionally distinct type of amyloid oligomer. J Biol Chem. 2009;284(7):4230–7. Available from: http://www.ncbi.nlm.nih.gov/pubmed/19098006

[212] Fändrich M. Oligomeric intermediates in amyloid formation: structure determination and mechanisms of toxicity. J Mol Biol. 2012;421(4–5):427–40. Available from: http://www.ncbi.nlm.nih.gov/pubmed/22248587

[213] Bartolini M, Bertucci C, Bolognesi ML, Cavalli A, Melchiorre C, Andrisano V. Insight into the kinetic of amyloid beta (1-42) peptide self-aggregation: elucidation of inhibitors' mechanism of action. Chembiochem. 2007;8(17):2152–61. Available from: http://www.ncbi.nlm.nih.gov/pubmed/17939148

[214] Tomaselli S, Esposito V, Vangone P, *et al.* The alpha-to-beta conformational transition of Alzheimer's Abeta-(1-42) peptide in aqueous media is reversible: a step by step conformational analysis suggests the location of beta conformation seeding. Chembiochem. 2006;7(2):257–67. Available from: http://www.ncbi.nlm.nih.gov/pubmed/16444756

[215] Greenfield NJ. Using circular dichroism spectra to estimate protein secondary structure Nat Protoc. Nature Publishing Group; 2007;1(6):2876–90. Available from: http://www.nature.com/doifinder/10.1038/nprot.2006.202 [http://dx.doi.org/10.1038/nprot.2006.202]

[216] Khurana R, Coleman C, Ionescu-Zanetti C, *et al.* Mechanism of thioflavin T binding to amyloid fibrils. J Struct Biol. 2005;151(3):229–38. Available from: http://www.ncbi.nlm.nih.gov/pubmed/16125973

[217] Abe H, Nakanishi H. Novel observation of a circular dichroism band originating from amyloid fibril Anal Sci. 2003;19(1):171–3. Available from: http://www.ncbi.nlm.nih.gov/pubmed/12558045 [http://dx.doi.org/10.2116/analsci.19.171]

[218] Ban T, Goto Y. Direct observation of amyloid growth monitored by total internal reflection fluorescence microscopy Methods Enzymol. 2006;413:91–102. Available from: http://www.ncbi.nlm.nih.gov/pubmed/17046392 [http://dx.doi.org/10.1016/S0076-6879(06)13005-0]

[219] LeVine H. Quantification of beta-sheet amyloid fibril structures with thioflavin T. Methods Enzymol. 1999;309:274–84. Available from: http://www.ncbi.nlm.nih.gov/ pubmed/10507030

[220] Kad NM, Thomson NH, Smith DP, Smith DA, Radford SE. β(2)-microglobulin and its deamidated variant, N17D form amyloid fibrils with a range of morphologies *in vitro*. J Mol Biol 2001; 313(3): 559-71.
[http://dx.doi.org/10.1006/jmbi.2001.5071] [PMID: 11676539]

[221] Wong HE, Kwon I. Xanthene food dye, as a modulator of Alzheimer's disease amyloid-beta peptide aggregation and the associated impaired neuronal cell function. PLoS One. 2011;6(10):e25752. http://www.ncbi.nlm.nih.gov/pubmed/21998691

[222] Ladiwala ARA, Dordick JS, Tessier PM. Aromatic small molecules remodel toxic soluble oligomers of amyloid beta through three independent pathways. J Biol Chem. 2011;286(5):3209–18. Available from: http://www.ncbi.nlm.nih.gov/pubmed/21098486

[223] Ryu J, Kanapathipillai M, Lentzen G, Park CB. Inhibition of beta-amyloid peptide aggregation and neurotoxicity by alpha-d-mannosylglycerate, a natural extremolyte Peptides. 2008;29(4):578–84. http://www.ncbi.nlm.nih.gov/pubmed/18304694

[224] Bhak G, Lee J-H, Hahn J-S, Paik SR. Granular assembly of alpha-synuclein leading to the accelerated amyloid fibril formation with shear stress. PLoS One. 2009;4(1):e4177. http://www.ncbi.nlm.nih.gov/pubmed/19137068

[225] Lee J-H, Bhak G, Lee S-G, Paik SR. Instantaneous amyloid fibril formation of alpha-synuclein from the oligomeric granular structures in the presence of hexane Biophys J. 2008;95(2):L16-8. Available from: http://www.ncbi.nlm.nih.gov/pubmed/18469076

[226] Ahmed M, Davis J, Aucoin D, *et al.* Structural conversion of neurotoxic amyloid-beta(1-42) oligomers to fibrils. Nat Struct Mol Biol. 2010;17(5):561–7. Available from: http://www.ncbi.nlm.nih.gov/pubmed/20383142

[227] Ladiwala ARA, Lin JC, Bale SS, *et al.* Resveratrol selectively remodels soluble oligomers and fibrils of amyloid Abeta into off-pathway conformers. J Biol Chem. 2010;285(31):24228–37. Available from: http://www.ncbi.nlm.nih.gov/pubmed/20511235

[228] Nilsson MR. Techniques to study amyloid fibril formation in vitro Methods. 2004;34(1):151–60. Available from: http://www.ncbi.nlm.nih.gov/pubmed/15283924
[http://dx.doi.org/10.1016/j.ymeth.2004.03.012]

[229] Maezawa I, Hong H-S, Liu R, *et al.* Congo red and thioflavin-T analogs detect Abeta oligomers. J Neurochem. 2008;104(2):457–68. Available from: http://www.ncbi.nlm.nih.gov/pubmed/17953662

[230] Reinke AA, Gestwicki JE. Insight into amyloid structure using chemical probes Chem Biol Drug Des. 2011;77(6):399–411. Available from: http://www.ncbi.nlm.nih.gov/ pubmed/21457473
[http://dx.doi.org/10.1111/j.1747-0285.2011.01110.x]

[231] Klunk WE, Jacob RF, Mason RP. Quantifying amyloid by congo red spectral shift assay Methods Enzymol. 1999;309:285–305. Available from: http://www.ncbi.nlm. nih.gov/pubmed/10507031
[http://dx.doi.org/10.1016/S0076-6879(99)09021-7]

[232] Waldo GS, Standish BM, Berendzen J, Terwilliger TC. Rapid protein-folding assay using green fluorescent protein Nat Biotechnol. 1999;17(7):691–5. Available from: http://www.ncbi.nlm.nih.gov/pubmed/10404163
[http://dx.doi.org/10.1038/10904]

[233] Kim W, Hecht MH. Mutations enhance the aggregation propensity of the Alzheimer's A beta peptide. J Mol Biol. 2008;377(2):565–74. Available from: http://www.ncbi.nlm.nih.gov/pubmed/18258258

[234] Ku SH, Park CB. Highly accelerated self-assembly and fibrillation of prion peptides on solid surfaces Langmuir. 2008;24(24):13822–7. Available from: http://www.ncbi.nlm.nih.gov/pubmed/19053635
[http://dx.doi.org/10.1021/la802931k]

[235] Hudson SA, Ecroyd H, Kee TW, Carver JA. The thioflavin T fluorescence assay for amyloid fibril detection can be biased by the presence of exogenous compounds FEBS J. 2009;276(20):5960–72. Available from: http://www.ncbi.nlm.nih.gov/pubmed/19754881 [http://dx.doi.org/10.1111/j.1742-4658.2009.07307.x]

[236] Bolognesi B, Kumita JR, Barros TP, *et al.* ANS binding reveals common features of cytotoxic amyloid species ACS Chem Biol. 2010;5(8):735–40. Available from: http://www.ncbi.nlm.nih.gov/pubmed/20550130 [http://dx.doi.org/10.1021/cb1001203]

[237] Sarroukh R, Cerf E, Derclaye S, *et al.* Transformation of amyloid β(1-40) oligomers into fibrils is characterized by a major change in secondary structure. Cell Mol Life Sci. 2011;68(8):1429–38. Available from: http://www.ncbi.nlm.nih.gov/pubmed/20853129

[238] Ha C, Park CB. Template-directed self-assembly and growth of insulin amyloid fibrils Biotechnol Bioeng. Wiley Subscription Services, Inc., A Wiley Company; 2005;90(7):848–55. Available from: http://doi.wiley.com/10.1002/bit.20486 [http://dx.doi.org/10.1002/bit.20486]

[239] Lindgren M, Hammarström P. Amyloid oligomers: spectroscopic characterization of amyloidogenic protein states FEBS J. 2010;277(6):1380–8. Available from: http://www.ncbi.nlm.nih.gov/pubmed/20148961 [http://dx.doi.org/10.1111/j.1742-4658.2010.07571.x]

[240] Friedman R. Aggregation of amyloids in a cellular context: modelling and experiment Biochem J. 2011;438(3):415–26. Available from: http://www.ncbi.nlm. nih.gov/pubmed/21867485 [http://dx.doi.org/10.1042/BJ20110369]

[241] Dasilva KA, Shaw JE, McLaurin J. Amyloid-beta fibrillogenesis: structural insight and therapeutic intervention Exp Neurol. 2010;223(2):311–21. Available from: http://www.ncbi.nlm.nih.gov/pubmed/19744483

[242] Gras SL, Waddington LJ, Goldie KN. Transmission electron microscopy of amyloid fibrils Methods Mol Biol. 2011;752:197–214. Available from: http://www.ncbi.nlm. nih.gov/pubmed/21713639 [http://dx.doi.org/10.1007/978-1-60327-223-0_13]

[243] Toyama BH, Weissman JS. Amyloid structure: conformational diversity and consequences Annu Rev Biochem. 2011;80:557–85. Available from: http://www.ncbi.nlm. nih.gov/pubmed/21456964 [http://dx.doi.org/10.1146/annurev-biochem-090908-120656]

[244] Langkilde AE, Vestergaard B. Methods for structural characterization of prefibrillar intermediates and amyloid fibrils FEBS Lett. 2009;583(16):2600–9. Available from: http://www.ncbi.nlm.nih.gov/pubmed/19481541 [http://dx.doi.org/10.1016/j.febslet.2009.05.040]

[245] Woods LA, Platt GW, Hellewell AL, *et al.* Ligand binding to distinct states diverts aggregation of an amyloid-forming protein Nat Chem Biol. 2011;7(10):730–9. Available from: http://www.ncbi.nlm.nih.gov/pubmed/21873994 [http://dx.doi.org/10.1038/nchembio.635]

[246] Chimon S, Shaibat MA, Jones CR, Calero DC, Aizezi B, Ishii Y. Evidence of fibril-like β-sheet structures in a neurotoxic amyloid intermediate of Alzheimer's β-amyloid Nat Struct Mol Biol. 2007;14(12):1157–64. Available from: http://www.ncbi.nlm.nih. gov/pubmed/18059284 [http://dx.doi.org/10.1038/nsmb1345]

[247] Lashuel HA, Wall JS. Molecular electron microscopy approaches to elucidating the mechanisms of protein fibrillogenesis Methods Mol Biol. 2005;299:81–101. Available from: http://www.ncbi.nlm.nih.gov/pubmed/15980597

[248] Stine WB, Dahlgren KN, Krafft GA, LaDu MJ. *In vitro* characterization of conditions for amyloid-beta peptide oligomerization and fibrillogenesis. J Biol Chem. 2003;278(13):11612–22. Available

from: http://www.ncbi.nlm.nih.gov/pubmed/12499373

[249] Blackley HKL, Sanders GHW, Davies MC, Roberts CJ, Tendler SJB, Wilkinson MJ. In-situ atomic force microscopy study of β-amyloid fibrillization. J Mol Biol 2000; 298(5): 833-40. [http://dx.doi.org/10.1006/jmbi.2000.3711] [PMID: 10801352]

CHAPTER 5

Intracellular Transport System in AD

Merari F.R. Ferrari*

Department of Genetics and Evolutionary Biology, Institute for Biosciences, University of São Paulo, São Paulo, Brazil

Abstract: The maintenance of intracellular trafficking is essential to neuron survival. Well-organized intracellular events contribute to synapse effectiveness and efficient communication between cells. Changes in microtubule trackers, vesicles, mitochondria or autophagosomes can lead to neurodegeneration. Protein aggregates containing amyloid-beta peptides and hyperphosphorylated tau are hallmarks of Alzheimer's disease and they impair intracellular trafficking. Moreover, dysfunction of intracellular transport might increase the formation of protein aggregates. In this chapter it is discussed the association between intracellular trafficking and Alzheimer's disease with emphasis in protein aggregation, cholesterol transport, molecular motors, rab proteins, autophagy, endoplasmic reticulum, mitochondria and calcium homeostasis.

Keywords: Actin, APOE, Anterograde Trafficking, Dynein, Dinactin, Endoplasmic Reticulum, Kinesin, Microtubules, Mitochondria, Miro, Rab Proteins, Retrograde Trafficking.

INTRACELLULAR TRAFFICKING DURING PROTEIN OLIGOMERIZATION AND AGGREGATION

Synaptic transmission depends upon well-structured axon terminals, which are dependent on axoplasmic flow, which mainly occurs in the presence of intact cytoskeleton and motor proteins.

Cytoskeleton network consists of three distinct classes of filaments: microfilaments (actin), microtubules and intermediate filaments. The role of the cytoskeleton is multifaceted, such as to provide stiffness and strength, to maintain cell shape and provide the trail on which organelles and vesicles are transported and anchored [1]. Two protein superfamily are known to use microtubules to transport cargoes: the kinesins and dyneins ATPases [2].

---

* **Corresponding author Merari F.R. Ferrari:** Departamento de Genetica e Biologia Evolutiva, Instituto de Biociencias, Universidade de São Paulo, Rua do Matao,277, Cidade Universitaria, São Paulo, SP, 05508-090, Brasil; Tel: +55 11 3091-8059; E-mail: merari@usp.br

Fernando A. Oliveira (Ed.)

Impairment of intracellular transport has been demonstrated before the occurrence of aggregates and neuron death [3 - 5]. Protein aggregation is a common feature of neurodegenerative diseases such as Parkinson's (PD) [6], Alzheimer's (AD) [7, 8], Amyotrophic Lateral Sclerosis (ALS), Huntington's and others. The occurrence of these aggregates are due to abnormal interactions between proteins that associate with each other, and with other molecules in the cell, ending up with insoluble bodies deposited throughout the brain, in either extra- and intracellular compartments.

Protein aggregates are widely related to pathological cellular processes during neurodegeneration. However, the presence of these aggregates in the brain of aged healthy individuals raises several questions regarding the real pathological role of protein inclusions [9], it strengthens the link between aging and neurode-generative diseases, though, as the aggregates are similar in each situation.

The presence of neurofibrillary tangles, which are mainly constituted of hyperphosphorylated and hyperacetylated tau protein, as well as the accumulation of protein in the form of plates or fibrils formed by amyloid-beta (Aß) peptide are features of the brain tissue of AD patients.

It has long been described a decrease in neuronal microtubule integrity during AD. Microtubules are in equilibrium with unpolymerized tubulin, the stability of the polymerized microtubules is due to association with tau, which is abnormally hyperphosphorylated in AD leading to tangle formation and destabilization of microtubules [10]. Tau is a neuron-specific phosphoprotein that stabilizes axonal microtubules driving neural polarization, growth and morphology of axon and axonal-dependent transport [11 - 13].

Dyneins and kinesins are molecular motors that transport cargoes toward cell body and synaptic terminals, respectively, through microtubule tracks. Tau concentration in microtubules is determinant for trafficking balance, since it modulates kinesin and dynein motors. Kinesin is inhibited more easily than dynein is by tau. Moreover, the microtubule-binding domain of tau is able to inhibit motor activity upon microtubules [11]. Fig. (**1**) illustrates trafficking upon axon microtubule and the importance of tau to maintain the integrity of microtubules.

Tau activity is mainly regulated by its phosphorylation of tyrosine, threonine and serine residues [14, 15], which represent 15% of the total residues of tau. Protein kinases such as GSK3β (glycogen synthase kinase 3 beta), cdk5 (Protein kinase cyclin dependent 5), PKA (protein kinase A), PKC (protein kinase C) and calmodulin have tau protein as substrate [16]. However, the level of tau phos-phorylation is also regulated by the activity of phosphatases PP1 (protein phosphatase 1), PP2A (protein phosphatase 2A) and Calcineurin [17].

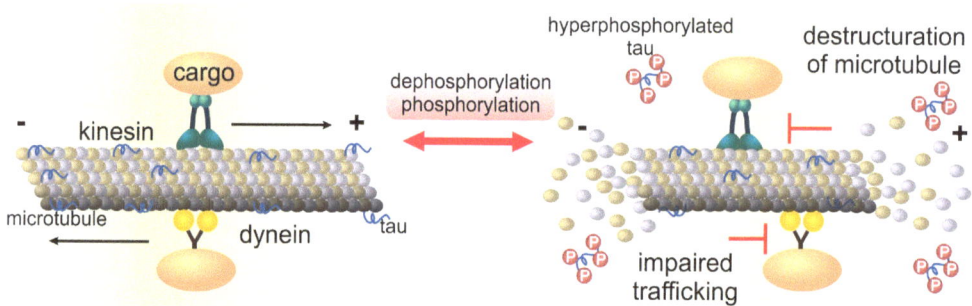

Fig. (1). Illustration representing axonal traffic associated with microtubule (MT) and motor proteins (dynein and kinesin) that promote bidirectional trafficking (anterograde, towards plus end; and retrograde, towards minus end). Tau stabilizes microtubules, which is important for axonal dynamics. During pathological conditions, hyperphosphorylation of tau promotes detachment of tau from microtubules resulting in dysfunction of microtubule dynamics and axonal trafficking. Modified from Ballatore *et al.* [18].

In AD, tau becomes hyperphosphorylated due to change in enzymatic activity of specific kinases and phosphatases. Tau hyperphosphorylation consequently induces its unbinding from microtubules and subsequent their destabilization, which is considered essential for AD etiology. In addition to microtubule destabilization, hyperphosphorylation of tau alters its tertiary structure rendering susceptibility to aggregation along with other constitutive proteins, lipids and nucleic acids [19, 20].

There is evidence that Aß peptide is also involved in hyperphosphorylation of tau. Production of Aß is considered one of the determining factors in the patho-physiology of AD disease [21], however its cytotoxicity is dependent on its action on tau protein [22, 23].

Overexpression of tau on neuroblastoma cell line, primary cortical neurons and retina ganglion cells selectively inhibit kinesin-mediated anterograde trafficking of mitochondria, causing prevalence of dynein-mediated retrograde mitochondrial transport and promoting accumulation of mitochondria in the cell body instead of locating also in the neuronal processes [24 - 26]. A study by Trinczek *et al.* [27] suggests that tau regulates the interaction of motor proteins (especially kinesins) with microtubules but not the speed of the mitochondrial transport. This hypo-thesis was reinforced by the same group that showed the increase of tau binding to microtubules compromising the mitochondrial transport axons; and that tau phos-phorylation mediated by MARK (a kinase that regulates the affinity of micro-tubule associated proteins –MAP– to microtubule) could remove the excess tau obstacles on the surface of microtubules clearing the way for motor proteins [28].

Interestingly, the decrease of tau expression prevents deficiency in axonal transport mediated by Aß peptide, indicating that the function of the peptide upon axonal traffic depends on tau [29]. The binding of tau to microtubules also improve interaction with motor proteins in order to regulate axonal traffic [30].

Thus, the disturbance of tau distribution in axons impairs axonal transport driving neurodegeneration. The raise of hyperphosphorylated tau levels leads to accumulation of APP-containing vesicles in the cell, removing them from the synapse, since the anterograde transport of APP is dependent upon kinesin and tau. The higher expenditure time of APP in the cell body due to slow traffic promoted by intracellular tau deficiency causes formation of toxic Aß peptides in the trans-Golgi network [31].

The idea that the protein aggregates would be the most toxic forms in neurodegenerative diseases has been challenged by studies showing that the oligomers of Aß and hyperphosphorylated tau exert greater cytotoxicity than aggregates [32]. It has long been proposed that hyperphosphorylated tau oligomers exert greater cytotoxic activity as it sequester non-hyperphosphorylated tau protein, it is postulated that aggregation of these proteins would inhibit this process [33]. Furthermore, experimental models of AD show that neuronal death occurs independently of the formation of protein aggregates, demonstrating that protein aggregation would not be the primary factor triggering neurodegenerative processes [3, 4, 34, 35].

Oligomers interact with motor proteins, cytoskeleton, membranes and organelles impairing their function (Fig. **2**). These interactions of oligomers with cellular compartments impair also lipid transport such as cholesterol.

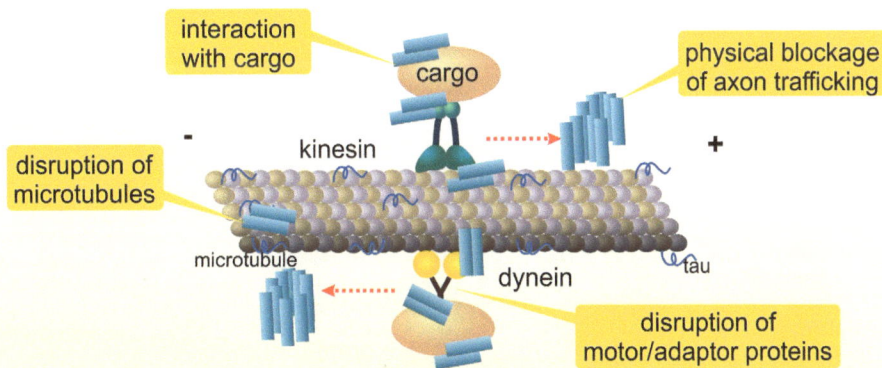

Fig. (2). Representative illustration of protein aggregates interaction with cargo, microtubule and motor proteins (kinesin, dynein). Major aggregates physically block trafficking in axon.

CHOLESTEROL TRANSPORT

The association between Alzheimer's disease and deposition of Aß peptides is linked to increased cellular cholesterol levels in the brain. In agreement with this, inhibition of cholesterol synthesis is correlated with decrease of Aß secretion.

Cholesterol is essential for the proper function of nervous system. Brain cholesterol is synthesized mainly by astrocytes and oligodendrocytes, as well as is taken up from blood.

Lipoprotein receptors are essential during synapse development and for signal transduction. These receptors play key roles in pathogenesis associated with Aß processing during the course of AD. The major genetic risk factor for late-onset AD is the ε4 isoform of apolipoprotein E (a cholesterol transport protein). There are three isoforms of ApoE: ε2 (ApoE2), ε3 (ApoE3) and ε4 (ApoE4). ApoE3 is the most prevalent isoform. Relative to ApoE3, ApoE4 is present in approximately 15%–20% of the population and is associated with increased risk of AD [36, 37]. In contrast, ApoE2 is protective against AD relative to ApoE3 and ApoE4 [38]. These isoforms have different conformational structure, which contribute to specificity in protein conformation, receptor binding, and endocytic trafficking [39].

Increased trafficking of APP to endosomes is considered pro-amyloidogenic, this is of special interest in AD brains where APP and BACE1 are colocalized to endosomes [40]. Interestingly, the probable mechanism underlying ApoE4 increased risk for AD is the colocalization of APP and BACE1 [41].

Dysfunction of endocytosis was confirmed in AD patients, who present enlarged endosomes as compared with age-matched control subjects [42]. Increased endosomal volume appears in the very beginning of AD and in the ApoeE4 carriers. However, it is still a matter of investigation the role of the different ApoE isoforms in the endocytic pathway, why the ApoE4 accelerates endocytosis and the other isoforms do not play a role in increasing Aß synthesis, or ApoE2 that even protects from AD [43].

Dysregulation of cholesterol transport is related also with reorganization of ER-membrane domains leading to increase of Aß biogenesis, which occurs because of the decrease in autophagy induced by ApoE4, mislocalization of lysosome hydrolases, defective lysosomal fusion and, as a consequence, accumulation of autophagic vacuoles containing undigested proteins such as APP and PSEN1 capable of generating Aß peptides [44].

RAB PROTEINS

Rab proteins are members of Ras superfamily of small G-proteins implicated in a variety of aspects of intracellular membrane trafficking processes [45]. Disorders of intracellular traffic are closely related to Rab proteins, since they are responsible for the formation of vesicles, motility among cellular compartments, docking, transport and fusion of mitochondria, recycling and autophagy [46].

Vesicles and organelles are recognized by Rab proteins before their anchoring and fusion of their membranes [47]. Rab proteins, in their active form, recruit effector proteins that perform various functions including recognition and preparation of vesicles to fusion [48].

The cycle of Rab is governed by factors such as guanine nucleotide exchange factor (GEF) that promotes switch between GDP state (inactive) and the GTP state, which is the active state of Rab, GTPase activating proteins (GAPs) switch the active state GTP to GDP state [49], and inhibitor of guanine nucleotide dissociation (GDIs) is responsible for blocking the dissociation of GDP [50]. Although Rab proteins are homologous proteins, because their binding sites amino are highly conserved, their modulatory factors are reasonably specific for each particular Rab [51].

Through the GDP-GTP cycle (inactive-active), Rab proteins function as modulators molecules of vesicular transport along the cytoskeleton, through the recruitment of specific motor proteins that ensure efficient connection and anchoring of vesicles in the target areas of the membrane [52]. Some Rabs appear to be more directly involved in neurodegenerative disorders, as following detailed.

Rab5 is a multifunctional protein that regulates the early stages of endocytosis, due to its interactions with effectors, which assist the activation of Rab 5, thereby regulating anchoring processes, fusion of endosomal membranes as well as endosomal mobility [53]. The regulation of the traffic and formation of endocytic vesicles also appears to be important for the formation of amyloid plaques [54]. Cataldo and collaborators [55] showed increased levels of Rab4, which is a protein related to endocytosis and recycling [56], and association between Rab5 and vesicles containing large amounts of Aß peptide in Alzheimer's disease indicating the unbalance of the endocytic pathway can be associated with the formation of protein aggregates.

Rab10 is also involved in vesicle trafficking and has been recently implicated in AD as it is found in hyperphorylated tau aggregates. Yan and colleagues [57] described the association between Rab10 phosphorylation and the possible implication for impaired trafficking during AD. Studies of genome sequencing also corroborate the association between Rab10 and AD. The single nucleotide polymorphism (SNP) rs142787485 in Rab10 was identified in resilient AD patients, who did not develop AD even when harboring the ApoE4 allele of lipoprotein receptor. That variant of Rab10 is associated with elevated protection against AD [58].

Disorder of vesicular traffic in Alzheimer's disease has been described for a long time, including the participation of Rab6 protein, which drives the transport between Golgi apparatus and endoplasmic reticulum, during formation of aggregates containing the Aß peptide [59]. The highest levels of Rab6 were found in neurons in stages that preceded the formation of hyperphosphorylated tau deposits and the formation of amyloid plaques in temporal cortex of individuals affected by Alzheimer's disease.

Rab6 is involved in directing vesicles, including those containing APP, from the endoplasmic reticulum to the Golgi, thus increasing Rab6 expression involves an increase in demand for retrograde traffic to the endoplasmic reticulum due to the accumulation in the Golgi during Alzheimer's disease. The Golgi apparatus undergoes serious consequences arising problems in intracellular transport that leads to fragmentation and may be a determining factor for irreversible neuronal death in cases of Alzheimer's and also amyotrophic lateral sclerosis [60].

Abnormalities of the cytoskeleton in Alzheimer's disease may slow down the exit of proteins from Golgi, resulting in accumulation of these proteins in Golgi. This was demonstrated in the Rab6 inhibition experiments extinguished amyloidogenic APP processing [59], suggesting that the dysfunction of Rab6 can delay the processing of APP and interfere with their physiology leading to the deposition of Aß. A better understanding of the role of Rab6 and endoplasmic reticulum stress for Alzheimer's disease can help the identification of specific targets for therapeutic intervention in the early stages of the disease [61].

Another important protein for cell maintenance is Rab32 that participates in the fission and fusion of mitochondria [62]. The presence of this organelle in specific neuron sites is critical for the modulation, dynamics and plasticity of synapse [63] and its dysfunction may lead to the onset of neurodegeneration [reviewed by 64], by means of change in traffic, fusion and fission of mitochondria [65].

There are numerous classes of Rab proteins known to participate in vesicular transport and organelles, vesicle fusion in different intracellular compartments and at the synaptic terminal, and endocytosis. This transport occurs through binding with cytoskeletal proteins, kinesins, dyneins, and proteins of the organelle to be transported [66]. However, the importance of these proteins in the formation of aggregates, and the chronological order of intracellular events that may contribute to neurological disorder are not properly characterized yet.

ANTEROGRADE TRAFFICKING

Kinesins are molecular motor proteins mainly responsible for anterograde trafficking, from cell body to periphery. Kinesin-1 is the anterograde motor of APP in axons.

APP is proposed to have a functional role linking kinesin-1 to axonal vesicles. This evidence may implicate kinesin-1-based transport in the development of Alzheimer's disease [67].

Decreased anterograde trafficking of APP-containing vesicles is an important factor to increase APP amyloidogenic processing, thus increasing Aß production in intracellular environment.

APP trafficking is dependent of kinesin. Variations in APP or tau affect mitochondrial and synaptic vesicle transport. It was also shown that axonal dysfunction might culminate in impaired synaptic plasticity, which is crucial for neuronal viability and function. Thus, changes in APP and tau expression may disturb axonal transport and alters APP processing, contributing to neurodegeneration in AD [68, 69].

GSK3β and Cdk5 are the major kinases responsible for tau phosphorylation, however these kinases also regulate kinesin-driven motility. In fact, it is proposed that misregulation of fast anterograde transport induced by an imbalance in specific kinase activities may represent an early step for neuronal pathology [70].

Pigino and colleagues [71] demonstrated that presenilin 1 (PSEN1) interacts with GSK3β phosphorylating kinesin light chains (KLC) and releasing kinesin-I from membrane-bound organelles and reducing kinesin-I driven motility. Mutations in PSEN1, related to AD, may impair kinesin-1-based trafficking by means of GSK3β.

Impaired Golgi function is also reported in AD, where its fragmentation accelerates Aß production [72]. In fact, Golgi apparatus is the primary organelle for vesicle anterograde trafficking, this organelle is responsible for protein modifications, sorting and trafficking. Golgi stress contributes to cell death after protein misfolding.

Reduction of presenilin or suppression of gamma-secretase activity substantially increases anterograde and retrograde velocities for APP vesicles, which is dependent of functional kinesin-1 and dynein motors. These findings suggest that a normal function of presenilin is to repress kinesin-1 and dynein motor activity during axonal transport of APP vesicles. This highlights a potential novel therapeutic pathway for early intervention, prior to neuronal loss and clinical manifestation of disease [73].

RETROGRADE TRAFFICKING

Retrograde trafficking is determined by microtubule-based molecular motors called dynein and its adaptor dynactin. These proteins carry cargoes towards cell body.

It is reported that disturbance of dynein not only disrupts retrograde trafficking of neurotrophins and also impairs anterograde trafficking of synaptic vesicles, since there is an increase of Rab3 expression [74].

Aging by itself attenuates the interaction between dynein-dynactin and disturbs endocytic pathways culminating with Aβ accumulation.

Dynein dysfunction induces axon swelling caused mainly by accumulation of neurofilaments, organelles and vesicles. These findings, together with the evidences of endocytic disturbance, corroborate that dynein dysfunction impairs neuronal activity, which may contribute to the development of AD [74].

Retrograde trafficking might be altered not only by impaired dynein-dynactin function, but also by dysfunction of Rab proteins [75]. Dynein dysfunction leads to endosomal accumulation of retromer-related proteins and APP. Moreover, knockdown of Rab7, Rab9, or Rab11 did not alter endogenous APP metabolism, such as what is observed in aged brains and in dynein-depleted cells. These findings suggest that dynein dysfunction can cause retromer deficiency and that concomitant disruption of retrograde trafficking may be the key factor underlying age-dependent Aβ pathology [75].

Impaired retrograde trafficking also contributes for tau pathology. Tau directly interacts with dynactin stabilizing the dynein-dynactin complex. Similarly, dysfunction of dynein-dynactin complex contributes to tau-induced pathology [76].

Association between impaired retrograde trafficking and tau expression promoted accumulation of synaptic proteins in axons, in the absence of synaptic failure, suggesting a pre-symptomatic phase of tauopathy. This evidence reinforces the occurrence of disturbed retrograde trafficking prior to cell failure.

Hyperphosphorylated tau decreases transport efficiency and leads to traffic jam because of microtubules disorganization. By increasing the ration of unbound/ bound microtubule axon microtubules become disorganized, impacting axonal trafficking of vesicles and organelles such as mitochondria [76].

MITOCHONDRIA TRAFFICKING AND BIOGENESIS

Mitochondria are organelles of fundamental importance for cellular homeostasis, for allocating the ATP synthesis machinery as well as for controlling and regulating the availability of intracellular Ca^{2+} and regulating apoptosis.

Mitochondrial function for cell maintenance is widely studied because these organelles are the power sources and participate in the homeostatic regulation of eukaryotic cells. Thus, it is postulated that mitochondrial dysfunction, including its traffic, can contribute to cytotoxicity, increased oxidative stress, energy deprivation and neurodegeneration [64].

Although a causative event for the deficiency of synapses during aging can not be definitely characterized by the multiple determinants of brain aging physiology, some experiments have demonstrated the importance of the presence of mitochondria in the synaptic terminal for modulation/dynamic of synapses and synaptic neuroplasticity [77].

Accumulation of nonfunctional mitochondria is characteristic of the aging process and neurodegenerative diseases. These accumulated mitochondria show structural changes in DNA and membranes, decrease of electron transport due to impairment of complexes I and IV of the respiratory chain resulting in decreased ATP synthesis, and accumulation of free radicals, which are claimed to drive brain senescence [78].

Brain aging is also marked by a decrease in the number of healthy mitochondria [79] and its persistent decreased membrane potential [80], which culminates in decrease of ATP synthesis and dysregulation of intracellular Ca^{2+} concentrations, leading to activation of caspases and cell death [81].

Interaction of Aβ peptides and fibrils with mitochondrial membranes inhibits mitochondrial dynamics but do not instantly affect its function. Concluding that inhibition of mitochondrial axonal trafficking is initiated by soluble Aβ and is exacerbated by fibrils [82]. This evidence indicates that restoration of mitochondrial axonal trafficking could be beneficial during early AD and might be an interesting therapeutic target to prevent worsening of AD symptoms.

Mitochondria biogenesis and degradation occur mainly in cell body, depending upon retrograde trafficking, the new organelle is then transported to the periphery through anterograde transport. Therefore, the mitochondrial membrane has motor protein binding sites and adapters that enable fast or slow anterograde and retrograde transport and anchoring [83].

For anterograde transport, kinesins 1 (KIF5) and 3 (KIF1B) associates with the adapter complex constituted by Milton (also known as TRAK1 or OIP106 and TRAK2 or GRIF1) and Miro (also called RHOT1 and RHOT2) proteins located in the mitochondrial outer membrane [84].

For retrograde transport, mitochondria bind to dynein and dynactin [85, 86]. Dynactin serves as an interface adaptor molecule that enables mitochondria to bind to cytoplasmic dynein, which in turn makes mitochondria linked to microtubule for organelle transport towards cell body.

Mitochondria have a specific anchoring mechanism that acts in places where the ATP and regulation of Ca^{2+} homeostasis are needed, such as in the presynaptic area, dendritic spines, growth cone and nodes of Ranvier. Kang and collaborators [87] demonstrated that syntaphilin participate of mitochondria anchoring. Chen *et al.* [88] also proposed that the light chain dynein 8 (LC8) can also regulate mitochondrial anchoring. Fig. (**3**) summarizes proteins involved in mitochondria dynamics in axon.

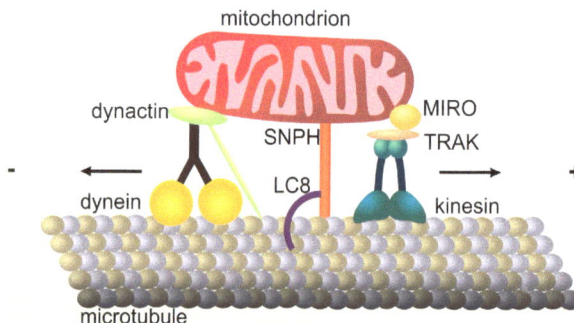

Fig. (3). Illustrative scheme depicting the role of molecular motors and accessory proteins related to anchoring, anterograde and retrograde trafficking of mitochondria. Modified from Cai and Sheng [94] and Chen *et al.* [88].

Mitochondria form a highly interconnected network throughout neuron and its dynamics involves continuously autophagic destruction, through macroautophagy process called mitophagy. Besides that, mitochondria maintenance also depends on fusion and fission processes, which alter their morphology and keep the quality of mitochondria [89, 90]. Deficits in fusion or fission machinery cause aggregation of organelle and loss of directed movement, which impair mitoch-ondria migration to neurites. Furthermore, investigations about impairment of fusion/fission revealed spontaneous generation of mtDNA mutations, which is linked with a set of neurodegenerative disorders [91 - 93].

During high metabolic activity or stress, fusion process increases density of cristae allowing maximization of ATP production [95, 96]. Whereas, fission process is important for mitochondria proliferation as well as for transportation of the organelle to regions with energy demands. In addition, this process is also involved in segregation of impaired mitochondria from network to degradation through mitophagy [96, 97]. Therefore, the balance between fission and fusion and mitophagy processes are essential to keep homeostasis. Particularly, aberrant fission has been shown to be involved in reduced mitochondria respiration, ATP (energy) depletion, increased ROS and release of pro-apoptotic factors during neurodegeneration [91, 98 - 101].

Thus, mitochondria dysfunction can significantly increase the amount of ROS in neurons, especially because about 0.2-2% of total oxygen, consumed in normal conditions, is naturally converted into free radicals in the mitochondria [102, 103].

Generation of energy by mitochondria also release unpaired electrons, mainly by the complexes I and III, facilitating the production of ROS which can accelerate aging even when antioxidant enzymes are activated [104 - 106]. Several studies have claimed that complex I disruption, increases ROS levels in mitochondria matrix and cytosol.

The electron transport chain is the source of 90% of ROS produced by the cells and is localized close to mtDNA, favoring mutations. Moreover, mtDNA is not protected by histones and its replication cycle occurs at high rate. Consequently, mutated mtDNA needs to be repaired quickly, otherwise, these mutations could be propagated causing somatic mosaicism, which is increased with age [107 - 109].

Compared to other tissues, brain is more susceptible to mtDNA mutations, leading to mitochondria dysfunction and consequently energy depletion. Decreased energy compromises repair of damaged mitochondria, crucial process to maintenance of quality of mitochondria, targeting mitochondria to degradation (mitophagy) [110]. Damaged or depolarized mitochondria cause electron leakage, generating excessive ROS and releasing pro-apoptotic factors such as cytochrome C to initiate cell death [111]. Besides that, Aß peptide interacts with complex IV that implies in ROS increasing.

Hyperphosphorylated tau and Aß peptide has been shown to interact with mitochondria membranes causing damage in the organelle including changes in mitochondria fission and morphology.

It has been demonstrated that disrupted trafficking of mitochondria, impairs ATP supply in specific sites such as synaptic terminal. Furthermore, generation of new/healthy mitochondria by fusion and fission processes at soma is impaired [112, 113].

Mitochondria quality control is essential to neuron survival. This process involves trafficking of organelle among neuron regions where energy is necessary and organelle return to be recycled/repaired, since fusion and fission processes occur preferentially at cell body. Anterograde mitochondria trafficking is axonal transportation from cell body to synaptic boutons. To be recycled or in cases of mitochondria dysfunction, the organelle needs to be retrogradely transported till cell body, where mitophagy involves lysosomes to degrade damaged mitochondria [114 - 116].

Since neurons are polarized cells and posses long axons, intracellular trafficking is crucial to neuronal survival, morphology and function [117]. Other studies demonstrated that during neurodegeneration alterations in motor proteins and, consequently, alterations in mitochondria trafficking, can occur [118].

Animal models of protein aggregation show that expression of anterograde and retrograde motor proteins were altered before protein aggregation, in addition, it was demonstrated that mitochondria trafficking was synchronized with expression of anterograde motor proteins and alteration in these proteins lead to specific changes in mitochondria trafficking [3, 4].

To transport mitochondria, motor proteins associate with the adaptor proteins TRAK (drosophila ortholog Milton) and Miro, which is attached to the outer mitochondria membrane, as illustrated before (Fig. **4**) [119].

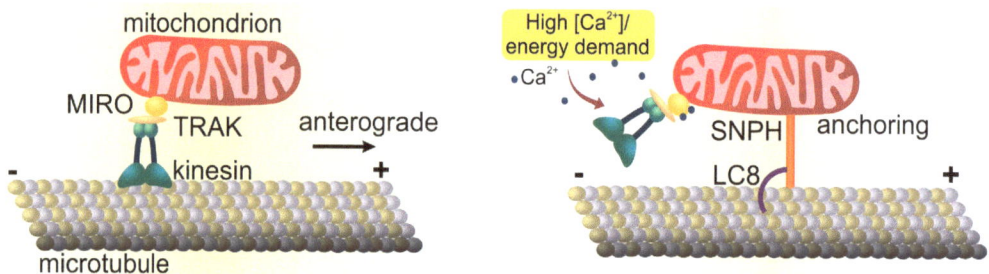

Fig. (4). Model of Ca^{2+}-dependent mitochondrial arrest. calcium binding to Miro EF-hands induces the release of the protein from the kinesin motors, determining the detachment of the mitochondrion from the microtubule tracks. Adapted from Devine *et al.* [119].

Interestingly, experiments changing Miro expression demonstrated that increase in Miro leads to increase in mitochondria transport, revealing that this protein can regulate mitochondria dynamics [120]. Recent data indicate that Miro acts at both microtubule and actin cytoskeleton, as well as coordinate anterograde and retrograde mitochondrial movements [121].

In addition, protein loss causes defective trafficking in both directions, suggesting that Miro is an adaptor for both anterograde transport through interaction with KIF5 and retrograde transport through interaction with dynein [122, 123]. Furthermore, investigations about mitochondria fragmentation and interconnectivity showed that non-functional Miro leads to mitochondria trafficking impairment and fragmentation, while overexpressed Miro increases mitochondria trafficking and also mitochondria interconnectivity, increasing mitochondria length in neurons [124].

Miro is a Ca^{+2} sensor containing 2 calcium-binding EF-hands. It has been shown increased calcium levels of calcium dissociate motor proteins from Miro and TRAK, blocking mitochondria trafficking, as exemplified in Fig. (**4**). This process is crucial to maintain mitochondria anchoring in specific sites of high demand of ATP is required, such as synapses. When ATP decreases, stationary mitochondria move to another site with low ATP levels. However, impairment of mitochondria trafficking can lead to organelle dysfunction where organelle is anchored, generating ROS [125 - 127].

It has been reported that Miro also interacts with Mfn (mitofusin) proteins, playing a role in mitochondria fusion. Intriguingly, mitochondria trafficking is decreased in knockout neurons for Mfn2, suggesting Miro and Mfn work together in mitochondria trafficking regulation [127]. It is known that Miro is associated with mitochondria outer membrane, coordinating mitochondria transport that has to move together with ER and stay close enough to this organelle in order to initiate mitochondria fusion or fission processes [128]. Once in contact, Mfn1 and Mfn2 interact with Miro and they are both required to axonal transport [129], suggesting association of these proteins and equilibrated trafficking are essential to fusion process.

Absence of Miro exacerbates mitophagy. Curiously, Mfn2 knockdown mouse present blocked mitophagy [130]. It has been shown that ER provides lipids to membrane formation of autophagic vacuole [131]. These lipids are transferred and accumulated in outer mitochondria membrane, and then they are transported to initiate the formation of vesicle and mitophagy [132]. However, alteration in Miro or Mfn proteins can disturb these processes, revealing that both proteins are needed to vesicle fusion and mitophagy.

Damaged mitochondria are targeted to mitophagy through PINK1 signaling. Parkin forms a complex with PINK1 in mitophagy process and ubiquitinates substrates of outer mitochondria membrane, including Miro triggering mitophagy. It has been suggested that Miro acts like a receptor for both proteins, since Miro interacts with PINK1 and Parkin allowing their association with outer mitochondria membrane. Moreover, damaged mitochondria require fast Miro ubiquitination dependent of Parkin. In addition, fibroblasts of patients carrying parkin mutations, showed altered Miro turnover, suggesting that Miro is intrinsically involved in regulation of fusion/fission and mitophagy events [133, 134].

Specificity of intracellular trafficking of organelles and among cellular compartments is strictly regulated by Rab GTPases. Besides that, Rabs are responsible to correctly attach motor proteins and cargoes, motility of cargoes and their delivery to correct destination as detailed earlier in this chapter.

Investigations about intracellular trafficking and autophagy dysfunction in neurodisorders, revealed that degradation *via* lysosome is crucial for maintenance of balanced axonal trafficking of vesicles and lysosomes. Further, impairment in intracellular trafficking leads to accumulation of lysosome vesicles causing axonal swelling and neurites dystrophy.

IMPAIRMENT OF AUTOPHAGY IN AD

Autophagy is related to a number of physiological processes, such as recycling of proteins and organelles, stress response, cell differentiation, programmed cell death, as well as pathological conditions, including neurodegeneration [135]. Intracellular trafficking is responsible for directing cargoes to degradation. Since disturbance of trafficking and presence of misfolded proteins are hallmarks of AD, there is evidence that these two systems are good targets for therapies against AD.

Lysosomal alterations appear in early stages of axon degeneration, and maintenance of function of these organelles may be important to slow the progression of neurodegenerative diseases [136]. Interestingly, there is an increase in autophagic activity during the beginning of aging in mice models of senescence, this autophagic activity then decreases with advancing age culminating with pathological cellular changes similar to the characteristics of sporadic Alzheimer's disease. Armstrong *et al.* [137] described possible molecular markers associated with lysosomal pathway, present in cerebrospinal fluid, which may be useful for the diagnosis of Alzheimer's disease.

The initial steps of macroautophagy signaling involve Ulk1/Beclin-1 complex that generates the lipid bilayer vesicles [138]. Beclin-1 plays a central role in the programming of cell survival, and its dysfunction may result in neurodegeneration [139]. The protein p62 participates in the macroautophagy, wherein p62 recognizes cargoes to be degraded and directs them to autophagosomes.

Autophagosomes then fuse with the lysosomes resulting in an autophagic body. LC3 protein, from the family of Atg8 proteins, is a microtubule-associated protein and also associates with autophagosome membrane. LC3-I is cytosolic and LC3-II is associated with the autophagic membrane. Two other members of Atg8 family are GABARAP and GATE-16 that are associated with the continued maturation of autophagosomes, after the action of LC3 [140]

The success of autophagy is closely related to intracellular traffic determined by specific proteins, among them are the Rab proteins, C9orf72 and histone deacetylase 6 (HDAC6).

Rab proteins are monomeric GTPases responsible for vesicle formation, mobility among cellular compartments, anchoring and transportation of organelles [141], as detailed earlier in this chapter. Dysfunction of these proteins cause extensive cell damage, for example, proteins accumulation in the endoplasmic reticulum, as well as failure in the degradation pathways [61].

Rab24 protein regulates the formation of autophagosomes, and participate in the retrograde traffic between the *cis* region of the Golgi complex and the endoplasmic reticulum, suggesting its involvement in the degradation process specially during protein aggregation [142].

The main function of Rab7 is to direct vesicles and organelles of the late endosome and autophagosomes to lysosomes [142]. Deficit in function of Rab7 were described in neurodegenerative diseases such as Charcot-Marie-Tooth disease and Alzheimer's disease resulting in impairment of cellular degradation [143, 144]. In addition, Rab7 seems to have a key role in the growth and neuronal maintenance, as part of the retrograde traffic of TrkA receptor, NGF (nerve growth factor). Dysfunction in traffic caused by the change of Rab7 can result in inhibition of cell growth and promote cell death [145].

Rab5, as mentioned earlier in this chapter, regulates the endocytosis, anchoring, trafficking and fusion of endosomal membranes [53]. In addition, mutated protein lead to accumulation of enlarged early and late endosome/phagosomes and defective regulation of trafficking of endosomes/phagosomes to lysosome involving Rab7 [146]. Rab5 has been suggested to be involved with trafficking of early endosomes/phagosomes. Whereas after vesicle maturation, Rab7 is responsible for coordinating fusion of late endosomes with autophagosomes [147].

Together, these findings indicate that Rab 5 is involved with formation and transportation of immature endosomes/phagosomes contributing to first steps of autophagy.

C9orf72 also appears to be associated with endosomes and regulates autophagy through interactions with Rab proteins, including Rab7 [148]. The function of this gene began to be evaluated when an intronic expansion GGGGCC hexanucleotide was identified, which leads to inhibition of gene expression in patients with amyotrophic lateral sclerosis, frontotemporal dementia and late-onset Alzheimer's disease [149, 150].

HDAC6 controls the merging of autophagosomes with lysosomes, operating together with p62, loss of this function is related to autophagosomes failure, protein aggregation and neurodegeneration [151, 152]. HDAC6 is also a molecular link between the proteasomal degradation and lysosomal system, which recovers the proteasomal system for directing polyubiquitinated proteins to lysosomal degradation [153]. However, recent studies demonstrated that there is an increase in the expression of HDAC6 in the hippocampus of AD patients [154], whereas inhibition of HDAC6 would improve memory by reducing tau deposition in animal models of AD [154, 155]

Maturation of autophagolysosomes as well as their retrograde trafficking are impaired in AD, causing a massive concentration of autophagic vesicles along degenerating neurites. Trafficking system is disturbed also because of the defected microtubules in Alzheimer's disease brains, since hyperphosphorylation of tau protein is responsible for dysfunction of neuronal cells microtubules. Ineffective degradation of autophagosomes ends up in generation of Aß peptides, because autophagic vacuoles hold amyloid precursor protein (APP) and secretases. The combination of raised autophagy induction and abnormal clearance of autophagic vacuoles creates circumstances that favor Aß peptide aggregation and accumulation in Alzheimer's disease.

Hippocampus of young PSEN1/APP mutant mice presents degenerative process underlying functional disturbance prior to neuronal loss. The early autophagy pathology is marked by increased LC3 levels, numerous autophagic vesicles and axonal swellings. Early neurodegeneration is accompanied by the presence of phosphorylated tau, along with decreased levels of kinesin-1 and dynein motor proteins, which, altogether, could be responsible for vesicle accumulation [156].

A specific autophagy pathway that degrades mitochondria is called mitophagy. It is well known that dysfunction in mitochondrial trafficking contributes to deficiency in mitochondrial quality control and biogenesis, which leads to increase in oxidative stress, PINK1 and Parkin are proteins associated with the labeling and targeting mitochondria for degradation.

Parkin-mediated mitophagy is induced in AD patient brains. Under AD-linked pathophysiological conditions, Parkin translocation predominantly occurs in the somatodendritic regions; such distribution is associated with reduced anterograde and increased retrograde transport of axonal mitochondria. Enhanced mitophagy was further confirmed in AD patient brains, accompanied with depletion of cytosolic Parkin over disease progression. This aberrant accumulation of dysfunctional mitochondria in AD-affected neurons is likely attributable to inadequate mitophagy capacity of eliminate those damaged mitochondria. Altogether, there is evidence that mitochondrial stress under pathophysiological conditions effectively triggers Parkin-dependent mitophagy [157].

The reduced number of mitochondria in axon is reported to implicate in tau phosphorylation. Using animal AD model expressing human tau, it was demonstrated that knockdown of TRAK or Miro (adaptor proteins essential for axonal transport of mitochondria), enhanced tau phosphorylation at an AD-related site Ser262. Tau phosphorylation at Ser262 has been reported to promote tau detachment from microtubules, which was confirmed by the increase of free tau. These evidence suggest that loss of axonal mitochondria may play an important role in tau phosphorylation and toxicity in the pathogenesis of AD [158].

PROPER INTRACELLULAR TRAFFICKING IS FUNDAMENTAL FOR CA²⁺ HOMEOSTASIS

Cell homeostasis is maintained by the equilibrium of organelles function and ionic balance. Disturbance of mitochondria, ER and calcium homeostasis is often related with AD.

Regulated mitochondria membrane potential is important to keep ER morphology. In cases of alteration in mitochondrial membrane potential, ER fragments and release calcium to cytosol, causing intracellular calcium elevation, leading to increased ROS levels. These findings suggest that both ER stress and mitochondria dysfunction contribute to neurodegeneration.

Moreover, it has been shown that both organelles are in close contact in synapses, promoting the calcium flow and synaptic activity [159, 160]. These studies strongly suggest that contact between mitochondria and ER is essential to neuron survival [159].

It has been reported that mitochondria fission process occurs near the contact sites with ER even in the absence of mitochondria fission factors. Besides that, MFN1 and MFN2, which are proteins related to mitochondria fusion, have their activity dependent of Miro1, that is a crucial protein associated with mitochondria trafficking and dynamics. Interestingly, Miro1 is located at sites of contact between ER and mitochondria.

Mitophagy process also seems to be dependent of mitochondria and ER membrane contact sites. Several ATG proteins, including ATG8 mammalian orthologs (LC3), are found at mitochondria and ER contact sites. Moreover, it has been demonstrated that in yeast or mammalians, mitochondria and ER contact sites forms a platform allowing mitophagosome biogenesis and mitochondria degradation [161, 162]

Stressed ER also generates ROS, decreasing reduced glutathione (GSH) levels and transferring excessive calcium to mitochondria, that also generates ROS. GSH is the main molecule responsible to keep ER and mitochondria redox state. In cases of accumulation of hyperphosphorylated tau in the ER, GSH is oxidized activating unfold protein response (UPR). In order to restore ER homeostasis, the protein IRE1α (inositol-requiring enzyme 1 alpha) activates UPR, which activates chaperons such as PDI (protein disulfide isomerase) that increases folding and secretion of proteins to be degraded, reestablishing ER redox state.

PDI is the main protein involved in folding protein machinery of ER. Moreover, the protein is found overexpressed in cases of ER stress, therefore, being one of the main markers of ER stress. During folding process PDI oxidizes proteins generating disulfides bonds in proteins and become reduced. The enzyme Ero1 (endoplasmic reticulum oxidoreductase 1) oxidizes PDI, reactivating the protein that becomes ready to another cycle of protein folding. Once reduced, the protein Ero1 transfer oxygen to molecular oxygen generating H_2O_2. Moreover, accumulated protein in ER favors calcium leakage to cytosol [163 - 166].

Increased cytoplasmic Ca^{2+} levels inhibits mitochondrial retrograde and anterograde transport; Miro has an important role in this inhibition [124, 167]. Miro proteins have 2 GTPase domains in N- and C- terminus and a pair of EF hands motifs where two molecules of Ca^{2+} binds [168, 169], as mentioned before.

Three different mechanisms of mitochondria anchoring by Ca^{2+} have been proposed: 1) increased Ca^{2+} would lead the motor domain of KIF5 to dissociate from microtubules and to interact with Miro on mitochondria; 2) there would be the inhibition of KIF5 interaction with Miro, uncoupling mitochondria from molecular motor; and 3) the dissociated KIF5 would interact with microtubule-bound Syntaphilin, which is a tethering protein, arresting mitochondria in the place where Ca^{2+} is elevated [120].

Miro would also play a key role in regulating Ca^{2+} levels in mitochondria matrix, this would determine the organelle transport because its possible Ca^{2+} overload [170]. Mitochondria also work as a calcium buffer, therefore, stocking calcium levels released from ER, consequently increasing its metabolism as well as generating ROS. Further, folding process requires high levels of ATP. Thereby, prolonged UPR activation promotes high levels of ROS.

Together these evidences indicate that the crosstalking between mitochondria and ER is important to keep homeostasis, but can also trigger cell death. ER stress may occur after excessive contingent of misfolded proteins that are formed in this organelle. The accumulation of protein aggregates in the brain of AD patients suggest that alterations in ER homeostasis is relevant for the neurodegenerative disease [171].

CONCLUDING REMARKS

The association between protein aggregation and impairment of intracellular trafficking during neurodegeneration is still a matter of investigation, however there is evidence that soluble misfolded proteins and their fibrils more toxic to intracellular trafficking than aggregates are. In AD tau and Aß peptide are the most toxic species.

Oligomers and fibrils of tau and Aß peptide impair anterograde and retrograde traffic of APP-containing vesicles and organelles such as mitochondria, which increase even more the synthesis of Aß inside cells, hyperphosphorylation of tau and disrupts ATP synthesis and Ca^{2+} homeostasis.

Plasma membrane and cholesterol dynamics is also related with increased amyloidogenic APP processing and hyperphosphorylation of tau. Accumulation of misfolded proteins overload autophagy system and impairs degradation of organelles such as old mitochondria, which elevates the levels of ROS generation.

Impaired trafficking culminates with ER and Golgi fragmentation that promotes signaling for cell death if maintained during prolonged period of time.

In conclusion, there is evidence that impairment of intracellular trafficking precedes cell death and intervention in order to rescue trafficking in early neurodegeneration may be of relevance to prevent the cognitive decline during the course of AD.

CONSENT FOR PUBLICATION

Not applicable.

CONFLICTS OF INTEREST

None declared

ACKNOWLEDGEMENT

None declared

REFERENCES

[1]   Horgan CP, McCaffrey MW. Rab GTPases and microtubule motors. Biochem Soc Trans 2011; 39(5): 1202-6.
      [http://dx.doi.org/10.1042/BST0391202] [PMID: 21936789]

[2]   Hirokawa N, Noda Y, Tanaka Y, Niwa S. Kinesin superfamily motor proteins and intracellular transport. Nat Rev Mol Cell Biol 2009; 10(10): 682-96.
      [http://dx.doi.org/10.1038/nrm2774] [PMID: 19773780]

[3]   Chaves RS, Melo TQ, D'Unhao AM.. Dynein c1h1, dynactin and syntaphilin expression in brain areas related to neurodegenerative diseases following exposure to rotenone. Acta Neurobiologiae Experimentalis 2013. no prelo

[4]   Melo TQ, D'Unhao AM, Martins SA. Rotenone-Dependent Changes of Anterograde Motor Protein Expression and Mitochondrial Mobility in Brain Areas Related to Neurodegenerative Diseases. Cell Mol Neurobiol 2012.
      [PMID: 23263842]

[5]   Orr AL, Li S, Wang CE, et al. N-terminal mutant huntingtin associates with mitochondria and impairs mitochondrial trafficking. J Neurosci 2008; 28(11): 2783-92.
      [http://dx.doi.org/10.1523/JNEUROSCI.0106-08.2008] [PMID: 18337408]

[6]   Gibb WR, Lees AJ. The relevance of the Lewy body to the pathogenesis of idiopathic Parkinson's disease. J Neurol Neurosurg Psychiatry 1988; 51(6): 745-52.
      [http://dx.doi.org/10.1136/jnnp.51.6.745] [PMID: 2841426]

[7]   Selkoe DJ. The deposition of amyloid proteins in the aging mammalian brain: implications for Alzheimer's disease. Ann Med 1989; 21(2): 73-6.
      [http://dx.doi.org/10.3109/07853898909149187] [PMID: 2504258]

[8]   Hardy J, Selkoe DJ. The amyloid hypothesis of Alzheimer's disease: progress and problems on the road to therapeutics. Science 2002; 297(5580): 353-6.
      [http://dx.doi.org/10.1126/science.1072994] [PMID: 12130773]

[9]   Dayan AD. Quantitative histological studies on the aged human brain. I. Senile plaques and neurofibrillary tangles in "normal" patients. Acta Neuropathol 1970; 16(2): 85-94.
      [http://dx.doi.org/10.1007/BF00687663] [PMID: 4919692]

[10] Terry RD. The cytoskeleton in Alzheimer disease. J Neural Transm Suppl 1998; 53: 141-5.
      [http://dx.doi.org/10.1007/978-3-7091-6467-9_12] [PMID: 9700652]

[11] Dixit R, Ross JL, Goldman YE, Holzbaur EL. Differential regulation of dynein and kinesin motor proteins by tau. Science 2008; 319(5866): 1086-9.
      [http://dx.doi.org/10.1126/science.1152993] [PMID: 18202255]

[12] Caceres A, Kosik KS. Inhibition of neurite polarity by tau antisense oligonucleotides in primary cerebellar neurons. Nature 1990; 343(6257): 461-3.
      [http://dx.doi.org/10.1038/343461a0] [PMID: 2105469]

[13] Esmaeli-Azad B, McCarty JH, Feinstein SC. Sense and antisense transfection analysis of tau function: tau influences net microtubule assembly, neurite outgrowth and neuritic stability. J Cell Sci 1994; 107

(Pt 4): 869-79.
[PMID: 8056843]

[14]   Williamson R, Scales T, Clark BR, *et al.* Rapid tyrosine phosphorylation of neuronal proteins including tau and focal adhesion kinase in response to amyloid-β peptide exposure: involvement of Src family protein kinases. J Neurosci 2002; 22(1): 10-20.
[http://dx.doi.org/10.1523/JNEUROSCI.22-01-00010.2002] [PMID: 11756483]

[15]   Grundke-Iqbal I, Iqbal K, Tung YC, Quinlan M, Wisniewski HM, Binder LI. Abnormal phosphorylation of the microtubule-associated protein tau (tau) in Alzheimer cytoskeletal pathology. Proc Natl Acad Sci USA 1986; 83(13): 4913-7.
[http://dx.doi.org/10.1073/pnas.83.13.4913] [PMID: 3088567]

[16]   Role of Tau Protein in Both Physiological and Pathological Conditions. 2004; 84: pp. 361-84.

[17]   Yamamoto H, Hasegawa M, Ono T, Tashima K, Ihara Y, Miyamoto E. Dephosphorylation of fetal-tau and paired helical filaments-tau by protein phosphatases 1 and 2A and calcineurin. J Biochem 1995; 118(6): 1224-31.
[http://dx.doi.org/10.1093/oxfordjournals.jbchem.a125011] [PMID: 8720139]

[18]   Ballatore C, Brunden KR, Huryn DM, Trojanowski JQ, Lee VM, Smith AB III. Microtubule stabilizing agents as potential treatment for Alzheimer's disease and related neurodegenerative tauopathies. J Med Chem 2012; 55(21): 8979-96.
[http://dx.doi.org/10.1021/jm301079z] [PMID: 23020671]

[19]   Churcher I. Tau therapeutic strategies for the treatment of Alzheimer's disease. Curr Top Med Chem 2006; 6(6): 579-95.
[http://dx.doi.org/10.2174/156802606776743057] [PMID: 16712493]

[20]   Alonso AC, Grundke-Iqbal I, Iqbal K. Alzheimer's disease hyperphosphorylated tau sequesters normal tau into tangles of filaments and disassembles microtubules. Nat Med 1996; 2(7): 783-7.
[http://dx.doi.org/10.1038/nm0796-783] [PMID: 8673924]

[21]   Haass C, Selkoe DJ. Soluble protein oligomers in neurodegeneration: lessons from the Alzheimer's amyloid beta-peptide. Nat Rev Mol Cell Biol 2007; 8(2): 101-12.
[http://dx.doi.org/10.1038/nrm2101] [PMID: 17245412]

[22]   Rapoport M, Dawson HN, Binder LI, Vitek MP, Ferreira A. Tau is essential to β -amyloid-induced neurotoxicity. Proc Natl Acad Sci USA 2002; 99(9): 6364-9.
[http://dx.doi.org/10.1073/pnas.092136199] [PMID: 11959919]

[23]   Shipton OA, Leitz JR, Dworzak J, *et al.* Tau protein is required for amyloid β-induced impairment of hippocampal long-term potentiation. J Neurosci 2011; 31(5): 1688-92.
[http://dx.doi.org/10.1523/JNEUROSCI.2610-10.2011] [PMID: 21289177]

[24]   Stamer K, Vogel R, Thies E, Mandelkow E, Mandelkow EM. Tau blocks traffic of organelles, neurofilaments, and APP vesicles in neurons and enhances oxidative stress. J Cell Biol 2002; 156(6): 1051-63.
[http://dx.doi.org/10.1083/jcb.200108057] [PMID: 11901170]

[25]   Dubey M, Chaudhury P, Kabiru H, Shea TB. Tau inhibits anterograde axonal transport and perturbs stability in growing axonal neurites in part by displacing kinesin cargo: neurofilaments attenuate tau-mediated neurite instability. Cell Motil Cytoskeleton 2008; 65(2): 89-99.
[http://dx.doi.org/10.1002/cm.20243] [PMID: 18000878]

[26]   Stoothoff W, Jones PB, Spires-Jones TL, *et al.* Differential effect of three-repeat and four-repeat tau on mitochondrial axonal transport. J Neurochem 2009; 111(2): 417-27.
[http://dx.doi.org/10.1111/j.1471-4159.2009.06316.x] [PMID: 19686388]

[27]   Trinczek B, Ebneth A, Mandelkow EM, Mandelkow E. Tau regulates the attachment/detachment but not the speed of motors in microtubule-dependent transport of single vesicles and organelles. J Cell Sci 1999; 112(Pt 14): 2355-67.

[PMID: 10381391]

[28]   Mandelkow EM, Thies E, Trinczek B, Biernat J, Mandelkow E. MARK/PAR1 kinase is a regulator of microtubule-dependent transport in axons. J Cell Biol 2004; 167(1): 99-110.
       [http://dx.doi.org/10.1083/jcb.200401085] [PMID: 15466480]

[29]   Vossel KA, Zhang K, Brodbeck J, *et al.* Tau reduction prevents Abeta-induced defects in axonal transport. Science 2010; 330(6001): 198.
       [http://dx.doi.org/10.1126/science.1194653] [PMID: 20829454]

[30]   Dixit R, Ross JL, Goldman YE, Holzbaur EL. Differential regulation of dynein and kinesin motor proteins by tau. Science 2008; 319(5866): 1086-9.
       [http://dx.doi.org/10.1126/science.1152993] [PMID: 18202255]

[31]   Mandelkow EM, Stamer K, Vogel R, Thies E, Mandelkow E. Clogging of axons by tau, inhibition of axonal traffic and starvation of synapses. Neurobiol Aging 2003; 24(8): 1079-85.
       [http://dx.doi.org/10.1016/j.neurobiolaging.2003.04.007] [PMID: 14643379]

[32]   Gispert-Sanchez S, Auburger G. The role of protein aggregates in neuronal pathology: guilty, innocent, or just trying to help? J Neural Transm Suppl 2006; (70): 111-7.
       [PMID: 17017517]

[33]   Alonso AdelC, Li B, Grundke-Iqbal I, Iqbal K. Polymerization of hyperphosphorylated tau into filaments eliminates its inhibitory activity. Proc Natl Acad Sci USA 2006; 103(23): 8864-9.
       [http://dx.doi.org/10.1073/pnas.0603214103] [PMID: 16735465]

[34]   Arrasate M, Mitra S, Schweitzer ES, Segal MR, Finkbeiner S. Inclusion body formation reduces levels of mutant huntingtin and the risk of neuronal death. Nature 2004; 431(7010): 805-10.
       [http://dx.doi.org/10.1038/nature02998] [PMID: 15483602]

[35]   Chaves RS, Melo TQ, Martins SA, Ferrari MF. Protein aggregation containing β-amyloid, α-synuclein and hyperphosphorylated τ in cultured cells of hippocampus, substantia nigra and locus coeruleus after rotenone exposure. BMC Neurosci 2010; 11: 144.
       [http://dx.doi.org/10.1186/1471-2202-11-144] [PMID: 21067569]

[36]   Corder EH, Saunders AM, Strittmatter WJ, *et al.* Gene dose of apolipoprotein E type 4 allele and the risk of Alzheimer's disease in late onset families. Science 1993; 261(5123): 921-3.
       [http://dx.doi.org/10.1126/science.8346443] [PMID: 8346443]

[37]   Schmechel DE, Saunders AM, Strittmatter WJ, *et al.* Increased amyloid beta-peptide deposition in cerebral cortex as a consequence of apolipoprotein E genotype in late-onset Alzheimer disease. Proc Natl Acad Sci USA 1993; 90(20): 9649-53.
       [http://dx.doi.org/10.1073/pnas.90.20.9649] [PMID: 8415756]

[38]   Corder EH, Saunders AM, Risch NJ, *et al.* Protective effect of apolipoprotein E type 2 allele for late onset Alzheimer disease. Nat Genet 1994; 7(2): 180-4.
       [http://dx.doi.org/10.1038/ng0694-180] [PMID: 7920638]

[39]   Kanekiyo T, Xu H, Bu G. ApoE and Aβ in Alzheimer's disease: accidental encounters or partners? Neuron 2014; 81(4): 740-54.
       [http://dx.doi.org/10.1016/j.neuron.2014.01.045] [PMID: 24559670]

[40]   Das U, Scott DA, Ganguly A, Koo EH, Tang Y, Roy S. Activity-induced convergence of APP and BACE-1 in acidic microdomains *via* an endocytosis-dependent pathway. Neuron 2013; 79(3): 447-60.
       [http://dx.doi.org/10.1016/j.neuron.2013.05.035] [PMID: 23931995]

[41]   Rhinn H, Fujita R, Qiang L, Cheng R, Lee JH, Abeliovich A. Integrative genomics identifies APOE ε4 effectors in Alzheimer's disease. Nature 2013; 500(7460): 45-50.
       [http://dx.doi.org/10.1038/nature12415] [PMID: 23883936]

[42]   Cataldo AM, Barnett JL, Pieroni C, Nixon RA. Increased neuronal endocytosis and protease delivery to early endosomes in sporadic Alzheimer's disease: neuropathologic evidence for a mechanism of increased beta-amyloidogenesis. J Neurosci 1997; 17(16): 6142-51.

[http://dx.doi.org/10.1523/JNEUROSCI.17-16-06142.1997] [PMID: 9236226]

[43]   Lane-Donovan C, Philips GT, Herz J. More than cholesterol transporters: lipoprotein receptors in CNS function and neurodegeneration. Neuron 2014; 83(4): 771-87.
[http://dx.doi.org/10.1016/j.neuron.2014.08.005] [PMID: 25144875]

[44]   Arenas F, Garcia-Ruiz C, Fernandez-Checa JC. Intracellular cholesterol trafficking and impact in neurodegeneration. Front Mol Neurosci 2017; 10: 382.
[http://dx.doi.org/10.3389/fnmol.2017.00382] [PMID: 29204109]

[45]   Kelly EE, Horgan CP, McCaffrey MW. Rab11 proteins in health and disease. Biochem Soc Trans 2012; 40(6): 1360-7.
[http://dx.doi.org/10.1042/BST20120157] [PMID: 23176481]

[46]   Stenmark H. Rab GTPases as coordinators of vesicle traffic. Nat Rev Mol Cell Biol 2009; 10(8): 513-25.
[http://dx.doi.org/10.1038/nrm2728] [PMID: 19603039]

[47]   Kornmann B, Currie E, Collins SR, *et al.* An ER-mitochondria tethering complex revealed by a synthetic biology screen. Science 2009; 325(5939): 477-81.
[http://dx.doi.org/10.1126/science.1175088] [PMID: 19556461]

[48]   Barbieri MA, Hoffenberg S, Roberts R, *et al.* Evidence for a symmetrical requirement for Rab5-GTP in *in vitro* endosome-endosome fusion. J Biol Chem 1998; 273(40): 25850-5.
[http://dx.doi.org/10.1074/jbc.273.40.25850] [PMID: 9748259]

[49]   Pan X, Eathiraj S, Munson M, Lambright DG. TBC-domain GAPs for Rab GTPases accelerate GTP hydrolysis by a dual-finger mechanism. Nature 2006; 442(7100): 303-6.
[http://dx.doi.org/10.1038/nature04847] [PMID: 16855591]

[50]   DerMardirossian C, Bokoch GM. GDIs: central regulatory molecules in Rho GTPase activation. Trends Cell Biol 2005; 15(7): 356-63.
[http://dx.doi.org/10.1016/j.tcb.2005.05.001] [PMID: 15921909]

[51]   Wang Y, Tang BL. SNAREs in neurons-beyond synaptic vesicle exocytosis (Review). Mol Membr Biol 2006; 23(5): 377-84. [Review].
[http://dx.doi.org/10.1080/09687860600776734] [PMID: 17060155]

[52]   Zhao C, Slevin JT, Whiteheart SW. Cellular functions of NSF: not just SNAPs and SNAREs. FEBS Lett 2007; 581(11): 2140-9.
[http://dx.doi.org/10.1016/j.febslet.2007.03.032] [PMID: 17397838]

[53]   Olchowik M, Miaczyńska M. [Effectors of GTPase Rab5 in endocytosis and signal transduction]. Postepy Biochem 2009; 55(2): 171-80. [Effectors of GTPase Rab5 in endocytosis and signal transduction].
[PMID: 19824473]

[54]   Haass C, Koo EH, Mellon A, Hung AY, Selkoe DJ. Targeting of cell-surface beta-amyloid precursor protein to lysosomes: alternative processing into amyloid-bearing fragments. Nature 1992; 357(6378): 500-3.
[http://dx.doi.org/10.1038/357500a0] [PMID: 1608449]

[55]   Cataldo AM, Peterhoff CM, Troncoso JC, Gomez-Isla T, Hyman BT, Nixon RA. Endocytic pathway abnormalities precede amyloid beta deposition in sporadic Alzheimer's disease and Down syndrome: differential effects of APOE genotype and presenilin mutations. Am J Pathol 2000; 157(1): 277-86.
[http://dx.doi.org/10.1016/S0002-9440(10)64538-5] [PMID: 10880397]

[56]   Stenmark H, Olkkonen VM. The Rab GTPase family. Genome Biol 2001; 2(5): REVIEWS3007.

[57]   Yan T, Wang L, Gao J, *et al.* Rab10 Phosphorylation is a Prominent Pathological Feature in Alzheimer's Disease. J Alzheimers Dis 2018; 63(1): 157-65.
[http://dx.doi.org/10.3233/JAD-180023] [PMID: 29562525]

[58]   Ridge PG, Karch CM, Hsu S, *et al*. Linkage, whole genome sequence, and biological data implicate variants in RAB10 in Alzheimer's disease resilience. Genome Med 2017; 9(1): 100.
[http://dx.doi.org/10.1186/s13073-017-0486-1] [PMID: 29183403]

[59]   McConlogue L, Castellano F, deWit C, Schenk D, Maltese WA. Differential effects of a Rab6 mutant on secretory *versus* amyloidogenic processing of Alzheimer's beta-amyloid precursor protein. J Biol Chem 1996; 271(3): 1343-8.
[http://dx.doi.org/10.1074/jbc.271.3.1343] [PMID: 8576122]

[60]   Gonatas NK, Stieber A, Gonatas JO. Fragmentation of the Golgi apparatus in neurodegenerative diseases and cell death. J Neurol Sci 2006; 246(1-2): 21-30.
[http://dx.doi.org/10.1016/j.jns.2006.01.019] [PMID: 16545397]

[61]   Scheper W, Hoozemans JJ, Hoogenraad CC, Rozemuller AJ, Eikelenboom P, Baas F. Rab6 is increased in Alzheimer's disease brain and correlates with endoplasmic reticulum stress. Neuropathol Appl Neurobiol 2007; 33(5): 523-32.
[PMID: 17573808]

[62]   Alto NM, Soderling J, Scott JD. Rab32 is an A-kinase anchoring protein and participates in mitochondrial dynamics. J Cell Biol 2002; 158(4): 659-68.
[http://dx.doi.org/10.1083/jcb.200204081] [PMID: 12186851]

[63]   Bertoni-Freddari C, Fattoretti P, Giorgetti B, *et al*. Preservation of mitochondrial volume homeostasis at the early stages of age-related synaptic deterioration. Ann N Y Acad Sci 2007; 1096: 138-46.
[http://dx.doi.org/10.1196/annals.1397.079] [PMID: 17405925]

[64]   Soane L, Kahraman S, Kristian T, Fiskum G. Mechanisms of impaired mitochondrial energy metabolism in acute and chronic neurodegenerative disorders. J Neurosci Res 2007; 85(15): 3407-15.
[http://dx.doi.org/10.1002/jnr.21498] [PMID: 17847081]

[65]   Van Laar VS, Berman SB. Mitochondrial dynamics in Parkinson's disease. Exp Neurol 2009; 218(2): 247-56.
[http://dx.doi.org/10.1016/j.expneurol.2009.03.019] [PMID: 19332061]

[66]   Hammer JA III, Wu XS. Rabs grab motors: defining the connections between Rab GTPases and motor proteins. Curr Opin Cell Biol 2002; 14(1): 69-75.
[http://dx.doi.org/10.1016/S0955-0674(01)00296-4] [PMID: 11792547]

[67]   Goldstein LS. Kinesin molecular motors: transport pathways, receptors, and human disease. Proc Natl Acad Sci USA 2001; 98(13): 6999-7003.
[http://dx.doi.org/10.1073/pnas.111145298] [PMID: 11416178]

[68]   Kins S, Lauther N, Szodorai A, Beyreuther K. Subcellular trafficking of the amyloid precursor protein gene family and its pathogenic role in Alzheimer's disease. Neurodegener Dis 2006; 3(4-5): 218-26.
[http://dx.doi.org/10.1159/000095259] [PMID: 17047360]

[69]   Pigino G, Morfini G, Atagi Y, *et al*. Disruption of fast axonal transport is a pathogenic mechanism for intraneuronal amyloid beta. Proc Natl Acad Sci USA 2009; 106(14): 5907-12.
[http://dx.doi.org/10.1073/pnas.0901229106] [PMID: 19321417]

[70]   Morfini G, Pigino G, Beffert U, Busciglio J, Brady ST. Fast axonal transport misregulation and Alzheimer's disease. Neuromolecular Med 2002; 2(2): 89-99.
[http://dx.doi.org/10.1385/NMM:2:2:089] [PMID: 12428805]

[71]   Pigino G, Morfini G, Pelsman A, Mattson MP, Brady ST, Busciglio J. Alzheimer's presenilin 1 mutations impair kinesin-based axonal transport. J Neurosci 2003; 23(11): 4499-508.
[http://dx.doi.org/10.1523/JNEUROSCI.23-11-04499.2003] [PMID: 12805290]

[72]   Joshi G, Wang Y. Golgi defects enhance APP amyloidogenic processing in Alzheimer's disease. BioEssays 2015; 37(3): 240-7.
[http://dx.doi.org/10.1002/bies.201400116] [PMID: 25546412]

[73]   Gunawardena S, Yang G, Goldstein LS. Presenilin controls kinesin-1 and dynein function during APP-vesicle transport *in vivo*. Hum Mol Genet 2013; 22(19): 3828-43.
[http://dx.doi.org/10.1093/hmg/ddt237] [PMID: 23710041]

[74]   Kimura N, Okabayashi S, Ono F. Dynein dysfunction disrupts intracellular vesicle trafficking bidirectionally and perturbs synaptic vesicle docking *via* endocytic disturbances a potential mechanism underlying age-dependent impairment of cognitive function. Am J Pathol 2012; 180(2): 550-61.
[http://dx.doi.org/10.1016/j.ajpath.2011.10.037] [PMID: 22182700]

[75]   Kimura N, Samura E, Suzuki K, Okabayashi S, Shimozawa N, Yasutomi Y. Dynein dysfunction reproduces age-dependent retromer deficiency: concomitant disruption of retrograde trafficking is required for alteration in beta-amyloid precursor protein metabolism. Am J Pathol 2016; 186(7): 1952-66.
[http://dx.doi.org/10.1016/j.ajpath.2016.03.006] [PMID: 27179390]

[76]   Butzlaff M, Hannan SB, Karsten P, *et al*. Impaired retrograde transport by the Dynein/Dynactin complex contributes to Tau-induced toxicity. Hum Mol Genet 2015; 24(13): 3623-37.
[http://dx.doi.org/10.1093/hmg/ddv107] [PMID: 25794683]

[77]   Bertoni-Freddari C, Fattoretti P, Giorgetti B, *et al*. Alterations of synaptic turnover rate in aging may trigger senile plaque formation and neurodegeneration. Ann N Y Acad Sci 2007; 1096: 128-37.
[http://dx.doi.org/10.1196/annals.1397.078] [PMID: 17405924]

[78]   Navarro A, Boveris A. Brain mitochondrial dysfunction in aging, neurodegeneration, and Parkinson's disease. Front Aging Neurosci 2010; 2: 2.
[PMID: 20890446]

[79]   Shankar SK. Biology of aging brain. Indian J Pathol Microbiol 2010; 53(4): 595-604.
[http://dx.doi.org/10.4103/0377-4929.71995] [PMID: 21045377]

[80]   Xiong J, Verkhratsky A, Toescu EC. Changes in mitochondrial status associated with altered Ca2+ homeostasis in aged cerebellar granule neurons in brain slices. J Neurosci 2002; 22(24): 10761-71.
[http://dx.doi.org/10.1523/JNEUROSCI.22-24-10761.2002] [PMID: 12486169]

[81]   Esiri MM. Ageing and the brain. J Pathol 2007; 211(2): 181-7.
[http://dx.doi.org/10.1002/path.2089] [PMID: 17200950]

[82]   Zhang L, Trushin S, Christensen TA, *et al*. Differential effect of amyloid beta peptides on mitochondrial axonal trafficking depends on their state of aggregation and binding to the plasma membrane. Neurobiol Dis 2018; 114: 1-16.
[http://dx.doi.org/10.1016/j.nbd.2018.02.003] [PMID: 29477640]

[83]   Hollenbeck PJ, Saxton WM. The axonal transport of mitochondria. J Cell Sci 2005; 118(Pt 23): 5411-9.
[http://dx.doi.org/10.1242/jcs.02745] [PMID: 16306220]

[84]   Nangaku M, Sato-Yoshitake R, Okada Y, *et al*. KIF1B, a novel microtubule plus end-directed monomeric motor protein for transport of mitochondria. Cell 1994; 79(7): 1209-20.
[http://dx.doi.org/10.1016/0092-8674(94)90012-4] [PMID: 7528108]

[85]   Chevalier-Larsen E, Holzbaur EL. Axonal transport and neurodegenerative disease. Biochim Biophys Acta 2006; 1762(11-12): 1094-108.
[http://dx.doi.org/10.1016/j.bbadis.2006.04.002] [PMID: 16730956]

[86]   Boldogh IR, Pon LA. Mitochondria on the move. Trends Cell Biol 2007; 17(10): 502-10.
[http://dx.doi.org/10.1016/j.tcb.2007.07.008] [PMID: 17804238]

[87]   Kang JS, Tian JH, Pan PY, *et al*. Docking of axonal mitochondria by syntaphilin controls their mobility and affects short-term facilitation. Cell 2008; 132(1): 137-48.
[http://dx.doi.org/10.1016/j.cell.2007.11.024] [PMID: 18191227]

[88]   Chen YM, Gerwin C, Sheng ZH. Dynein light chain LC8 regulates syntaphilin-mediated

mitochondrial docking in axons. J Neurosci 2009; 29(30): 9429-38.
[http://dx.doi.org/10.1523/JNEUROSCI.1472-09.2009] [PMID: 19641106]

[89]   van der Bliek AM, Shen Q, Kawajiri S. Mechanisms of mitochondrial fission and fusion. Cold Spring
        Harb Perspect Biol 2013; 5(6): a011072.
        [http://dx.doi.org/10.1101/cshperspect.a011072] [PMID: 23732471]

[90]   Bereiter-Hahn J, Vöth M. Dynamics of mitochondria in living cells: shape changes, dislocations,
        fusion, and fission of mitochondria. Microsc Res Tech 1994; 27(3): 198-219.
        [http://dx.doi.org/10.1002/jemt.1070270303] [PMID: 8204911]

[91]   Chen H, Chan DC. Mitochondrial dynamics--fusion, fission, movement, and mitophagy--in
        neurodegenerative diseases. Hum Mol Genet 2009; 18(R2): R169-76.
        [http://dx.doi.org/10.1093/hmg/ddp326] [PMID: 19808793]

[92]   Chen H, Detmer SA, Ewald AJ, Griffin EE, Fraser SE, Chan DC. Mitofusins Mfn1 and Mfn2
        coordinately regulate mitochondrial fusion and are essential for embryonic development. J Cell Biol
        2003; 160(2): 189-200.
        [http://dx.doi.org/10.1083/jcb.200211046] [PMID: 12527753]

[93]   Becker T, Gebert M, Pfanner N, van der Laan M. Biogenesis of mitochondrial membrane proteins.
        Curr Opin Cell Biol 2009; 21(4): 484-93.
        [http://dx.doi.org/10.1016/j.ceb.2009.04.002] [PMID: 19423316]

[94]   Cai Q, Sheng Z-H. Moving or stopping mitochondria: Miro as a traffic cop by sensing calcium.
        Neuron 2009; 61(4): 493-6.
        [http://dx.doi.org/10.1016/j.neuron.2009.02.003] [PMID: 19249268]

[95]   Westermann B. Bioenergetic role of mitochondrial fusion and fission. Biochim Biophys Acta 2012;
        1817(10): 1833-8.
        [http://dx.doi.org/10.1016/j.bbabio.2012.02.033] [PMID: 22409868]

[96]   Youle RJ, van der Bliek AM. Mitochondrial fission, fusion, and stress. Science 2012; 337(6098):
        1062-5.
        [http://dx.doi.org/10.1126/science.1219855] [PMID: 22936770]

[97]   Otera H, Ishihara N, Mihara K. New insights into the function and regulation of mitochondrial fission.
        Biochim Biophys Acta 2013; 1833(5): 1256-68.
        [http://dx.doi.org/10.1016/j.bbamcr.2013.02.002] [PMID: 23434681]

[98]   Detmer SA, Chan DC. Functions and dysfunctions of mitochondrial dynamics. Nat Rev Mol Cell Biol
        2007; 8(11): 870-9.
        [http://dx.doi.org/10.1038/nrm2275] [PMID: 17928812]

[99]   Song W, Bossy B, Martin OJ, *et al.* Assessing mitochondrial morphology and dynamics using
        fluorescence wide-field microscopy and 3D image processing. Methods 2008; 46(4): 295-303.
        [http://dx.doi.org/10.1016/j.ymeth.2008.10.003] [PMID: 18952177]

[100]   Jahani-Asl A, Pilon-Larose K, Xu W, *et al.* The mitochondrial inner membrane GTPase, optic atrophy
        1 (Opa1), restores mitochondrial morphology and promotes neuronal survival following excitotoxicity.
        J Biol Chem 2011; 286(6): 4772-82.
        [http://dx.doi.org/10.1074/jbc.M110.167155] [PMID: 21041314]

[101]   Chen H, Chomyn A, Chan DC. Disruption of fusion results in mitochondrial heterogeneity and
        dysfunction. J Biol Chem 2005; 280(28): 26185-92.
        [http://dx.doi.org/10.1074/jbc.M503062200] [PMID: 15899901]

[102]   Richter C. Reactive oxygen and DNA damage in mitochondria. Mutat Res 1992; 275(3-6): 249-55.
        [http://dx.doi.org/10.1016/0921-8734(92)90029-O] [PMID: 1383767]

[103]   Maharjan S, Sakai Y, Hoseki J. Screening of dietary antioxidants against mitochondria-mediated
        oxidative stress by visualization of intracellular redox state. Biosci Biotechnol Biochem 2016; 80(4):
        726-34.

[http://dx.doi.org/10.1080/09168451.2015.1123607] [PMID: 26967637]

[104] Scialò F, Sriram A, Fernández-Ayala D, *et al.* Mitochondrial ROS Produced *via* Reverse Electron Transport Extend Animal Lifespan. Cell Metab 2016; 23(4): 725-34.
[http://dx.doi.org/10.1016/j.cmet.2016.03.009] [PMID: 27076081]

[105] Lenaz G, Tioli G, Falasca AI, Genova ML. Complex I function in mitochondrial supercomplexes. Biochim Biophys Acta 2016; 1857(7): 991-1000.
[http://dx.doi.org/10.1016/j.bbabio.2016.01.013] [PMID: 26820434]

[106] Forkink M, Basit F, Teixeira J, Swarts HG, Koopman WJ, Willems PH. Complex I and complex III inhibition specifically increase cytosolic hydrogen peroxide levels without inducing oxidative stress in HEK293 cells. Redox Biol 2015; 6: 607-16.
[http://dx.doi.org/10.1016/j.redox.2015.09.003] [PMID: 26516986]

[107] Leman G, Gueguen N, Desquiret-Dumas V, *et al.* Assembly defects induce oxidative stress in inherited mitochondrial complex I deficiency. Int J Biochem Cell Biol 2015; 65: 91-103.
[http://dx.doi.org/10.1016/j.biocel.2015.05.017] [PMID: 26024641]

[108] Fayet G, Jansson M, Sternberg D, *et al.* Ageing muscle: clonal expansions of mitochondrial DNA point mutations and deletions cause focal impairment of mitochondrial function. Neuromuscul Disord 2002; 12(5): 484-93.
[http://dx.doi.org/10.1016/S0960-8966(01)00332-7] [PMID: 12031622]

[109] Wang D, Kreutzer DA, Essigmann JM. Mutagenicity and repair of oxidative DNA damage: insights from studies using defined lesions. Mutat Res 1998; 400(1-2): 99-115.
[http://dx.doi.org/10.1016/S0027-5107(98)00066-9] [PMID: 9685598]

[110] Lauri A, Pompilio G, Capogrossi MC. The mitochondrial genome in aging and senescence. Ageing Res Rev 2014; 18: 1-15.
[http://dx.doi.org/10.1016/j.arr.2014.07.001] [PMID: 25042573]

[111] Brustovetsky N, Brustovetsky T, Jemmerson R, Dubinsky JM. Calcium-induced cytochrome c release from CNS mitochondria is associated with the permeability transition and rupture of the outer membrane. J Neurochem 2002; 80(2): 207-18.
[http://dx.doi.org/10.1046/j.0022-3042.2001.00671.x] [PMID: 11902111]

[112] Nguyen TT, Oh SS, Weaver D, *et al.* Loss of Miro1-directed mitochondrial movement results in a novel murine model for neuron disease. Proc Natl Acad Sci USA 2014; 111(35): E3631-40.
[http://dx.doi.org/10.1073/pnas.1402449111] [PMID: 25136135]

[113] Billingsley ML, Kincaid RL. Regulated phosphorylation and dephosphorylation of tau protein: effects on microtubule interaction, intracellular trafficking and neurodegeneration. Biochem J 1997; 323(Pt 3): 577-91.
[http://dx.doi.org/10.1042/bj3230577] [PMID: 9169588]

[114] Florenzano F. Localization of axonal motor molecules machinery in neurodegenerative disorders. Int J Mol Sci 2012; 13(4): 5195-206.
[http://dx.doi.org/10.3390/ijms13045195] [PMID: 22606038]

[115] Brookes PS, Yoon Y, Robotham JL, Anders MW, Sheu SS. Calcium, ATP, and ROS: a mitochondrial love-hate triangle. Am J Physiol Cell Physiol 2004; 287(4): C817-33.
[http://dx.doi.org/10.1152/ajpcell.00139.2004] [PMID: 15355853]

[116] Gumeni S, Trougakos IP. Cross Talk of Proteostasis and Mitostasis in Cellular Homeodynamics, Ageing, and Disease. Oxid Med Cell Longev 2016; 2016: 4587691.
[http://dx.doi.org/10.1155/2016/4587691] [PMID: 26977249]

[117] Hirokawa N, Noda Y. Intracellular transport and kinesin superfamily proteins, KIFs: structure, function, and dynamics. Physiol Rev 2008; 88(3): 1089-118.
[http://dx.doi.org/10.1152/physrev.00023.2007] [PMID: 18626067]

[118] Cooper O, Seo H, Andrabi S, *et al.* Pharmacological rescue of mitochondrial deficits in iPSC-derived

neural cells from patients with familial Parkinson's disease. Sci Transl Med 2012; 4(141): 141ra90.
[http://dx.doi.org/10.1126/scitranslmed.3003985] [PMID: 22764206]

[119]   Devine MJ, Birsa N, Kittler JT. Miro sculpts mitochondrial dynamics in neuronal health and disease. Neurobiol Dis 2016; 90: 27-34.
[http://dx.doi.org/10.1016/j.nbd.2015.12.008] [PMID: 26707701]

[120]   Chen Y, Sheng Z-H. Kinesin-1-syntaphilin coupling mediates activity-dependent regulation of axonal mitochondrial transport. J Cell Biol 2013; 202(2): 351-64.
[http://dx.doi.org/10.1083/jcb.201302040] [PMID: 23857772]

[121]   López-Doménech G, Covill-Cooke C, Ivankovic D, *et al.* Miro proteins coordinate microtubule- and actin-dependent mitochondrial transport and distribution. EMBO J 2018; 37(3): 321-36.
[http://dx.doi.org/10.15252/embj.201696380] [PMID: 29311115]

[122]   Russo GJ, Louie K, Wellington A, *et al.* Drosophila Miro is required for both anterograde and retrograde axonal mitochondrial transport. J Neurosci 2009; 29(17): 5443-55.
[http://dx.doi.org/10.1523/JNEUROSCI.5417-08.2009] [PMID: 19403812]

[123]   Guo J, Yang Z, Song W, *et al.* Nudel contributes to microtubule anchoring at the mother centriole and is involved in both dynein-dependent and -independent centrosomal protein assembly. Mol Biol Cell 2006; 17(2): 680-9.
[http://dx.doi.org/10.1091/mbc.e05-04-0360] [PMID: 16291865]

[124]   Macaskill AF, Rinholm JE, Twelvetrees AE, *et al.* Miro1 is a calcium sensor for glutamate receptor-dependent localization of mitochondria at synapses. Neuron 2009; 61(4): 541-55.
[http://dx.doi.org/10.1016/j.neuron.2009.01.030] [PMID: 19249275]

[125]   Klosowiak JL, Focia PJ, Chakravarthy S, Landahl EC, Freymann DM, Rice SE. Structural coupling of the EF hand and C-terminal GTPase domains in the mitochondrial protein Miro. EMBO Rep 2013; 14 (11): 968-74.
[http://dx.doi.org/10.1038/embor.2013.151] [PMID: 24071720]

[126]   Mironov SL. ADP regulates movements of mitochondria in neurons. Biophys J 2007; 92(8): 2944-52.
[http://dx.doi.org/10.1529/biophysj.106.092981] [PMID: 17277190]

[127]   Saotome M, Safiulina D, Szabadkai G, *et al.* Bidirectional Ca2+-dependent control of mitochondrial dynamics by the Miro GTPase. Proc Natl Acad Sci USA 2008; 105(52): 20728-33.
[http://dx.doi.org/10.1073/pnas.0808953105] [PMID: 19098100]

[128]   Friedman JR, Lackner LL, West M, DiBenedetto JR, Nunnari J, Voeltz GK. ER tubules mark sites of mitochondrial division. Science 2011; 334(6054): 358-62.
[http://dx.doi.org/10.1126/science.1207385] [PMID: 21885730]

[129]   Misko A, Jiang S, Wegorzewska I, Milbrandt J, Baloh RH. Mitofusin 2 is necessary for transport of axonal mitochondria and interacts with the Miro/Milton complex. J Neurosci 2010; 30(12): 4232-40.
[http://dx.doi.org/10.1523/JNEUROSCI.6248-09.2010] [PMID: 20335458]

[130]   Liu W, Tian F, Kurata T, Morimoto N, Abe K. Dynamic changes of mitochondrial fusion and fission proteins after transient cerebral ischemia in mice. J Neurosci Res 2012; 90(6): 1183-9.
[http://dx.doi.org/10.1002/jnr.23016] [PMID: 22345048]

[131]   Axe EL, Walker SA, Manifava M, *et al.* Autophagosome formation from membrane compartments enriched in phosphatidylinositol 3-phosphate and dynamically connected to the endoplasmic reticulum. J Cell Biol 2008; 182(4): 685-701.
[http://dx.doi.org/10.1083/jcb.200803137] [PMID: 18725538]

[132]   Hailey DW, Rambold AS, Satpute-Krishnan P, *et al.* Mitochondria supply membranes for autophagosome biogenesis during starvation. Cell 2010; 141(4): 656-67.
[http://dx.doi.org/10.1016/j.cell.2010.04.009] [PMID: 20478256]

[133]   Birsa N, Norkett R, Wauer T, *et al.* Lysine 27 ubiquitination of the mitochondrial transport protein Miro is dependent on serine 65 of the Parkin ubiquitin ligase. J Biol Chem 2014; 289(21): 14569-82.

[http://dx.doi.org/10.1074/jbc.M114.563031] [PMID: 24671417]

[134] Kazlauskaite A, Kondapalli C, Gourlay R, *et al.* Parkin is activated by PINK1-dependent phosphorylation of ubiquitin at Ser65. Biochem J 2014; 460(1): 127-39.
[http://dx.doi.org/10.1042/BJ20140334] [PMID: 24660806]

[135] Rami A. Review: autophagy in neurodegeneration: firefighter and/or incendiarist? Neuropathol Appl Neurobiol 2009; 35(5): 449-61.
[http://dx.doi.org/10.1111/j.1365-2990.2009.01034.x] [PMID: 19555462]

[136] Zheng J, Yan T, Feng Y, Zhai Q. Involvement of lysosomes in the early stages of axon degeneration. Neurochem Int 2010; 56(3): 516-21.
[http://dx.doi.org/10.1016/j.neuint.2009.12.012] [PMID: 20036294]

[137] Armstrong A, Mattsson N, Appelqvist H, *et al.* Lysosomal network proteins as potential novel CSF biomarkers for Alzheimer's disease. Neuromolecular Med 2014; 16(1): 150-60.
[http://dx.doi.org/10.1007/s12017-013-8269-3] [PMID: 24101586]

[138] Tanida I. Autophagosome Formation and Molecular Mechanism of Autophagy. Antioxid Redox Signal 2010.
[PMID: 20712405]

[139] Kang R, Zeh HJ, Lotze MT, Tang D. The Beclin 1 network regulates autophagy and apoptosis. Cell Death Differ 2011; 18(4): 571-80.
[http://dx.doi.org/10.1038/cdd.2010.191] [PMID: 21311563]

[140] Weidberg H, Shvets E, Shpilka T, Shimron F, Shinder V, Elazar Z. LC3 and GATE-16/GABARAP subfamilies are both essential yet act differently in autophagosome biogenesis. EMBO J 2010; 29(11): 1792-802.
[http://dx.doi.org/10.1038/emboj.2010.74] [PMID: 20418806]

[141] Zhen Y, Stenmark H. Cellular functions of Rab GTPases at a glance. J Cell Sci 2015; 128(17): 3171-6.
[http://dx.doi.org/10.1242/jcs.166074] [PMID: 26272922]

[142] Ao X, Zou L, Wu Y. Regulation of autophagy by the Rab GTPase network. Cell Death Differ 2014; 21(3): 348-58.
[http://dx.doi.org/10.1038/cdd.2013.187] [PMID: 24440914]

[143] Verhoeven K, De Jonghe P, Coen K, *et al.* Mutations in the small GTP-ase late endosomal protein RAB7 cause Charcot-Marie-Tooth type 2B neuropathy. Am J Hum Genet 2003; 72(3): 722-7.
[http://dx.doi.org/10.1086/367847] [PMID: 12545426]

[144] Cataldo AM, Mathews PM, Boiteau AB, *et al.* Down syndrome fibroblast model of Alzheimer-related endosome pathology: accelerated endocytosis promotes late endocytic defects. Am J Pathol 2008; 173(2): 370-84.
[http://dx.doi.org/10.2353/ajpath.2008.071053] [PMID: 18535180]

[145] Deinhardt K, Salinas S, Verastegui C, *et al.* Rab5 and Rab7 control endocytic sorting along the axonal retrograde transport pathway. Neuron 2006; 52(2): 293-305.
[http://dx.doi.org/10.1016/j.neuron.2006.08.018] [PMID: 17046692]

[146] Girard E, Chmiest D, Fournier N, *et al.* Rab7 is functionally required for selective cargo sorting at the early endosome. Traffic 2014; 15(3): 309-26.
[http://dx.doi.org/10.1111/tra.12143] [PMID: 24329906]

[147] Wang Z, Miao G, Xue X, *et al.* The Vici Syndrome Protein EPG5 Is a Rab7 Effector that Determines the Fusion Specificity of Autophagosomes with Late Endosomes/Lysosomes. Mol Cell 2016; 63(5): 781-95.
[http://dx.doi.org/10.1016/j.molcel.2016.08.021] [PMID: 27588602]

[148] Farg MA, Sundaramoorthy V, Sultana JM, *et al.* C9ORF72, implicated in amytrophic lateral sclerosis and frontotemporal dementia, regulates endosomal trafficking. Hum Mol Genet 2014; 23(13): 3579--.
[http://dx.doi.org/10.1093/hmg/ddu068] [PMID: 24549040]

[149] DeJesus-Hernandez M, Mackenzie IR, Boeve BF, *et al.* Expanded GGGGCC hexanucleotide repeat in noncoding region of C9ORF72 causes chromosome 9p-linked FTD and ALS. Neuron 2011; 72(2): 245-56.
[http://dx.doi.org/10.1016/j.neuron.2011.09.011] [PMID: 21944778]

[150] Harms M, Benitez BA, Cairns N, *et al.* C9orf72 hexanucleotide repeat expansions in clinical Alzheimer disease. JAMA Neurol 2013; 70(6): 736-41.
[http://dx.doi.org/10.1001/2013.jamaneurol.537] [PMID: 23588422]

[151] Yan J, Seibenhener ML, Calderilla-Barbosa L, *et al.* SQSTM1/p62 interacts with HDAC6 and regulates deacetylase activity. PLoS One 2013; 8(9): e76016.
[http://dx.doi.org/10.1371/journal.pone.0076016] [PMID: 24086678]

[152] Lee JY, Koga H, Kawaguchi Y, *et al.* HDAC6 controls autophagosome maturation essential for ubiquitin-selective quality-control autophagy. EMBO J 2010; 29(5): 969-80.
[http://dx.doi.org/10.1038/emboj.2009.405] [PMID: 20075865]

[153] Shaid S, Brandts CH, Serve H, Dikic I. Ubiquitination and selective autophagy. Cell Death Differ 2013; 20(1): 21-30.
[http://dx.doi.org/10.1038/cdd.2012.72] [PMID: 22722335]

[154] Zhang L, Sheng S, Qin C. The role of HDAC6 in Alzheimer's disease. J Alzheimers Dis 2013; 33(2): 283-95.
[http://dx.doi.org/10.3233/JAD-2012-120727] [PMID: 22936009]

[155] Selenica ML, Benner L, Housley SB, *et al.* Histone deacetylase 6 inhibition improves memory and reduces total tau levels in a mouse model of tau deposition. Alzheimers Res Ther 2014; 6(1): 12.
[http://dx.doi.org/10.1186/alzrt241] [PMID: 24576665]

[156] Sanchez-Varo R, Trujillo-Estrada L, Sanchez-Mejias E, *et al.* Abnormal accumulation of autophagic vesicles correlates with axonal and synaptic pathology in young Alzheimer's mice hippocampus. Acta Neuropathol 2012; 123(1): 53-70.
[http://dx.doi.org/10.1007/s00401-011-0896-x] [PMID: 22020633]

[157] Ye X, Sun X, Starovoytov V, Cai Q. Parkin-mediated mitophagy in mutant hAPP neurons and Alzheimer's disease patient brains. Hum Mol Genet 2015; 24(10): 2938-51.
[http://dx.doi.org/10.1093/hmg/ddv056] [PMID: 25678552]

[158] Iijima-Ando K, Sekiya M, Maruko-Otake A, *et al.* Loss of axonal mitochondria promotes tau-mediated neurodegeneration and Alzheimer's disease-related tau phosphorylation *via* PAR-1. PLoS Genet 2012; 8(8): e1002918.
[http://dx.doi.org/10.1371/journal.pgen.1002918] [PMID: 22952452]

[159] Krols M, Bultynck G, Janssens S. ER-Mitochondria contact sites: A new regulator of cellular calcium flux comes into play. J Cell Biol 2016; 214(4): 367-70.
[http://dx.doi.org/10.1083/jcb.201607124] [PMID: 27528654]

[160] Mironov SL, Symonchuk N. ER vesicles and mitochondria move and communicate at synapses. J Cell Sci 2006; 119(Pt 23): 4926-34.
[http://dx.doi.org/10.1242/jcs.03254] [PMID: 17105774]

[161] Böckler S, Westermann B. ER-mitochondria contacts as sites of mitophagosome formation. Autophagy 2014; 10(7): 1346-7.
[http://dx.doi.org/10.4161/auto.28981] [PMID: 24905224]

[162] Hamasaki M, Furuta N, Matsuda A, *et al.* Autophagosomes form at ER-mitochondria contact sites. Nature 2013; 495(7441): 389-93.
[http://dx.doi.org/10.1038/nature11910] [PMID: 23455425]

[163] Feissner RF, Skalska J, Gaum WE, Sheu SS. Crosstalk signaling between mitochondrial Ca2+ and ROS. Front Biosci 2009; 14: 1197-218.
[http://dx.doi.org/10.2741/3303] [PMID: 19273125]

[164] Malhotra JD, Kaufman RJ. The endoplasmic reticulum and the unfolded protein response. Semin Cell Dev Biol 2007; 18(6): 716-31.
[http://dx.doi.org/10.1016/j.semcdb.2007.09.003] [PMID: 18023214]

[165] Tu BP, Weissman JS. Oxidative protein folding in eukaryotes: mechanisms and consequences. J Cell Biol 2004; 164(3): 341-6.
[http://dx.doi.org/10.1083/jcb.200311055] [PMID: 14757749]

[166] Haynes CM, Titus EA, Cooper AA. Degradation of misfolded proteins prevents ER-derived oxidative stress and cell death. Mol Cell 2004; 15(5): 767-76.
[http://dx.doi.org/10.1016/j.molcel.2004.08.025] [PMID: 15350220]

[167] Wang X, Schwarz TL. The mechanism of Ca^{2+}-dependent regulation of kinesin-mediated mitochondrial motility. Cell 2009; 136(1): 163-74.
[http://dx.doi.org/10.1016/j.cell.2008.11.046] [PMID: 19135897]

[168] Fransson A, Ruusala A, Aspenström P. Atypical Rho GTPases have roles in mitochondrial homeostasis and apoptosis. J Biol Chem 2003; 278(8): 6495-502.
[http://dx.doi.org/10.1074/jbc.M208609200] [PMID: 12482879]

[169] Frederick RL, McCaffery JM, Cunningham KW, Okamoto K, Shaw JM. Yeast Miro GTPase, Gem1p, regulates mitochondrial morphology *via* a novel pathway. J Cell Biol 2004; 167(1): 87-98.
[http://dx.doi.org/10.1083/jcb.200405100] [PMID: 15479738]

[170] Chang KT, Niescier RF, Min KT. Mitochondrial matrix Ca^{2+} as an intrinsic signal regulating mitochondrial motility in axons. Proc Natl Acad Sci USA 2011; 108(37): 15456-61.
[http://dx.doi.org/10.1073/pnas.1106862108] [PMID: 21876166]

[171] Plácido AI, Pereira CM, Duarte AI, *et al.* The role of endoplasmic reticulum in amyloid precursor protein processing and trafficking: implications for Alzheimer's disease. Biochim Biophys Acta 2014; 1842(9): 1444-53.
[http://dx.doi.org/10.1016/j.bbadis.2014.05.003] [PMID: 24832819]

CHAPTER 6

Alzheimer's Disease and Oxidative Stress

Andrea R. Vasconcelos[#], Paula F. Kinoshita[#], Cristoforo Scavone and **Elisa M. Kawamoto***

Pharmacology Department, Instituto de Ciências Biomédicas, Universidade de São Paulo, São Paulo, Brazil

Abstract: Alzheimer's disease is a neurodegenerative disorder with no cure and not completely understood mechanisms. This devastating disease is one of the main causes of dementia in elderly people worldwide. Among different mechanisms of neuronal death associated to Alzheimer's disease, oxidative stress can be considered as one of the most studied. Several data from literature in this field have shown that oxidative stress seems to be a critical step in the neurodegenerative course of the disease. Clinical trials using antioxidants have described conflicting results, some of them supporting the importance of the use of antioxidant compounds to ameliorate disease's symptoms and the others showing negative results in terms of beneficial effects of antioxidant therapy in the disease progression.

Keywords: Alzeimer's Disease, Antioxidants, Neurodegeneration, Oxidative stress.

INTRODUCTION

Alzheimer's disease (AD), the main cause of senile dementia in western societies, is a neurodegenerative disease associated with memory and cognitive dysfunction due to synaptic loss and neuronal cell death [1, 2]. By 2040, it is estimated that 80 million people worldwide will suffer from dementia, 60% of whom will be classed as AD [3].

Classically, such neurodegenerative processes are thought to arise as a consequence of an increase in amyloid-beta peptide (Aβ)-associated senile plaques and hyperphosphorylated tau-associated neurofibrillary tangles [4, 5]. However, while considerably investigated, the mechanism underlying the pathophysiology of AD has still to be elucidated. Accumulating evidence indicates that oxidative stress is important in the aetiology and course of AD,

---

* **Corresponding author Elisa Mitiko Kawamoto:** Department of Pharmacology, Institute of Biomedical Science-ICB-1, Avenida Professor Lineu Prestes, 1524, University of São Paulo, São Paulo 05508-900, Brazil; Tel: 55-1--2648-1379/55-11-3091-7325; E-mail: kawamotoe@gmail.com
\# The authors contributed equally to the work.

Fernando A. Oliveira (Ed.)

perhaps especially in the late-onset sporadic forms of the disease [6 - 8]. Interestingly, the brain has a high demand of oxygen, which corresponds to 20% of the total body consumption, and modest antioxidant defenses, which render the brain more sensitive to oxidative stress and neurodegeneration [9].

Oxidative stress arises from an increase in the oxidant/antioxidant ratio due to an augmentation in reactive oxygen species (ROS) production and/or impaired antioxidant synthesis. Such increases in ROS can also be strongly linked to mitochondrial dysfunction, given that these organelles produce significant levels of ROS during normal functioning.

Increased ROS is associated with free radical damage to membranes and DNA, with detrimental consequences on cellular functioning and survival. This process can become a cumulative cycle of damage, because oxidative stress can destroy biomolecules that can increase even more ROS levels [10]. Thus, the levels of antioxidants and antioxidant enzyme activity must be appropriate to counteract the damaging oxidative stress effects.

However, it should be emphasized that ROS generally need to be present in low levels and cannot be fully eliminated [10]. ROS are an important part of normal cell functioning, being necessary to induce plasticity changes arising from different cellular challenges, while exceeding levels of ROS have deleterious effects [11].

ALZHEIMER'S DISEASE AND OXIDATIVE STRESS

The brain is susceptible to ROS-induced oxidative stress, due primarily to its high demand of energy, and therefore its need for oxygen and mitochondrial activity. Neuronal cells have also high lipid and iron content and less antioxidant enzymes in comparison with other tissues, which makes the brain a relevant target for oxidative stress [12].

Increased oxidative stress is generally enhanced over normal aging, in association with decreased antioxidant defenses and neurogenesis [13, 14]. Both oxygen, in the form of ROS, and nitrogen, in the form of reactive nitrogen species (RNS), can produce damaging reactive species. ROS and RNS can be variably reactive, with the hydroxyl radical (OH$\cdot$) being highly reactive, whilst hydrogen peroxide (H_2O_2), not actually a free radical, is less so [15], although it can be rapidly converted to the more damaging free radical, superoxide (O_2^-). In association with increased nitric oxide (NO$\cdot$) levels, a major source of RNS, O_2^- can form other reactive species, including peroxynitrite (ONOO$^-$). Both ROS and RNS can damage essential cell elements, such as proteins, lipids and nucleic acids [16 - 18], with such increased levels of oxidative and nitrosative stress (O&NS) contributing

contributing to further ROS and RNS production [19].

An extensive array of data, centrally and systemically, shows protein nitrosylation and lipid peroxidation to be increased in AD [20 - 22]. Due to this clear link between oxidative stress and AD, recent studies are attempting to establish reliable O&NS biomarkers to help in the early AD diagnosis [23]. 4-hydroxy-nonenal (HNE) is a product, and widely used indicant of lipid peroxidation. This oxidative stress biomarker is produced in the brain by the peroxidation of arachidonic acid and is highly reactive. HNE is increased in AD brains, including the early stages [24, 25]. Other indicants of O&NS, in both the early and late AD stages, include protein carbonyls and protein nitration [26, 27]. Such raised levels of ROS and RNS are often accompanied with a decrease in antioxidant defenses in AD, leading to an increase in the total oxidative capacity [28].

It should be noted that increased O&NS is linked to a wide array of other pathophysiological changes in AD, including DNA damage, leading to the induction of the DNA repair response system, including poly (ADP-ribose) polymerase-1 (PARP1), which requires nicotinamide (NAD$^+$). By reducing NAD$^+$ levels, PARP1 upregulation decreases the induction of sirtuins. This may be relevant in AD, as sirtuin-1, known as the longevity protein, is an important regulator of peroxisome proliferator-activated receptor gamma coactivator 1-alpha (PGC-1α), known as the master mitochondria regulator.

RNA is more susceptible to oxidative insults since is a single-stranded structure and is not protected by specific proteins such histones for DNA. Even though oxidative damage in RNA is less lethal than mutations in the DNA, it is involved in degeneration especially associated with aging. This corroborates the fact that oxidative RNA damage is present in the common neurodegenerative diseases such as AD. Oxidative damage occurs on in protein-coding RNAs and in non-coding RNAs, which will disrupt the regulation of gene expression and modified proteins. Studies showed that oxidative RNA damage is present in early-stage of neurodegenerative disorders suggesting that oxidative RNA damage is relevant to the onset and/or development of AD [29].

Increased O&NS may also be linked to an array of other protein changes and pathophysiological processes that are known to be altered in AD. This also includes increased levels of autoimmune responses that can arise from the lipid peroxidation driving the creation of neo-epitopes, because of the immune system not recognising the new amino acid patterns from inside the newly exposed inner leaf of the lipid bilayer membrane. As such, O&NS is an important link to many of the pathophysiological processes associated with AD.

CAUSES OF OXIDATIVE STRESS DURING AD

Loss of Antioxidant Defenses

Under normal circumstances, RNS and ROS can be kept at physiological concentrations by endogenous and dietary antioxidants, such as glutathione (GSH), as well as the antioxidant enzymes, including glutaredoxins, catalase, thioredoxins, glutathione peroxidase (GPx), glutathione reductase (GR) and superoxide dismutase (SOD). These antioxidant systems are located in various subcellular compartments and are frequently complementary [15]. However, in neurodegenerative processes, these antioxidant systems can be insufficient in controlling the increased ROS production [30], which, as can occur in AD, may arise from their downregulation or loss of function, resulting in a pro-oxidative state [28, 31].

GSH is highly and ubiquitously expressed. Increased H_2O_2 leads to the induction of GPx, which reduces H_2O_2 by oxidizing GSH into glutathione disulphide (GSSG), allowing the GSH/GSSG ratio to be a good marker for oxidative challenge [32]. In AD erythrocytes, this ratio is lowered, likely as a consequence of increased GPx activity [33], although mixed results are also evident [34]. The activity of SOD1 has also been found to be lower in frontal lobes of AD patients [35], suggesting that regional variations in central antioxidant enzyme activity may be relevant in AD. Accordingly, when compared to healthy controls, circulating SOD and GPx activities were lower not only in AD patients, but also in individuals with mild cognitive impairment, a prodromal stage of AD, supporting the notion that oxidative stress is an early sign of AD progression [36, 37].

As indicated above, such increases in O&NS may drive an array of the pathophysiological processes evident in AD, including processes that are relevant to mitochondria regulation, in turn contributing as to how antioxidant dysregulation can lead to neuronal apoptosis [15, 18].

Mitochondria Dysfunction

Due to the activity of the electron transport chain in its inner membrane during oxidative phosphorylation-driven energy production in the form of adenosine triphosphate (ATP), mitochondria become a major source of ROS generation. A significant percentage of cellular H_2O_2 arises from mitochondria, which can be rapidly be converted to O_2^-, due, in part, to the leakage of electrons during energy production [38, 39].

Oxidative damage also has a high impact in proteins that are involved in mitochondria ATP production and glycolysis, because this impairment in metabolism leads to even more ROS production. The consequent lower levels of ATP can cause increased mitochondria activity resulting in higher ROS production and electron leakage, creating a positive feedback loop of oxidative stress and damage [18]. Such suboptimal mitochondrial functioning and consequent increased ROS and decreased ATP production, have been proposed as critical to the pathogenesis of AD [40].

Mitochondria dysfunction is present in the early stages and course of AD [41]. Many parameters of mitochondria functioning are altered, including energy metabolism and calcium homeostasis, as well as the expression of proteins and mitochondrial DNA [14, 42, 43]. Glucose metabolism correlates with cognition and wider functioning in AD, as well as being a measurement that allows for the monitoring of disease development [44]. In addition, the energy metabolism genes, such as the subunits of the mitochondrial electron transport chain, have also been shown to be decreased in the AD posterior cingulate cortex, a region affected in the early stages of AD [45].

The low glucose metabolism in the AD brain is also related to the decrease of important enzymes in the mitochondrial electron transport chain, such as pyruvate dehydrogenase, alpha-ketoglutarate dehydrogenase complex and cytochrome oxidase. There is a correlation between the decrease of the activity of these proteins and the clinical presentation, as well as the amount of Aβ plaques [46].

AD brains also show higher levels of mitochondrial DNA (mtDNA) oxidation, *versus* age-matched controls, in association with higher mutation levels [47, 48]. mtDNA are more vulnerable to oxidative damage [49] because of their proximity to sites of ROS generation, coupled to the lack of protective histone proteins in mtDNA. Such mutations affect not only mitochondrial functioning, but also the number of mitochondria [14]. Mitochondria numbers are lower in AD brains, *versus* age-matched controls, with higher levels of mitochondrial DNA and proteins evident in the cytoplasm [50]. Interestingly, the mitochondrial size is also increased in AD brain, due to the impairment in fusion and fission dynamics by the abnormal expression of proteins involved in these processes [51].

Dihydrosphingosine phosphate lyase (DPL1) is a protein mostly expressed in the cytoplasm, being recruited to mitochondria during the process of fission. DPL1 is increased in AD and may also be relevant to wider aspects of AD pathophysiology, as it can also interact with Aβ and phosphorylated tau. Excessive fission may also increase O&NS in AD brain [52].

Calcium is an important cell signalling second messenger, which, when dysregulated, can make neurons more vulnerable to neurodegeneration, including AD-associated processes [53]. ROS resulted from mitochondria damage can also alter calcium homeostasis, leading to an inability of the endoplasmic reticulum to adequately buffer calcium. This can be significantly detrimental to cell signaling and survival [54]. In fact, calcium related-enzymes are increased in AD patients [55].

It should be emphasized that mitochondria are an important target in apoptosis, with ROS able to activate the caspases, which, in turn, induce pro-apoptotic proteins, such as Bax, to translocate to the mitochondrial membrane, thereby inducing the formation of the mitochondrial membrane permeability transition pore, resulting in the release of cytochrome c [56]. Although there is still some controversy as to the role of these processes in AD, caspase 3 is relevant to neurofibrillary tangle formation [57].

Amyloid Beta (Aβ) Peptide

Other possible sources of oxidative stress include the Aβ peptide, which can induce augmented production of ROS and mitochondrial impairment, consequently aggravating the pro-oxidative status [41, 58]. It has been observed that brain regions that have a higher expression of Aβ present more protein oxidation and lipid peroxidation in comparison to cerebellum, considered an Aβ-poor region [59]. In amyloid plaques, the majority of Aβ contains a sulfoxide modification of methionine, indicating lipid peroxidation as one of the first stages of neurodegeneration [60]. Furthermore, when inserted into lipid bilayer membranes, Aβ can induce oxidative stress that results in lipid peroxidation, leading to nucleic acid and protein damage [58, 61]. Proteins are highly vulnerable to oxidative damage, which results in the irreversible modification of structure and shape. These alterations include unfolding, aggregation and detachment of subunits, which ultimately results in the loss of function [62].

In both AD patients and transgenic mice, Aβ was shown to interact with a mitochondrial enzyme, Aβ-binding alcohol dehydrogenase (ABAD) [63], causing mitochondrial dysfunction, increased ROS production and eventually apoptosis [64]. Apoptosis is the main type of cell death during AD progression, which, as indicated above, is linked to increased O&NS, as seen in AD models [65]. The treatment of AD fibroblasts with Aβ peptide results in the oxidation of the anti-apoptotic proteins vimentin and heat shock protein 60 (HSP60). Likewise, it was shown that neuroblastoma cells treated with Aβ (1-42) show evidence of increased oxidation of the anti-apoptotic proteins glutaredoxin-1 (GRX-1) and thioredoxin-1 (TRX-1) [66]. Moreover, higher levels of the pro-apoptotic protein, p53, and its oxidized form, have been detected in the AD brain [67], which ultimately contributes to increased apoptosis [68]. Overall, the induction of Aβ will contribute to the increased oxidant status in AD.

Glutamatergic Signalling Dysfunction

Glial pathology and neurotransmitter system dysfunction contribute to the pathophysiology of an array of central nervous system (CNS) diseases [69, 70]. Astrocytes play numerous and complex roles, including regulating synaptic transmission, nutrient supply to neurons, controlling vasodilation and regulating blood-brain barrier permeability, as well as producing responses to injury and immune defense [71 - 73]. Recent works indicate that the glutamatergic system is a potential target for treatment of a variety of neuropsychiatric diseases [69, 74 - 78]. Glutamate is the major excitatory neurotransmitter in the mammalian CNS and is an important driver of brain plasticity processes [79 - 82]. However, excess glutamate contributes to numerous acute and chronic brain pathologies, including neurodegenerative diseases, brain trauma, seizures, and cerebral ischemic injury [83 - 86].

Glutamate exerts its excitatory function by activating the ionotropic, N-methyl-D-Aspartate receptor (NMDAR), α-amino-3-hydroxy-5-methyl-4-isoxazole-propionic acid (AMPA) receptor and kainate receptor, as well as the metabotropic (coupled to G proteins) glutamate receptors [87]. Astrocytes play an essential role in glutamate recycling. Glutamate uptake is predominantly *via* astrocytes [73], with glutamine synthetase (GS), which convert glutamate to glutamine, being an exclusively astrocytic enzyme [88, 89].

Astrocytes play an important role during excitatory synaptic activity since they promote a fine regulation of the glutamate extracellular levels at nanomolar concentrations, which are dependent on the electrochemical gradient generated by Na,K-ATPase [90 - 92]. Astrocytes uptake glutamate *via* glutamate aspartate transporter (GLAST or EAAT1) and glutamate transporter 1 (GLT-1 or EAAT2). EAAT1 and EAAT2 are the most important and predominant kind of glutamate transporters in astrocytes [93 - 95] and were found to be impaired in AD [96]. Therefore, changes in the Na,K-ATPase ionic and electrochemical gradient, such as those arising from mutations in the ATP1A2 gene, is closely related to astrocyte modulation of glutamatergic activity [97, 98].

The control of glutamate is essential for life, because low levels of this neurotransmitter compromise the neuronal cell survival while its excess leads to excitotoxicity. The excitotoxicity is a result of the increase of intracellular calcium mostly by the increased NMDAR activity that at pathological level leads to impairment of synaptic function and neuronal cell death. Calcium has an important interplay with ROS and this pathological calcium increasing leads to an increase in ROS [99, 100]. One pathway involved in this process is the increase in neuronal nitric oxide synthase (nNOS) that creates O&NS. In AD, the glutamate availability and the NMDAR function are impaired, which leads to more oxidative stress and consequently more neuronal damage and cell death [101].

Corroborating these notions, studies have demonstrated that AD is in fact associated with astrocytes dysfunction due to the abnormal Aβ production, resulting in the dysregulation of astrocyte-dependent processes, including glutamate transport, Aβ clearance and energy metabolism, which ultimately can intensify oxidative stress, as observed in Fig. (**1**) [102].

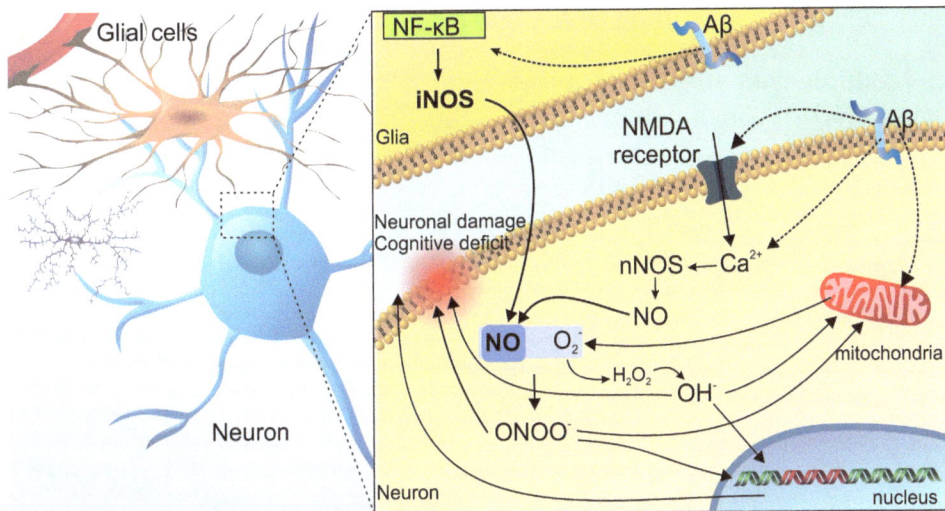

Fig. (1). Illustration of an oxidative stress scenario in Alzheimer's disease brain. Amyloid-β (Aβ) can cause mitochondrial damage, which in turn can release a large amount of superoxide anion (O_2^-) which in combination with nitric oxide (NO) produces peroxynitrite anion ($ONOO^-$), leading to DNA, protein and lipid, as well as mitochondrial damage, thereby contributing to neurodegenerative processes. NO can come from activation of nNOS following glutamatergic receptor activation and/or from iNOS activated by the transcription factor NF-κB. The glutamate (Glu) uptake is impaired and there is an increase in Glu amount in the synaptic cleft. Metals like zinc (Zn), copper (Cu) and iron (Fe) can also interact with Aβ and promote ROS production. Abbreviations: Amyloid-β (Aβ), calcium (Ca^{2+}) copper (Cu), cyclic GMP (cGMP), glutamate (Glu), hydrogen peroxide (H_2O_2), hydroxyl anion (OH^-), inducible nitric oxide synthase (iNOS), iron (Fe), N-Methyl-D-Aspartate (NMDA), neuronal nitric oxide synthase (nNOS), nitric oxide (NO), peroxynitrite anion ($ONOO^-$), protein kinase dependent of cGMP (PKG), superoxide anion (O_2^-), superoxide dismutase (SOD), zinc (Zn).

Neuroinflammation

Aging is associated with an increased susceptibility to almost all medical conditions, including a number of neurodegenerative disorders, such as AD. Aging is generally considered to be a multifactorial process, involving an array of inter-system interactions, including of the immune system and the CNS, with alterations in sirtuins and mitochondrial functioning changing the nature of such interactions [103, 104]. As such, immune inflammatory activity is intimately linked to neurodegenerative processes, including in AD [105]. Chronic inflammation is increased in aging and neurodegenerative conditions, which is widely believed to increase central inflammatory processes, including microglia activation and inflammatory cytokines, like interleukin-1β (IL-1β) and tumor necrosis factor-α (TNF-α) as well as intercellular adhesion molecule 1 in microglia and neurons [103, 105]. Such increases in microglia TNF-α can induce the β-secretase, BACE1, leading to the synthesis of Aβ [106]. As such, microglia activation can contribute to some of the classical pathophysiological changes in the AD brain. Microglia activation has also been associated with glutamate release, which in turn can activate NMDA receptors leading to NO synthesis.

NO is produced from its precursor L-arginine. This production is regulated by NO synthases (NOS), which requires O_2^- and NADPH as co-substrates, with citrulline generated as a co-product. There are three isoforms of NOS which are encoded by distinct genes. NOS-3 and NOS-1 were first identified in endothelial cells and neurons, respectively, and therefore often referred to as eNOS and nNOS. Those two isoforms are expressed constitutively and once stimulated by agonists increase intracellular calcium. However, the other isoform, NOS-2, is transcriptionally regulated, and does not depend on calcium for its activity [107]. NO reacts with the superoxide anion to form peroxynitrite anion (ONOO⁻), a free radical that can lead to the production of the highly reactive hydroxyl radical (OH•), a significant contributor to cell death. NO produced by Ca^{2+}-calmoduli--dependent activation of nNOS can also activate soluble guanylyl cyclase (sGC), by the synthesis of cyclic guanosine monophosphate (cGMP), which acts as a second messenger [108], indicating that NO is significant regulator of wider intracellular pathways.

Aβ peptide and a systemic inflammatory reaction increase glutamate release in synaptic cleft and activate NMDA receptors, leading to nuclear factor kappa-light-chain-enhancer of activated B cells (NF-κB)-induced NOS expression [109 - 111]. Glutamate and NMDA can activate NF-κB in primary neuronal cultures [112, 113]. NF-κB is a transcription factor that is present in many cell types, including microglia, astrocytes, immune cells and neurons [114]. NF-κB can modulate hundreds of genes, including many that are associated with inflammatory responses, such as pro-inflammatory cytokines (*e.g.* IL-1β and TNFα) as well as inducible NOS. This transcription factor is therefore a key regulator of brain inflammatory processes, and thereby a modulator of the development and course of neurodegenerative processes [115 - 117].

Na,K-ATPase activity can also be modulated by glutamate, *via* NMDA receptor activation and NO production, which leads to cyclic GMP-PKG activation [118, 119]. Alterations on the cyclic GMP–PKG pathway are linked to the decline in α2/3-Na,K-ATPase activity in the CNS, which is related to aging [120]. The decrease in cyclic GMP levels is related to the aging process and connected to the rise in NOS activity and oxidative stress in the CNS as well as in rodent and human platelets and erythrocytes [121], which can be related to neurodegenerative processes [122].

Metals-induced Oxidative Stress

O&NS in AD can also be triggered by the presence of metals, such as copper and iron [65, 123]. These metals are capable of ROS production catalysis regardless of the binding state. They can be reduced by reducing agents such as ascorbate and glutathione and also react with peroxides and form superoxide and hydroxyl radicals. However, they are present in antioxidant enzymes like cooper in SOD1 and iron in catalase [9]. Levels of copper, iron and zinc are altered in some brain regions in AD [124], although not in the brain as a whole [125]. Plasma zinc levels are decreased over the course of aging, even more so in AD patients [126]. Interestingly, the brain is an organ with a high concentration of these metals, primarily due to their need during metabolism and enzymatic activity [127]. Aβ can also bind to metals such as copper, zinc and iron, which can promote Aβ oligomer formation and can also increase the ROS production [128, 129]. There is also an interaction between copper and amyloid precursor protein (APP) [130, 131], with copper able to control APP expression and its trafficking within the cell [132, 133]. APP can also control the levels of copper, suggesting reciprocated interactions in the course of AD [134]. Iron also acts to regulate APP [135, 136].

Copper and iron also have a redox potential by Fenton's and Haber-Weiss reactions, with iron interacting with hydrogen peroxide to produce ROS [113]. In contrast, zinc is inert, but its levels must be maintained as it plays an essential role in the folding and maintenance of protein structure. The zinc transporter, ZnT3, is decreased over the course of aging, contributing to memory and learning impairments [137]. It seems that treatment with zinc can contribute to normal copper levels, which are also impaired in AD [138]. As such, alterations in metals, including over the course of aging, can contribute to the suspected pathophysiology of AD.

Although the neurotoxic role of aluminium in AD is controversial, aluminium chloride does facilitate lipid peroxidation by iron, leading to a Fenton's reaction dysregulation, which increases ROS and decreases antioxidant enzyme levels and activities [139].

The levels of metals can be controlled by metallothioneins (MT), which are small proteins rich in cysteine that can bind to metals and can buffer high metal concentrations by sequestration [140]. Of the different MT isoforms, MT1 and MT2 are elevated in AD, likely due to raised metals levels [141]. MT3 is highly expressed in the brain, and can interact with the Aβ-copper complex, with MT3 being decreased in the AD brain [142]. Furthermore, recent studies showed that chelators, which can also bind to metals, result in decreased Aβ toxicity and oxidative stress *in vitro,* suggesting that chelation therapy may possibly be a novel therapeutic intervention for AD in the future [143, 144].

ANTIOXIDANT THERAPIES IN ALZHEIMER'S DISEASE

Given the important role played by O&NS in AD, many clinical trials have evaluated the efficacy of antioxidant therapies in AD, with mixed results. In this section, such antioxidant therapies in AD patients are reviewed.

Most studies indicate the relevance of a healthy lifestyle to diseases prevention across a host of medical conditions, especially aging-associated chronic disorders, such as cancer and neurodegenerative diseases. More specifically, the consumption of vegetables and fruits, which can contain appreciable amounts of antioxidants, can be neuroprotective [145]. A wide array of different antioxidants have been used in the management of AD, mostly in AD transgenic animal models, including: vitamin (vit)E, vitC, carotenoids, lipoic acid, coenzyme Q10, melatonin, estrogen, glutathione, N-acetylcysteine and polyphenols, as well as phytochemicals, such as *Ginkgo biloba*, berberine, palmatine, curcumin, caffeine and omega-3 polyunsaturated fatty acid [146]. Here we focus on vitamins, polyphenols and natural products, as they have been more extensively studied. Their main effects are summarized in Fig. (**2**).

Vitamins

Tocopherol, together with tocotrienol and tocomonoenol, are vitE species. Tocopherol in turn can be divided into α-, β-, γ- and δ-tocopherol. Sunflower and olive oils are typical sources of α-tocopherol, with γ-tocopherol being more highly present in corn and soybean oils [147]. As such, dietary factors can significantly influence not only the level, but also species of vitE.

VitE is a good source of antioxidants. However, it has been suggested that more investigation is needed, especially regarding its long-term effects, before its utilization in AD. For example, an *in vitro* study showed that tocopherols can increase Aβ production and decrease Aβ degradation by insulin degrading enzyme (IDE), and it seems that other Aβ-degrading enzymes could be affected by tocopherols [147]. These effects require further investigation, especially *in vivo* studies, across a host of physiological processes thought to be relevant in AD.

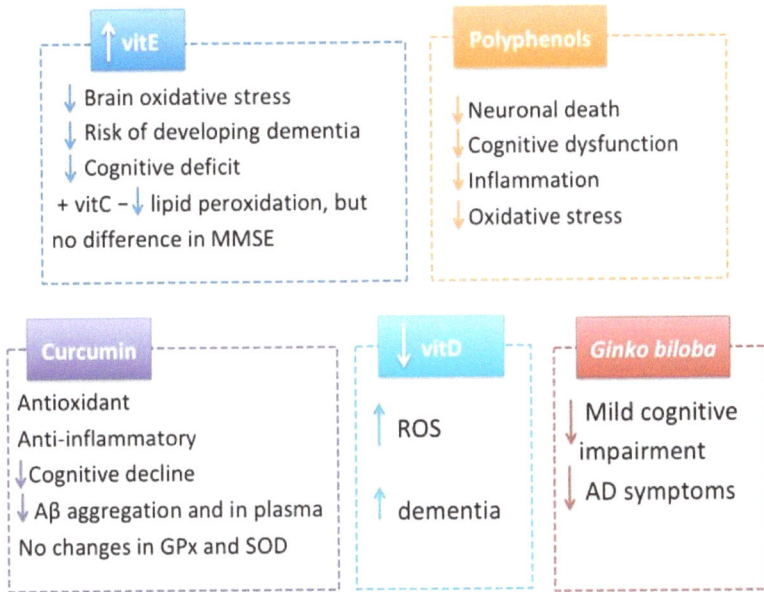

Fig. (2). Important antioxidants studied so far that could be used in therapeutic strategies for Alzheimer's disease treatment. Most of them decrease the cognitive deficit and the risk of developing dementia. Polyphenols and curcumin have also an anti-inflammatory property. Curcumin also decreases Amyloid-β (Aβ) aggregation and the plasma levels of Aβ. Abbreviations: Alzheimer's disease (AD), Amyloid-β (Aβ), glutathione peroxidase (GPx), Mini-Mental State Examination (MMSE), reactive oxygen species (ROS), superoxide dismutase (SOD), vitamin C (vitC), vitamin D (vitD).

In *in vivo* study, it has been shown that vitE reduces Aβ formation only when vitE is given to the young AD transgenic mice, or else before the deposition of Aβ-plaques. VitE administration to old animals was not able to reduce Aβ levels, although in both age groups, vitE decreased brain oxidative stress status, suggesting the importance of the temporal initiation of vitE administration, being earlier, seems better [148]. Human studies indicate that high vitE plasma concentrations can reduce the risk of developing dementia, including AD, over the course of aging [149, 150]. When all 8 vitE species were added to the diet of people aged 65 years old or plus, a slower rate of cognitive deficit was observed, including a reduced risk of AD developing [151].

Conversely, the supplementation with vitE (400 I.U./day) or selenium (200 µg/day), used alone or in combination, was not able to prevent dementia in elderly men [152]. Another study assessed the effects of vitE (400 I.U./day) and vitC (1,000 mg/day) supplementation in AD patients. Results showed that, after one year of treatment, although there was a reduction in lipid peroxidation measured in the cerebrospinal fluid (CSF), there was no difference in the clinical course of the disease, as indicated by the Mini-Mental State Examination (MMSE) score to test cognitive function [153]. A clinical, double blind, placebo-controlled trial evaluated AD treatment with α-tocopherol (800 I.U./day), vitamin C (500 mg/day), α-lipoic acid (900 mg/day) and coenzyme Q (1200 mg/day) for 16 weeks. This study also reported a reduction in CSF lipid peroxidation levels, although there was no alteration in Aβ42, tau and hyperphosphorylated-tau levels. Unexpectedly, MMSE score showed faster cognitive decline for patients receiving the antioxidant therapy, when compared to the placebo treated group [154]. Generally, most studies investigating vitE effects indicate a positive effect regarding neuroprotection against cognitive decline, but only when the vitE is diet derived and not when given a synthetic supplementation, perhaps as a consequence of an increased mixture of more vitE species when diet derived [155, 156]. However, a recent study in humans showed that γ-tocopherol and not α-tocopherol was associated with lower Aβ deposit and less damage from neurofibrillary tangles [157]. Overall, there are some mixed results as to the benefits that can be derived from vitE in AD, with dietary vitE being more beneficial than supplementation.

Vitamin D (vitD) also has an important role in the control of ROS levels, because it activates Nrf2 that increases the cellular antioxidants which could help to decrease abnormal ROS levels [158]. Low concentrations of vitD in humans might also contribute to the development of dementia [159]. In fact, a recent study has shown that patients with mild cognitive impairment and AD had lower serum concentration of vitD when compared to healthy subjects. The results support the adoption of serum vitD levels as an AD biomarker and the use of this vitamin to supplement AD patients [160].

Polyphenols and Natural Compounds

Polyphenols are abundant in a range of foods, being defined by the presence of different types of compounds containing phenol rings. Flavonoids, one of the largest polyphenolic groups, are often present in human foods. Flavonoids are divided into the following subtypes: flavanols (epicatechin, present in green tea), flavonols (quercetin, present in *Ginkgo biloba*), anthocyanins (cyaniding, present in colorful fruits), flavones (tangeritin, present in tangerine), isoflavones (genistein, present in soybean) and flavanones (hesperidin, found in citrus fruits) [161, 162]. Flavonoids can also act as phytoestrogens, having estrogenic activities [163]. Red wine is an example of a mix of different classes of polyphenolic compounds, with red wine shown to have antioxidant activity *in vitro* [164 - 166]. White wine polyphenols have also been shown to promote beneficial effects against oxidative stress and AD neuropathology in mice model [167].

Polyphenols, in general, protect the brain from neuronal death [168] and cognitive dysfunction induced by Aβ deposition as evidenced in AD animal models [169 - 171], with some of this beneficial effect suggested to arise from its antioxidant capacity *per se*, or from distally connected neuroprotective signaling pathways, such as AMP-activated protein kinase and sirtuin-1 [172 - 174].

Emerging *in vivo* and *in vitro* studies have shown that the polyphenol resveratrol, mostly present in grapes and red wine, is effective in counteracting oxidative stress and inflammation induced by Aβ. This compound was also shown to decrease Aβ production and aggregation and increase its clearance, suggesting that it might be beneficial for AD patients [175]. In fact, a recent clinical trial with 119 AD subjects showed that resveratrol treatment (up to 2 g daily, for 1 year) promoted anti-inflammatory effects, mitigated Aβ levels reduction in plasma and CSF (a sign of AD progression) and counteracted cognitive and functional decline, measured by MMSE and activities of daily living (ADL) scores, respectively [176].

Another polyphenolic flavonoid named anthocyanins, which can be found in vegetables, fruits and flowers, also has an antioxidant effect in streptozotocin (STZ) model. This model induces sporadic dementia of Alzheimer's type (SDAT) that can improve behavioral and in biochemical alterations by anthocyanins [177].

Curcumin, a naturally occurring biphenolic compound derived from tumeric (*Curcuma longa* plant), has antioxidant and anti-inflammatory properties, in turn, counteracting cognitive decline and preventing Aβ aggregation [178 - 180]. Studies in a transgenic murine AD model showed promising results with Begum *et al.* [181] showing that curcumin decreases oxidative stress and Aβ plaque deposition in these transgenic mice. Furthermore, mice fed with this compound for 1 month presented improved performance in behavioral tests to evaluate cognition [182].

These findings encouraged tests with curcumin in clinical trials, which did not show a positive effect. In a double-blind, randomized, placebo-controlled clinical trial, AD patients were supplemented with 1 or 4 g of daily curcumin for 6 months. There were no changes in circulating levels of Aβ (1-40) and F2-isoprostane, or in cognition (measured by the MMSE score). However, biomarkers were measured only in blood, which may not necessarily be correlated to CSF levels [183].

Another double-blind, randomized clinical trial done in mild to moderate AD patients treated with 2 or 4 g of a curcuminoid mixture for 24 weeks, also measured CSF biomarkers, again finding no significant difference in comparison to placebo for levels of Aβ (1-40 and 1-42), F2-isoprostanes, tau, hyper-phosphorylated-tau, and cognition. Furthermore, the study reported low bioavailability of this compound [184]. Interestingly, curcumin in its lipidated form tested in middle-aged people (80 mg/day, four weeks) resulted in increased antioxidant markers in saliva and catalase activity in the plasma, although no changes were found in GPx and SOD activities. Furthermore, there was a significant decrease in plasma Aβ (1-40) levels. In conclusion, the study suggested a better bioavailability of curcumin in its lipidated form [185]. Overall, the promise of curcumin in the modulation of AD has not been fulfilled, although more extensive investigation of methods to increase its bioavailability, especially centrally, is required.

Ginkgo biloba is a herbal preparation and EGb761 is its most used extract in randomized clinical trials, composed from 24% ginkgo flavonoids and 6% terpenoids [186]. Studies using AD animal models have been shown anti-inflammatory effects of *Ginkgo biloba* extract EGb 761, coupled to an amelioration of cognitive deficits [187, 188].

Recently, two meta-analyses investigated the use of *Ginkgo biloba* in clinical trials with AD patients. In one study, the systematic review concluded that *Ginkgo biloba* extract EGb761 seems to be safe and moderately effective in the treatment of AD patients with moderate psychological symptoms [189]. Another meta-analysis investigated the utility of *Ginkgo biloba* to treat mild cognitive impairment (MCI) and AD, concluding that although this phytochemical seems to be beneficial in improving cognitive dysfunction in MCI and AD, further research is necessary as to its safety and efficacy in humans [190]. A randomized clinical trial with more than 300 elderly people with intact cognition or a mild deficit indicated that *Ginkgo biloba* extracts could not be recommended for the prevention of dementia [191].

CONCLUDING REMARKS

Oxidative stress is a result of the abnormal increase in ROS and is one of the main mechanisms involved in AD. The oxidative stress can be a result of the impairment of many different systems such as mitochondria dysfunction, Aβ overproduction and decrease in Aβ degradation, loss of antioxidant defences, glutamatergic signaling dysfunction, neuroinflammation and altered levels of metals. Despite the potential involvement of oxidative stress in AD, the treatment of the disease using antioxidants is still controversial according to the clinical trials performed so far. Table **1** and Fig. (**3**) summarize the main conclusions of the chapter.

Table 1. Summary table of major conclusions.

Section	Major Conclusions
AD and oxidative stress	- Oxidative stress occurs due to an imbalance between free radicals' production and the body's antioxidant defenses. - The brain is highly susceptible to oxidative damage mainly due to its high energy demand. - During aging, there is an increase in oxidative stress levels and reduction of antioxidant defenses. - There is a clear link between AD and oxidative stress, which ultimately results in cell death.
Causes of oxidative stress during AD	- AD is associated with loss of antioxidant defenses (*e.g.*, reduced antioxidant enzymes activities), which aggravate oxidative stress. - Mitochondria are a major source of ROS and their dysfunction accounts for increased oxidative stress in AD. - Aβ can also exacerbate AD-related pro-oxidative status directly (*e.g.*, inducing lipid peroxidation when inserted into membranes) or indirectly (*e.g.*, promoting mitochondria dysfunction). - In AD, there is an increase of glutamatergic signaling and decrease in glutamate clearance due to astrocyte dysfunction, resulting in excitotoxicity and free radicals' production. - Metals, like copper, zinc and iron, can also generate free radicals, contributing to AD pathogenesis.
Antioxidant therapies in AD	- Due to the key role played by oxidative stress in AD pathogenesis, many antioxidant therapies were tested but no clear beneficial effect was proved. - Supplementation with vitamins (especially vitE and vitD) seems to be beneficial against AD, but mixed results indicate that further studies are necessary. - Polyphenolic compounds (especially resveratrol, *Ginkgo biloba* and curcumin) were shown to have strong antioxidant properties and exert promising positive effects in AD, preventing cognitive impairment and Aβ toxicity.

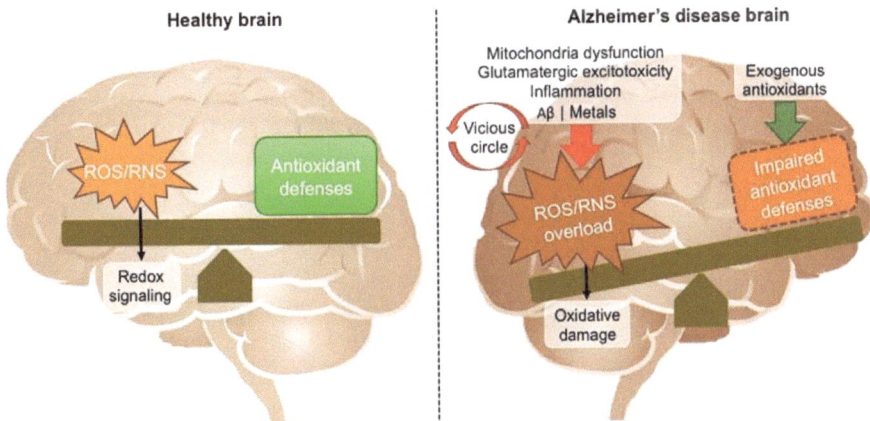

Fig. (3). Comparison of oxidative stress status in healthy brain and Alzheimer's disease brain. In healthy brain, free radicals are kept under physiological levels by antioxidant defenses, being important for cellular redox signaling. On the other hand, Alzheimer's disease brain presents excessive amounts of ROS and RNS and dysfunctional antioxidant defenses, resulting in oxidative damage and neuronal cell death. Free radicals' levels are exacerbated by many factors, including: (1) mitochondria dysfunction, (2) glutamate-induced excitotoxicity, (2) increased inflammation, (3) elevated levels of Aβ aggregates and (4) impaired metal ion homeostasis. All these factors are exacerbated by and contribute to oxidative stress, resulting in a vicious circle. Hence, oxidative stress is closely linked to AD neuropathology and disease progression. Abbreviations: Amyloid-β (Aβ), glutathione reactive oxygen species (ROS), reactive nitrogen species (RNS).

CONSENT FOR PUBLICATION

Not applicable.

CONFLICT OF INTEREST

The authors declare that they have no competing interests.

ACKNOWLEDGEMENTS

We thank George Anderson, CRC Scotland & London for English Editing. C.S. was supported by grants from São Paulo Research Foundation (FAPESP #2014/05026-0), Conselho Nacional de Desenvolvimento Científico e Tecnológico (CNPq #2011/04327-9), and Neuroscience Research Support Centers (NAPNA). From FAPESP, P.F.K. was supported by grant #2014/01435-3, A.R.V was supported by grant #2011/12255-8, and E.M.K. was supported by young investigator grant #2011/21308-8.

REFERENCES

[1]   Katzman R, Saitoh T. Advances in Alzheimer's disease. FASEB J 1991; 5(3): 278-86.
       [http://dx.doi.org/10.1096/fasebj.5.3.2001787] [PMID: 2001787]

[2]   Braak H, Braak E. Morphological criteria for the recognition of Alzheimer's disease and the distribution pattern of cortical changes related to this disorder. Neurobiol Aging 1994; 15(3): 355-6.
       [http://dx.doi.org/10.1016/0197-4580(94)90032-9] [PMID: 7936061]

[3]   Trovato A, Siracusa R, Di Paola R, *et al.* Redox modulation of cellular stress response and lipoxin A4 expression by Hericium Erinaceus in rat brain: relevance to Alzheimer's disease pathogenesis. Immun Ageing 2016; 13: 23.
       [http://dx.doi.org/10.1186/s12979-016-0078-8] [PMID: 27398086]

[4]   Selkoe DJ. Alzheimer's disease: a central role for amyloid. J Neuropathol Exp Neurol 1994; 53(5): 438-47.
       [http://dx.doi.org/10.1097/00005072-199409000-00003] [PMID: 8083687]

[5]   Arriagada PV, Growdon JH, Hedley-Whyte ET, Hyman BT. Neurofibrillary tangles but not senile plaques parallel duration and severity of Alzheimer's disease. Neurology 1992; 42(3 Pt 1): 631-9.
       [http://dx.doi.org/10.1212/WNL.42.3.631] [PMID: 1549228]

[6]   Smith MA, Rottkamp CA, Nunomura A, Raina AK, Perry G. Oxidative stress in Alzheimer's disease. Biochim Biophys Acta 2000; 1502(1): 139-44.
       [http://dx.doi.org/10.1016/S0925-4439(00)00040-5] [PMID: 10899439]

[7]   Migliore L, Fontana I, Trippi F, *et al.* Oxidative DNA damage in peripheral leukocytes of mild cognitive impairment and AD patients. Neurobiol Aging 2005; 26(5): 567-73.

[http://dx.doi.org/10.1016/j.neurobiolaging.2004.07.016] [PMID: 15708428]

[8]   Guidi I, Galimberti D, Lonati S, *et al.* Oxidative imbalance in patients with mild cognitive impairment and Alzheimer's disease. Neurobiol Aging 2006; 27(2): 262-9.
[http://dx.doi.org/10.1016/j.neurobiolaging.2005.01.001] [PMID: 16399211]

[9]   Halliwell B. Oxidative stress and neurodegeneration: where are we now? J Neurochem 2006; 97(6): 1634-58.
[http://dx.doi.org/10.1111/j.1471-4159.2006.03907.x] [PMID: 16805774]

[10]   Cheignon C, Tomas M, Bonnefont-Rousselot D, Faller P, Hureau C, Collin F. Oxidative stress and the amyloid beta peptide in Alzheimer's disease. Redox Biol 2018; 14: 450-64.
[http://dx.doi.org/10.1016/j.redox.2017.10.014] [PMID: 29080524]

[11]   Schieber M, Chandel NS. ROS function in redox signaling and oxidative stress. Curr Biol 2014; 24(1 0): R453-62.
[http://dx.doi.org/10.1016/j.cub.2014.03.034] [PMID: 24845678]

[12]   Ahmad W, Ijaz B, Shabbiri K, Ahmed F, Rehman S. Oxidative toxicity in diabetes and Alzheimer's disease: mechanisms behind ROS/ RNS generation. J Biomed Sci 2017; 24(1): 76.
[http://dx.doi.org/10.1186/s12929-017-0379-z] [PMID: 28927401]

[13]   Uttara B, Singh AV, Zamboni P, Mahajan RT. Oxidative stress and neurodegenerative diseases: a review of upstream and downstream antioxidant therapeutic options. Curr Neuropharmacol 2009; 7(1): 65-74.
[http://dx.doi.org/10.2174/157015909787602823] [PMID: 19721819]

[14]   Wang X, Wang W, Li L, Perry G, Lee HG, Zhu X. Oxidative stress and mitochondrial dysfunction in Alzheimer's disease. Biochim Biophys Acta 2014; 1842(8): 1240-7.
[http://dx.doi.org/10.1016/j.bbadis.2013.10.015] [PMID: 24189435]

[15]   Dai DF, Chiao YA, Marcinek DJ, Szeto HH, Rabinovitch PS. Mitochondrial oxidative stress in aging and healthspan. Longev Healthspan 2014; 3: 6.
[http://dx.doi.org/10.1186/2046-2395-3-6] [PMID: 24860647]

[16]   Mecocci P, MacGarvey U, Beal MF. Oxidative damage to mitochondrial DNA is increased in Alzheimer's disease. Ann Neurol 1994; 36(5): 747-51.
[http://dx.doi.org/10.1002/ana.410360510] [PMID: 7979220]

[17]   Butterfield DA, Bader Lange ML, Sultana R. Involvements of the lipid peroxidation product, HNE, in the pathogenesis and progression of Alzheimer's disease. Biochim Biophys Acta 2010; 1801(8): 924--.
[http://dx.doi.org/10.1016/j.bbalip.2010.02.005] [PMID: 20176130]

[18]   Tramutola A, Lanzillotta C, Perluigi M, Butterfield DA. Oxidative stress, protein modification and Alzheimer disease. Brain Res Bull 2017; 133: 88-96.
[http://dx.doi.org/10.1016/j.brainresbull.2016.06.005] [PMID: 27316747]

[19]   Doorn JA, Petersen DR. Covalent adduction of nucleophilic amino acids by 4-hydroxynonenal and 4-oxononenal. Chem Biol Interact 2003; 143-144: 93-100.
[http://dx.doi.org/10.1016/S0009-2797(02)00178-3] [PMID: 12604193]

[20]   Markesbery WR, Lovell MA. Four-hydroxynonenal, a product of lipid peroxidation, is increased in the brain in Alzheimer's disease. Neurobiol Aging 1998; 19(1): 33-6.
[http://dx.doi.org/10.1016/S0197-4580(98)00009-8] [PMID: 9562500]

[21]   Dildar K, Sinem F, Gökhan E, Orhan Y, Filiz M. Serum nitrosative stress levels are increased in Alzheimer disease but not in vascular dementia. Alzheimer Dis Assoc Disord 2010; 24(2): 194-7.
[http://dx.doi.org/10.1097/WAD.0b013e3181c53d0d] [PMID: 20505437]

[22]   Sultana R, Mecocci P, Mangialasche F, Cecchetti R, Baglioni M, Butterfield DA. Increased protein and lipid oxidative damage in mitochondria isolated from lymphocytes from patients with Alzheimer's disease: insights into the role of oxidative stress in Alzheimer's disease and initial investigations into a potential biomarker for this dementing disorder. J Alzheimers Dis 2011; 24(1): 77-84.

[http://dx.doi.org/10.3233/JAD-2011-101425] [PMID: 21383494]

[23]   García-Blanco A, Baquero M, Vento M, Gil E, Bataller L, Cháfer-Pericás C. Potential oxidative stress biomarkers of mild cognitive impairment due to Alzheimer disease. J Neurol Sci 2017; 373: 295-302.
[http://dx.doi.org/10.1016/j.jns.2017.01.020] [PMID: 28131209]

[24]   Bradley MA, Xiong-Fister S, Markesbery WR, Lovell MA. Elevated 4-hydroxyhexenal in Alzheimer's disease (AD) progression. Neurobiol Aging 2012; 33(6): 1034-44.
[http://dx.doi.org/10.1016/j.neurobiolaging.2010.08.016] [PMID: 20965613]

[25]   Di Domenico F, Tramutola A, Butterfield DA. Role of 4-hydroxy-2-nonenal (HNE) in the pathogenesis of alzheimer disease and other selected age-related neurodegenerative disorders. Free Radic Biol Med 2017; 111: 253-61.
[http://dx.doi.org/10.1016/j.freeradbiomed.2016.10.490] [PMID: 27789292]

[26]   Perluigi M, Sultana R, Cenini G, *et al.* Redox proteomics identification of 4-hydroxynonenal-modified brain proteins in Alzheimer's disease: Role of lipid peroxidation in Alzheimer's disease pathogenesis. Proteomics Clin Appl 2009; 3(6): 682-93.
[http://dx.doi.org/10.1002/prca.200800161] [PMID: 20333275]

[27]   Aluise CD, Robinson RA, Cai J, Pierce WM, Markesbery WR, Butterfield DA. Redox proteomics analysis of brains from subjects with amnestic mild cognitive impairment compared to brains from subjects with preclinical Alzheimer's disease: insights into memory loss in MCI. J Alzheimers Dis 2011; 23(2): 257-69.
[http://dx.doi.org/10.3233/JAD-2010-101083] [PMID: 20930294]

[28]   Kim TS, Pae CU, Yoon SJ, *et al.* Decreased plasma antioxidants in patients with Alzheimer's disease. Int J Geriatr Psychiatry 2006; 21(4): 344-8.
[http://dx.doi.org/10.1002/gps.1469] [PMID: 16534775]

[29]   Nunomura A, Hofer T, Moreira PI, Castellani RJ, Smith MA, Perry G. RNA oxidation in Alzheimer disease and related neurodegenerative disorders. Acta Neuropathol 2009; 118(1): 151-66.
[http://dx.doi.org/10.1007/s00401-009-0508-1] [PMID: 19271225]

[30]   Chen X, Guo C, Kong J. Oxidative stress in neurodegenerative diseases. Neural Regen Res 2012; 7(5): 376-85.
[PMID: 25774178]

[31]   Sinclair AJ, Bayer AJ, Johnston J, Warner C, Maxwell SR. Altered plasma antioxidant status in subjects with Alzheimer's disease and vascular dementia. Int J Geriatr Psychiatry 1998; 13(12): 840-5.
[http://dx.doi.org/10.1002/(SICI)1099-1166(1998120)13:12<840::AID-GPS877>3.0.CO;2-R] [PMID: 9884908]

[32]   Owen JB, Butterfield DA. Measurement of oxidized/reduced glutathione ratio. Methods Mol Biol 2010; 648: 269-77.
[http://dx.doi.org/10.1007/978-1-60761-756-3_18] [PMID: 20700719]

[33]   Martín-Aragón S, Bermejo-Bescós P, Benedí J, *et al.* Metalloproteinase's activity and oxidative stress in mild cognitive impairment and Alzheimer's disease. Neurochem Res 2009; 34(2): 373-8.
[http://dx.doi.org/10.1007/s11064-008-9789-3] [PMID: 18618244]

[34]   Bermejo P, Martín-Aragón S, Benedí J, *et al.* Peripheral levels of glutathione and protein oxidation as markers in the development of Alzheimer's disease from Mild Cognitive Impairment. Free Radic Res 2008; 42(2): 162-70.
[http://dx.doi.org/10.1080/10715760701861373] [PMID: 18297609]

[35]   Marcus DL, Thomas C, Rodriguez C, *et al.* Increased peroxidation and reduced antioxidant enzyme activity in Alzheimer's disease. Exp Neurol 1998; 150(1): 40-4.
[http://dx.doi.org/10.1006/exnr.1997.6750] [PMID: 9514828]

[36]   Rinaldi P, Polidori MC, Metastasio A, *et al.* Plasma antioxidants are similarly depleted in mild cognitive impairment and in Alzheimer's disease. Neurobiol Aging 2003; 24(7): 915-9.

[http://dx.doi.org/10.1016/S0197-4580(03)00031-9] [PMID: 12928050]

[37] Padurariu M, Ciobica A, Hritcu L, Stoica B, Bild W, Stefanescu C. Changes of some oxidative stress markers in the serum of patients with mild cognitive impairment and Alzheimer's disease. Neurosci Lett 2010; 469(1): 6-10.
[http://dx.doi.org/10.1016/j.neulet.2009.11.033] [PMID: 19914330]

[38] Koopman WJ, Nijtmans LG, Dieteren CE, *et al.* Mammalian mitochondrial complex I: biogenesis, regulation, and reactive oxygen species generation. Antioxid Redox Signal 2010; 12(12): 1431-70.
[http://dx.doi.org/10.1089/ars.2009.2743] [PMID: 19803744]

[39] Ray PD, Huang BW, Tsuji Y. Reactive oxygen species (ROS) homeostasis and redox regulation in cellular signaling. Cell Signal 2012; 24(5): 981-90.
[http://dx.doi.org/10.1016/j.cellsig.2012.01.008] [PMID: 22286106]

[40] Reiss AB, Arain HA, Stecker MM, Siegart NM, Kasselman LJ. Amyloid toxicity in Alzheimer's disease. Rev Neurosci 2018; /j/revneuro.ahead-of-print/revneuro-2017-0063/revneuro-2017-0063.xml.
[PMID: 29447116]

[41] Reiss AB, Arain HA, Stecker MM, Siegart NM, Kasselman LJ. Amyloid toxicity in Alzheimer's disease. Rev Neurosci 2018; /j/revneuro.ahead-of-print/revneuro-2017-0063/revneuro-2017-0063.xml.
[PMID: 29447116]

[42] Moreira PI, Carvalho C, Zhu X, Smith MA, Perry G. Mitochondrial dysfunction is a trigger of Alzheimer's disease pathophysiology. Biochim Biophys Acta 2010; 1802(1): 2-10.
[http://dx.doi.org/10.1016/j.bbadis.2009.10.006] [PMID: 19853658]

[43] Yu H, Lin X, Wang D, *et al.* Mitochondrial molecular abnormalities revealed by proteomic analysis of hippocampal organelles of mice triple transgenic for alzheimer disease. Front Mol Neurosci 2018; 11: 74.
[http://dx.doi.org/10.3389/fnmol.2018.00074] [PMID: 29593495]

[44] Sun J, Feng X, Liang D, Duan Y, Lei H. Down-regulation of energy metabolism in Alzheimer's disease is a protective response of neurons to the microenvironment. J Alzheimers Dis 2012; 28(2): 389-402.
[http://dx.doi.org/10.3233/JAD-2011-111313] [PMID: 22008267]

[45] Liang WS, Reiman EM, Valla J, *et al.* Alzheimer's disease is associated with reduced expression of energy metabolism genes in posterior cingulate neurons. Proc Natl Acad Sci USA 2008; 105(11): 4441-6.
[http://dx.doi.org/10.1073/pnas.0709259105] [PMID: 18332434]

[46] Gibson GE, Sheu KF, Blass JP. Abnormalities of mitochondrial enzymes in Alzheimer disease. J Neural Transm (Vienna) 1998; 105(8-9): 855-70.
[http://dx.doi.org/10.1007/s007020050099] [PMID: 9869323]

[47] Corral-Debrinski M, Horton T, Lott MT, *et al.* Marked changes in mitochondrial DNA deletion levels in Alzheimer brains. Genomics 1994; 23(2): 471-6.
[http://dx.doi.org/10.1006/geno.1994.1525] [PMID: 7835898]

[48] Coskun PE, Wyrembak J, Derbereva O, *et al.* Systemic mitochondrial dysfunction and the etiology of Alzheimer's disease and down syndrome dementia. J Alzheimers Dis 2010; 20 (Suppl. 2): S293-310.
[http://dx.doi.org/10.3233/JAD-2010-100351] [PMID: 20463402]

[49] Guo C, Sun L, Chen X, Zhang D. Oxidative stress, mitochondrial damage and neurodegenerative diseases. Neural Regen Res 2013; 8(21): 2003-14.
[PMID: 25206509]

[50] Zhao Y, Zhao B. Oxidative stress and the pathogenesis of Alzheimer's disease. Oxid Med Cell Longev 2013; 2013: 316523.
[http://dx.doi.org/10.1155/2013/316523] [PMID: 23983897]

[51] Wang X, Su B, Lee HG, *et al.* Impaired balance of mitochondrial fission and fusion in Alzheimer's

disease. J Neurosci 2009; 29(28): 9090-103.
[http://dx.doi.org/10.1523/JNEUROSCI.1357-09.2009] [PMID: 19605646]

[52]   Manczak M, Reddy PH. Abnormal interaction between the mitochondrial fission protein Drp1 and hyperphosphorylated tau in Alzheimer's disease neurons: implications for mitochondrial dysfunction and neuronal damage. Hum Mol Genet 2012; 21(11): 2538-47.
[http://dx.doi.org/10.1093/hmg/dds072] [PMID: 22367970]

[53]   Wojda U, Salinska E, Kuznicki J. Calcium ions in neuronal degeneration. IUBMB Life 2008; 60(9): 575-90.
[http://dx.doi.org/10.1002/iub.91] [PMID: 18478527]

[54]   Yan Y, Wei CL, Zhang WR, Cheng HP, Liu J. Cross-talk between calcium and reactive oxygen species signaling. Acta Pharmacol Sin 2006; 27(7): 821-6.
[http://dx.doi.org/10.1111/j.1745-7254.2006.00390.x] [PMID: 16787564]

[55]   Ghosh A, Giese KP. Calcium/calmodulin-dependent kinase II and Alzheimer's disease. Mol Brain 2015; 8(1): 78.
[http://dx.doi.org/10.1186/s13041-015-0166-2] [PMID: 26603284]

[56]   Khan SM, Cassarino DS, Abramova NN, *et al.* Alzheimer's disease cybrids replicate beta-amyloid abnormalities through cell death pathways. Ann Neurol 2000; 48(2): 148-55.
[http://dx.doi.org/10.1002/1531-8249(200008)48:2<148::AID-ANA3>3.0.CO;2-7] [PMID: 10939564]

[57]   Rissman RA, Poon WW, Blurton-Jones M, *et al.* Caspase-cleavage of tau is an early event in Alzheimer disease tangle pathology. J Clin Invest 2004; 114(1): 121-30.
[http://dx.doi.org/10.1172/JCI200420640] [PMID: 15232619]

[58]   Butterfield DA, Drake J, Pocernich C, Castegna A. Evidence of oxidative damage in Alzheimer's disease brain: central role for amyloid beta-peptide. Trends Mol Med 2001; 7(12): 548-54.
[http://dx.doi.org/10.1016/S1471-4914(01)02173-6] [PMID: 11733217]

[59]   Butterfield DA. The 2013 SFRBM discovery award: selected discoveries from the butterfield laboratory of oxidative stress and its sequela in brain in cognitive disorders exemplified by Alzheimer disease and chemotherapy induced cognitive impairment. Free Radic Biol Med 2014; 74: 157-74.
[http://dx.doi.org/10.1016/j.freeradbiomed.2014.06.006] [PMID: 24996204]

[60]   Boutte AM, Woltjer RL, Zimmerman LJ, *et al.* Selectively increased oxidative modifications mapped to detergent-insoluble forms of Abeta and beta-III tubulin in Alzheimer's disease. FASEB J 2006; 20 (9): 1473-83.
[http://dx.doi.org/10.1096/fj.06-5920com] [PMID: 16816122]

[61]   Butterfield DA. Amyloid beta-peptide (1-42)-induced oxidative stress and neurotoxicity: implications for neurodegeneration in Alzheimer's disease brain. A review. Free Radic Res 2002; 36(12): 1307-13.
[http://dx.doi.org/10.1080/1071576021000049890] [PMID: 12607822]

[62]   Dean RT, Fu S, Stocker R, Davies MJ. Biochemistry and pathology of radical-mediated protein oxidation. Biochem J 1997; 324(Pt 1): 1-18.
[http://dx.doi.org/10.1042/bj3240001] [PMID: 9164834]

[63]   Lustbader JW, Cirilli M, Lin C, *et al.* ABAD directly links Abeta to mitochondrial toxicity in Alzheimer's disease. Science 2004; 304(5669): 448-52.
[http://dx.doi.org/10.1126/science.1091230] [PMID: 15087549]

[64]   Takuma K, Yao J, Huang J, *et al.* ABAD enhances Abeta-induced cell stress *via* mitochondrial dysfunction. FASEB J 2005; 19(6): 597-8.
[http://dx.doi.org/10.1096/fj.04-2582fje] [PMID: 15665036]

[65]   Persson T, Popescu BO, Cedazo-Minguez A. Oxidative stress in Alzheimer's disease: why did antioxidant therapy fail? Oxid Med Cell Longev 2014; 2014: 427318.
[http://dx.doi.org/10.1155/2014/427318] [PMID: 24669288]

[66]   Akterin S, Cowburn RF, Miranda-Vizuete A, *et al.* Involvement of glutaredoxin-1 and thioredoxin-1

in beta-amyloid toxicity and Alzheimer's disease. Cell Death Differ 2006; 13(9): 1454-65.
[http://dx.doi.org/10.1038/sj.cdd.4401818] [PMID: 16311508]

[67]   Cenini G, Sultana R, Memo M, Butterfield DA. Elevated levels of pro-apoptotic p53 and its oxidative modification by the lipid peroxidation product, HNE, in brain from subjects with amnestic mild cognitive impairment and Alzheimer's disease. J Cell Mol Med 2008; 12(3): 987-94.
[http://dx.doi.org/10.1111/j.1582-4934.2008.00163.x] [PMID: 18494939]

[68]   Sharma A, Sharma R, Chaudhary P, *et al.* 4-Hydroxynonenal induces p53-mediated apoptosis in retinal pigment epithelial cells. Arch Biochem Biophys 2008; 480(2): 85-94.
[http://dx.doi.org/10.1016/j.abb.2008.09.016] [PMID: 18930016]

[69]   Sanacora G, Rothman DL, Mason G, Krystal JH. Clinical studies implementing glutamate neurotransmission in mood disorders. Ann N Y Acad Sci 2003; 1003: 292-308.
[http://dx.doi.org/10.1196/annals.1300.018] [PMID: 14684453]

[70]   Krystal JH, Tolin DF, Sanacora G, *et al.* Neuroplasticity as a target for the pharmacotherapy of anxiety disorders, mood disorders, and schizophrenia. Drug Discov Today 2009; 14(13-14): 690-7.
[http://dx.doi.org/10.1016/j.drudis.2009.05.002] [PMID: 19460458]

[71]   Pekny M, Nilsson M. Astrocyte activation and reactive gliosis. Glia 2005; 50(4): 427-34.
[http://dx.doi.org/10.1002/glia.20207] [PMID: 15846805]

[72]   Pellerin L, Bouzier-Sore AK, Aubert A, *et al.* Activity-dependent regulation of energy metabolism by astrocytes: an update. Glia 2007; 55(12): 1251-62.
[http://dx.doi.org/10.1002/glia.20528] [PMID: 17659524]

[73]   Bélanger M, Magistretti PJ. The role of astroglia in neuroprotection. Dialogues Clin Neurosci 2009; 11(3): 281-95.
[PMID: 19877496]

[74]   Chojnacka-Wójcik E, Kłodzinska A, Pilc A. Glutamate receptor ligands as anxiolytics. Curr Opin Investig Drugs 2001; 2(8): 1112-9.
[PMID: 11892923]

[75]   Cryan JF, Kelly PH, Neijt HC, Sansig G, Flor PJ, van Der Putten H. Antidepressant and anxiolytic-like effects in mice lacking the group III metabotropic glutamate receptor mGluR7. Eur J Neurosci 2003; 17(11): 2409-17.
[http://dx.doi.org/10.1046/j.1460-9568.2003.02667.x] [PMID: 12814372]

[76]   Bergink V, van Megen HJ, Westenberg HG. Glutamate and anxiety. Eur Neuropsychopharmacol 2004; 14(3): 175-83.
[http://dx.doi.org/10.1016/S0924-977X(03)00100-7] [PMID: 15056476]

[77]   Palucha A, Pilc A. Metabotropic glutamate receptor ligands as possible anxiolytic and antidepressant drugs. Pharmacol Ther 2007; 115(1): 116-47.
[http://dx.doi.org/10.1016/j.pharmthera.2007.04.007] [PMID: 17582504]

[78]   Kapus GL, Gacsályi I, Vegh M, *et al.* Antagonism of AMPA receptors produces anxiolytic-like behavior in rodents: effects of GYKI 52466 and its novel analogues. Psychopharmacology (Berl) 2008; 198(2): 231-41.
[http://dx.doi.org/10.1007/s00213-008-1121-z] [PMID: 18363046]

[79]   Ozawa S. [Ca2+ permeation through the ionotropic glutamate receptor]. Tanpakushitsu Kakusan Koso 1998; 43(12) (Suppl.): 1589-95. [Ca2+ permeation through the ionotropic glutamate receptor].
[PMID: 9788157]

[80]   Segovia G, Porras A, Del Arco A, Mora F. Glutamatergic neurotransmission in aging: a critical perspective. Mech Ageing Dev 2001; 122(1): 1-29.
[http://dx.doi.org/10.1016/S0047-6374(00)00225-6] [PMID: 11163621]

[81]   Izquierdo I, Bevilaqua LR, Rossato JI, Bonini JS, Medina JH, Cammarota M. Different molecular cascades in different sites of the brain control memory consolidation. Trends Neurosci 2006; 29(9):

496-505.
[http://dx.doi.org/10.1016/j.tins.2006.07.005] [PMID: 16872686]

[82]   Schmidt AP, Böhmer AE, Leke R, *et al.* Antinociceptive effects of intracerebroventricular administration of guanine-based purines in mice: evidences for the mechanism of action. Brain Res 2008; 1234: 50-8.
[http://dx.doi.org/10.1016/j.brainres.2008.07.091] [PMID: 18708036]

[83]   Lipton SA, Rosenberg PA. Excitatory amino acids as a final common pathway for neurologic disorders. N Engl J Med 1994; 330(9): 613-22.
[http://dx.doi.org/10.1056/NEJM199403033300907] [PMID: 7905600]

[84]   Meldrum BS. The role of glutamate in epilepsy and other CNS disorders. Neurology 1994; 44(11) (Suppl. 8): S14-23.
[PMID: 7970002]

[85]   Maragakis NJ, Rothstein JD. Mechanisms of Disease: astrocytes in neurodegenerative disease. Nat Clin Pract Neurol 2006; 2(12): 679-89.
[http://dx.doi.org/10.1038/ncpneuro0355] [PMID: 17117171]

[86]   Sheldon AL, Robinson MB. The role of glutamate transporters in neurodegenerative diseases and potential opportunities for intervention. Neurochem Int 2007; 51(6-7): 333-55.
[http://dx.doi.org/10.1016/j.neuint.2007.03.012] [PMID: 17517448]

[87]   Kew JN, Kemp JA. Ionotropic and metabotropic glutamate receptor structure and pharmacology. Psychopharmacology (Berl) 2005; 179(1): 4-29.
[http://dx.doi.org/10.1007/s00213-005-2200-z] [PMID: 15731895]

[88]   Gjessing LR, Gjesdahl P, Sjaastad O. The free amino acids in human cerebrospinal fluid. J Neurochem 1972; 19(7): 1807-8.
[http://dx.doi.org/10.1111/j.1471-4159.1972.tb06226.x] [PMID: 5042475]

[89]   Danbolt NC. Glutamate uptake. Prog Neurobiol 2001; 65(1): 1-105.
[http://dx.doi.org/10.1016/S0301-0082(00)00067-8] [PMID: 11369436]

[90]   Chatton JY, Marquet P, Magistretti PJ. A quantitative analysis of L-glutamate-regulated Na+ dynamics in mouse cortical astrocytes: implications for cellular bioenergetics. Eur J Neurosci 2000; 12(11): 3843-53.
[http://dx.doi.org/10.1046/j.1460-9568.2000.00269.x] [PMID: 11069579]

[91]   Anderson CM, Swanson RA. Astrocyte glutamate transport: review of properties, regulation, and physiological functions. Glia 2000; 32(1): 1-14.
[http://dx.doi.org/10.1002/1098-1136(200010)32:1<1::AID-GLIA10>3.0.CO;2-W] [PMID: 10975906]

[92]   Kanner BI. Structure and function of sodium-coupled GABA and glutamate transporters. J Membr Biol 2006; 213(2): 89-100.
[http://dx.doi.org/10.1007/s00232-006-0877-5] [PMID: 17417704]

[93]   Rothstein JD, Dykes-Hoberg M, Pardo CA, *et al.* Knockout of glutamate transporters reveals a major role for astroglial transport in excitotoxicity and clearance of glutamate. Neuron 1996; 16(3): 675-86.
[http://dx.doi.org/10.1016/S0896-6273(00)80086-0] [PMID: 8785064]

[94]   Dunlop J. Glutamate-based therapeutic approaches: targeting the glutamate transport system. Curr Opin Pharmacol 2006; 6(1): 103-7.
[http://dx.doi.org/10.1016/j.coph.2005.09.004] [PMID: 16368269]

[95]   Matos M, Augusto E, Agostinho P, Cunha RA, Chen JF. Antagonistic interaction between adenosine A2A receptors and Na+/K+-ATPase-α2 controlling glutamate uptake in astrocytes. J Neurosci 2013; 33(47): 18492-502.
[http://dx.doi.org/10.1523/JNEUROSCI.1828-13.2013] [PMID: 24259572]

[96]   Zhang LN, Sun YJ, Wang LX, Gao ZB. Glutamate Transporters/Na(+), K(+)-ATPase Involving in the Neuroprotective Effect as a Potential Regulatory Target of Glutamate Uptake. Mol Neurobiol 2016;

53(2): 1124-31.
[http://dx.doi.org/10.1007/s12035-014-9071-4] [PMID: 25586061]

[97]   Bøttger P, Glerup S, Gesslein B, *et al.* Glutamate-system defects behind psychiatric manifestations in a familial hemiplegic migraine type 2 disease-mutation mouse model. Sci Rep 2016; 6: 22047.
[http://dx.doi.org/10.1038/srep22047] [PMID: 26911348]

[98]   Kinoshita PF, Leite JA, Orellana AM, *et al.* The Influence of Na(+), K(+)-ATPase on Glutamate Signaling in Neurodegenerative Diseases and Senescence. Front Physiol 2016; 7: 195.
[http://dx.doi.org/10.3389/fphys.2016.00195] [PMID: 27313535]

[99]   Wang R, Reddy PH. Role of Glutamate and NMDA Receptors in Alzheimer's Disease. J Alzheimers Dis 2017; 57(4): 1041-8.
[http://dx.doi.org/10.3233/JAD-160763] [PMID: 27662322]

[100]   Görlach A, Bertram K, Hudecova S, Krizanova O. Calcium and ROS: A mutual interplay. Redox Biol 2015; 6: 260-71.
[http://dx.doi.org/10.1016/j.redox.2015.08.010] [PMID: 26296072]

[101]   Girouard H, Wang G, Gallo EF, *et al.* NMDA receptor activation increases free radical production through nitric oxide and NOX2. J Neurosci 2009; 29(8): 2545-52.
[http://dx.doi.org/10.1523/JNEUROSCI.0133-09.2009] [PMID: 19244529]

[102]   Acosta C, Anderson HD, Anderson CM. Astrocyte dysfunction in Alzheimer disease. J Neurosci Res 2017; 95(12): 2430-47.
[http://dx.doi.org/10.1002/jnr.24075] [PMID: 28467650]

[103]   Orellana AM, Vasconcelos AR, Leite JA, *et al.* Age-related neuroinflammation and changes in AKT-GSK-3β and WNT/ β-CATENIN signaling in rat hippocampus. Aging (Albany NY) 2015; 7(12): 1094-111.
[http://dx.doi.org/10.18632/aging.100853] [PMID: 26647069]

[104]   van de Ven RAH, Santos D, Haigis MC. Mitochondrial sirtuins and molecular mechanisms of aging. Trends Mol Med 2017; 23(4): 320-31.
[http://dx.doi.org/10.1016/j.molmed.2017.02.005] [PMID: 28285806]

[105]   Aisen PS, Davis KL. Inflammatory mechanisms in Alzheimer's disease: implications for therapy. Am J Psychiatry 1994; 151(8): 1105-13.
[http://dx.doi.org/10.1176/ajp.151.8.1105] [PMID: 7518651]

[106]   Cheng X, He P, Lee T, Yao H, Li R, Shen Y. High activities of BACE1 in brains with mild cognitive impairment. Am J Pathol 2014; 184(1): 141-7.
[http://dx.doi.org/10.1016/j.ajpath.2013.10.002] [PMID: 24332014]

[107]   Knowles RG, Moncada S. Nitric oxide synthases in mammals. Biochem J 1994; 298(Pt 2): 249-58.
[http://dx.doi.org/10.1042/bj2980249] [PMID: 7510950]

[108]   Lipton SA, Choi YB, Pan ZH, *et al.* A redox-based mechanism for the neuroprotective and neuro-destructive effects of nitric oxide and related nitroso-compounds. Nature 1993; 364(6438): 626-32.
[http://dx.doi.org/10.1038/364626a0] [PMID: 8394509]

[109]   Glezer I, Munhoz CD, Kawamoto EM, Marcourakis T, Avellar MC, Scavone C. MK-801 and 7-Ni atte- nuate the activation of brain NF-kappa B induced by LPS. Neuropharmacology 2003; 45(8): 1120-9.
[http://dx.doi.org/10.1016/S0028-3908(03)00279-X] [PMID: 14614955]

[110]   Huang WT, Niu KC, Chang CK, Lin MT, Chang CP. Curcumin inhibits the increase of glutamate, hydroxyl radicals and PGE2 in the hypothalamus and reduces fever during LPS-induced systemic inflammation in rabbits. Eur J Pharmacol 2008; 593(1-3): 105-11.
[http://dx.doi.org/10.1016/j.ejphar.2008.07.017] [PMID: 18664365]

[111]   Kawamoto EM, Lepsch LB, Boaventura MF, *et al.* Amyloid beta-peptide activates nuclear factor-kappaB through an N-methyl-D-aspartate signaling pathway in cultured cerebellar cells. J Neurosci

Res 2008; 86(4): 845-60.
[http://dx.doi.org/10.1002/jnr.21548] [PMID: 17969100]

[112] Kaltschmidt C, Kaltschmidt B, Baeuerle PA. Stimulation of ionotropic glutamate receptors activates transcription factor NF-kappa B in primary neurons. Proc Natl Acad Sci USA 1995; 92(21): 9618-22.
[http://dx.doi.org/10.1073/pnas.92.21.9618] [PMID: 7568184]

[113] Guerrini L, Blasi F, Denis-Donini S. Synaptic activation of NF-kappa B by glutamate in cerebellar granule neurons *in vitro*. Proc Natl Acad Sci USA 1995; 92(20): 9077-81.
[http://dx.doi.org/10.1073/pnas.92.20.9077] [PMID: 7568076]

[114] Kaltschmidt C, Kaltschmidt B, Neumann H, Wekerle H, Baeuerle PA. Constitutive NF-kappa B activity in neurons. Mol Cell Biol 1994; 14(6): 3981-92.
[http://dx.doi.org/10.1128/MCB.14.6.3981] [PMID: 8196637]

[115] Mattson MP, Camandola S. NF-kappaB in neuronal plasticity and neurodegenerative disorders. J Clin Invest 2001; 107(3): 247-54.
[http://dx.doi.org/10.1172/JCI11916] [PMID: 11160145]

[116] O'Neill LA, Kaltschmidt C. NF-kappa B: a crucial transcription factor for glial and neuronal cell function. Trends Neurosci 1997; 20(6): 252-8.
[http://dx.doi.org/10.1016/S0166-2236(96)01035-1] [PMID: 9185306]

[117] Mattson MP, Meffert MK. Roles for NF-kappaB in nerve cell survival, plasticity, and disease. Cell Death Differ 2006; 13(5): 852-60.
[http://dx.doi.org/10.1038/sj.cdd.4401837] [PMID: 16397579]

[118] Scavone C, Munhoz CD, Kawamoto EM, *et al.* Age-related changes in cyclic GMP and PKG-stimulated cerebellar Na,K-ATPase activity. Neurobiol Aging 2005; 26(6): 907-16.
[http://dx.doi.org/10.1016/j.neurobiolaging.2004.08.013] [PMID: 15718050]

[119] Munhoz CD, Kawamoto EM, de Sá Lima L, *et al.* Glutamate modulates sodium-potassium-ATPase through cyclic GMP and cyclic GMP-dependent protein kinase in rat striatum. Cell Biochem Funct 2005; 23(2): 115-23.
[http://dx.doi.org/10.1002/cbf.1217] [PMID: 15624118]

[120] Kawamoto EM, Munhoz CD, Lepsch LB, *et al.* Age-related changes in cerebellar phosphatase-1 reduce Na,K-ATPase activity. Neurobiol Aging 2008; 29(11): 1712-20.
[http://dx.doi.org/10.1016/j.neurobiolaging.2007.04.008] [PMID: 17537548]

[121] Kawamoto EM, Munhoz CD, Glezer I, *et al.* Oxidative state in platelets and erythrocytes in aging and Alzheimer's disease. Neurobiol Aging 2005; 26(6): 857-64.
[http://dx.doi.org/10.1016/j.neurobiolaging.2004.08.011] [PMID: 15718044]

[122] Mattson MP, Liu D. Energetics and oxidative stress in synaptic plasticity and neurodegenerative disorders. Neuromolecular Med 2002; 2(2): 215-31.
[http://dx.doi.org/10.1385/NMM:2:2:215] [PMID: 12428812]

[123] Hsu HW, Bondy SC, Kitazawa M. Environmental and dietary exposure to copper and its cellular mechanisms linking to Alzheimer disease. Toxicol Sci 2018; 163(2): 338-45.
[http://dx.doi.org/10.1093/toxsci/kfy025] [PMID: 29409005]

[124] Greenough MA, Camakaris J, Bush AI. Metal dyshomeostasis and oxidative stress in Alzheimer's disease. Neurochem Int 2013; 62(5): 540-55.
[http://dx.doi.org/10.1016/j.neuint.2012.08.014] [PMID: 22982299]

[125] Schrag M, Mueller C, Oyoyo U, Smith MA, Kirsch WM. Iron, zinc and copper in the Alzheimer's disease brain: a quantitative meta-analysis. Some insight on the influence of citation bias on scientific opinion. Prog Neurobiol 2011; 94(3): 296-306.
[http://dx.doi.org/10.1016/j.pneurobio.2011.05.001] [PMID: 21600264]

[126] Ravaglia G, Forti P, Maioli F, *et al.* Blood micronutrient and thyroid hormone concentrations in the oldest-old. J Clin Endocrinol Metab 2000; 85(6): 2260-5.

[http://dx.doi.org/10.1210/jcem.85.6.6627] [PMID: 10852460]

[127] Popescu BF, Nichol H. Mapping brain metals to evaluate therapies for neurodegenerative disease. CNS Neurosci Ther 2011; 17(4): 256-68.
[http://dx.doi.org/10.1111/j.1755-5949.2010.00149.x] [PMID: 20553312]

[128] Miura T, Suzuki K, Kohata N, Takeuchi H. Metal binding modes of Alzheimer's amyloid beta-peptide in insoluble aggregates and soluble complexes. Biochemistry 2000; 39(23): 7024-31.
[http://dx.doi.org/10.1021/bi0002479] [PMID: 10841784]

[129] Dong J, Atwood CS, Anderson VE, *et al.* Metal binding and oxidation of amyloid-beta within isolated senile plaque cores: Raman microscopic evidence. Biochemistry 2003; 42(10): 2768-73.
[http://dx.doi.org/10.1021/bi0272151] [PMID: 12627941]

[130] Barnham KJ, McKinstry WJ, Multhaup G, *et al.* Structure of the Alzheimer's disease amyloid precursor protein copper binding domain. A regulator of neuronal copper homeostasis. J Biol Chem 2003; 278(19): 17401-7.
[http://dx.doi.org/10.1074/jbc.M300629200] [PMID: 12611883]

[131] Cheignon C, Jones M, Atrián-Blasco E, *et al.* Identification of key structural features of the elusive Cu-Aβ complex that generates ROS in Alzheimer's disease. Chem Sci (Camb) 2017; 8(7): 5107-18.
[http://dx.doi.org/10.1039/C7SC00809K] [PMID: 28970897]

[132] Bellingham SA, Lahiri DK, Maloney B, La Fontaine S, Multhaup G, Camakaris J. Copper depletion down-regulates expression of the Alzheimer's disease amyloid-beta precursor protein gene. J Biol Chem 2004; 279(19): 20378-86.
[http://dx.doi.org/10.1074/jbc.M400805200] [PMID: 14985339]

[133] Acevedo KM, Hung YH, Dalziel AH, *et al.* Copper promotes the trafficking of the amyloid precursor protein. J Biol Chem 2011; 286(10): 8252-62.
[http://dx.doi.org/10.1074/jbc.M110.128512] [PMID: 21177866]

[134] Singh I, Sagare AP, Coma M, *et al.* Low levels of copper disrupt brain amyloid-β homeostasis by altering its production and clearance. Proc Natl Acad Sci USA 2013; 110(36): 14771-6.
[http://dx.doi.org/10.1073/pnas.1302212110] [PMID: 23959870]

[135] Rogers JT, Bush AI, Cho HH, *et al.* Iron and the translation of the amyloid precursor protein (APP) and ferritin mRNAs: riboregulation against neural oxidative damage in Alzheimer's disease. Biochem Soc Trans 2008; 36(Pt 6): 1282-7.
[http://dx.doi.org/10.1042/BST0361282] [PMID: 19021541]

[136] Rogers JT, Randall JD, Cahill CM, *et al.* An iron-responsive element type II in the 5'-untranslated region of the Alzheimer's amyloid precursor protein transcript. J Biol Chem 2002; 277(47): 45518-28.
[http://dx.doi.org/10.1074/jbc.M207435200] [PMID: 12198135]

[137] Adlard PA, Parncutt JM, Finkelstein DI, Bush AI. Cognitive loss in zinc transporter-3 knock-out mice: a phenocopy for the synaptic and memory deficits of Alzheimer's disease? J Neurosci 2010; 30(5): 1631-6.
[http://dx.doi.org/10.1523/JNEUROSCI.5255-09.2010] [PMID: 20130173]

[138] Ventriglia M, Brewer GJ, Simonelli I, *et al.* Zinc in Alzheimer's Disease: A Meta-Analysis of Serum, Plasma, and Cerebrospinal Fluid Studies. J Alzheimers Dis 2015; 46(1): 75-87.
[http://dx.doi.org/10.3233/JAD-141296] [PMID: 25697706]

[139] Tomljenovic L. Aluminum and Alzheimer's disease: after a century of controversy, is there a plausible link? J Alzheimers Dis 2011; 23(4): 567-98.
[http://dx.doi.org/10.3233/JAD-2010-101494] [PMID: 21157018]

[140] Hidalgo J, Aschner M, Zatta P, Vasák M. Roles of the metallothionein family of proteins in the central nervous system. Brain Res Bull 2001; 55(2): 133-45.
[http://dx.doi.org/10.1016/S0361-9230(01)00452-X] [PMID: 11470309]

[141] Zambenedetti P, Giordano R, Zatta P. Metallothioneins are highly expressed in astrocytes and

microcapillaries in Alzheimer's disease. J Chem Neuroanat 1998; 15(1): 21-6.
[http://dx.doi.org/10.1016/S0891-0618(98)00024-6] [PMID: 9710146]

[142]   Yu WH, Lukiw WJ, Bergeron C, Niznik HB, Fraser PE. Metallothionein III is reduced in Alzheimer's disease. Brain Res 2001; 894(1): 37-45.
[http://dx.doi.org/10.1016/S0006-8993(00)03196-6] [PMID: 11245813]

[143]   D'Acunto CW, Kaplánek R, Gbelcová H, *et al.* Metallomics for alzheimer's disease treatment: Use of new generation of chelators combining metal-cation binding and transport properties. Eur J Med Chem 2018; 150: 140-55.
[http://dx.doi.org/10.1016/j.ejmech.2018.02.084] [PMID: 29525434]

[144]   Zhang W, Huang D, Huang M, *et al.* Preparation of tetradentate copper chelators as potential anti-alzheimer agents. ChemMedChem 2018; 13(7): 684-704.
[http://dx.doi.org/10.1002/cmdc.201700734] [PMID: 29420864]

[145]   Albarracin SL, Stab B, Casas Z, *et al.* Effects of natural antioxidants in neurodegenerative disease. Nutr Neurosci 2012; 15(1): 1-9.
[http://dx.doi.org/10.1179/1476830511Y.0000000028] [PMID: 22305647]

[146]   Mecocci P, Polidori MC. Antioxidant clinical trials in mild cognitive impairment and Alzheimer's disease. Biochim Biophys Acta 2012; 1822(5): 631-8.
[http://dx.doi.org/10.1016/j.bbadis.2011.10.006] [PMID: 22019723]

[147]   Grimm MO, Lehmann J, Mett J, *et al.* Impact of Vitamin D on amyloid precursor protein processing and amyloid-β peptide degradation in Alzheimer's disease. Neurodegener Dis 2014; 13(2-3): 75-81.
[http://dx.doi.org/10.1159/000355462] [PMID: 24192346]

[148]   Sung S, Yao Y, Uryu K, *et al.* Early vitamin E supplementation in young but not aged mice reduces Abeta levels and amyloid deposition in a transgenic model of Alzheimer's disease. FASEB J 2004; 18 (2): 323-5.
[http://dx.doi.org/10.1096/fj.03-0961fje] [PMID: 14656990]

[149]   Mangialasche F, Kivipelto M, Mecocci P, *et al.* High plasma levels of vitamin E forms and reduced Alzheimer's disease risk in advanced age. J Alzheimers Dis 2010; 20(4): 1029-37.
[http://dx.doi.org/10.3233/JAD-2010-091450] [PMID: 20413888]

[150]   Mangialasche F, Solomon A, Kåreholt I, *et al.* Serum levels of vitamin E forms and risk of cognitive impairment in a Finnish cohort of older adults. Exp Gerontol 2013; 48(12): 1428-35.
[http://dx.doi.org/10.1016/j.exger.2013.09.006] [PMID: 24113154]

[151]   Morris MC, Evans DA, Tangney CC, *et al.* Relation of the tocopherol forms to incident Alzheimer disease and to cognitive change. Am J Clin Nutr 2005; 81(2): 508-14.
[http://dx.doi.org/10.1093/ajcn.81.2.508] [PMID: 15699242]

[152]   Kryscio RJ, Abner EL, Caban-Holt A, *et al.* Association of antioxidant supplement use and dementia in the prevention of alzheimer's disease by vitamin e and selenium trial (PREADViSE). JAMA Neurol 2017; 74(5): 567-73.
[http://dx.doi.org/10.1001/jamaneurol.2016.5778] [PMID: 28319243]

[153]   Arlt S, Müller-Thomsen T, Beisiegel U, Kontush A. Effect of one-year vitamin C- and E-supplementation on cerebrospinal fluid oxidation parameters and clinical course in Alzheimer's disease. Neurochem Res 2012; 37(12): 2706-14.
[http://dx.doi.org/10.1007/s11064-012-0860-8] [PMID: 22878647]

[154]   Galasko DR, Peskind E, Clark CM, *et al.* Antioxidants for Alzheimer disease: a randomized clinical trial with cerebrospinal fluid biomarker measures. Arch Neurol 2012; 69(7): 836-41.
[http://dx.doi.org/10.1001/archneurol.2012.85] [PMID: 22431837]

[155]   Morris MC, Evans DA, Bienias JL, *et al.* Dietary intake of antioxidant nutrients and the risk of incident Alzheimer disease in a biracial community study. JAMA 2002; 287(24): 3230-7.
[http://dx.doi.org/10.1001/jama.287.24.3230] [PMID: 12076219]

[156] Engelhart MJ, Geerlings MI, Ruitenberg A, *et al.* Dietary intake of antioxidants and risk of Alzheimer disease. JAMA 2002; 287(24): 3223-9.
[http://dx.doi.org/10.1001/jama.287.24.3223] [PMID: 12076218]

[157] Morris MC, Schneider JA, Li H, *et al.* Brain tocopherols related to Alzheimer's disease neuropathology in humans. Alzheimers Dement 2015; 11(1): 32-9.
[http://dx.doi.org/10.1016/j.jalz.2013.12.015] [PMID: 24589434]

[158] Berridge MJ. Vitamin D deficiency accelerates ageing and age-related diseases: a novel hypothesis. J Physiol 2017; 595(22): 6825-36.
[http://dx.doi.org/10.1113/JP274887] [PMID: 28949008]

[159] Sommer I, Griebler U, Kien C, *et al.* Vitamin D deficiency as a risk factor for dementia: a systematic review and meta-analysis. BMC Geriatr 2017; 17(1): 16.
[http://dx.doi.org/10.1186/s12877-016-0405-0] [PMID: 28086755]

[160] Ouma S, Suenaga M, Bölükbaşı Hatip FF, Hatip-Al-Khatib I, Tsuboi Y, Matsunaga Y. Serum vitamin D in patients with mild cognitive impairment and Alzheimer's disease. Brain Behav 2018; 8(3): e00936.
[http://dx.doi.org/10.1002/brb3.936] [PMID: 29541546]

[161] Schaffer S, Asseburg H, Kuntz S, Muller WE, Eckert GP. Effects of polyphenols on brain ageing and Alzheimer's disease: focus on mitochondria. Mol Neurobiol 2012; 46(1): 161-78.
[http://dx.doi.org/10.1007/s12035-012-8282-9] [PMID: 22706880]

[162] Caruana M, Cauchi R, Vassallo N. Putative role of red wine polyphenols against brain pathology in alzheimer's and parkinson's disease. Front Nutr 2016; 3: 31.
[http://dx.doi.org/10.3389/fnut.2016.00031] [PMID: 27570766]

[163] Lampe JW. Isoflavonoid and lignan phytoestrogens as dietary biomarkers. J Nutr 2003; 133 (Suppl. 3): 956S-64S.
[http://dx.doi.org/10.1093/jn/133.3.956S] [PMID: 12612182]

[164] Bastianetto S, Zheng WH, Quirion R. Neuroprotective abilities of resveratrol and other red wine constituents against nitric oxide-related toxicity in cultured hippocampal neurons. Br J Pharmacol 2000; 131(4): 711-20.
[http://dx.doi.org/10.1038/sj.bjp.0703626] [PMID: 11030720]

[165] Marambaud P, Zhao H, Davies P. Resveratrol promotes clearance of Alzheimer's disease amyloid-beta peptides. J Biol Chem 2005; 280(45): 37377-82.
[http://dx.doi.org/10.1074/jbc.M508246200] [PMID: 16162502]

[166] Martín S, González-Burgos E, Carretero ME, Gómez-Serranillos MP. Protective effects of Merlot red wine extract and its major polyphenols in PC12 cells under oxidative stress conditions. J Food Sci 2013; 78(1): H112-8.
[http://dx.doi.org/10.1111/1750-3841.12000] [PMID: 23278327]

[167] Mendes D, Oliveira MM, Moreira PI, *et al.* Beneficial effects of white wine polyphenols-enriched diet on Alzheimer's disease-like pathology. J Nutr Biochem 2018; 55: 165-77.
[http://dx.doi.org/10.1016/j.jnutbio.2018.02.001] [PMID: 29525608]

[168] Sureda A, Xavier C, Tejada S. Neuroprotective effects of flavonoid compounds on neuronal death associated to Alzheimer's disease. Curr Med Chem 2017.
[http://dx.doi.org/10.2174/0929867325666171226103237] [PMID: 29278202]

[169] Fernández-Fernández L, Comes G, Bolea I, *et al.* LMN diet, rich in polyphenols and polyunsaturated fatty acids, improves mouse cognitive decline associated with aging and Alzheimer's disease. Behav Brain Res 2012; 228(2): 261-71.
[http://dx.doi.org/10.1016/j.bbr.2011.11.014] [PMID: 22119712]

[170] Grossi C, Rigacci S, Ambrosini S, *et al.* The polyphenol oleuropein aglycone protects TgCRND8 mice against Aß plaque pathology. PLoS One 2013; 8(8): e71702.

[http://dx.doi.org/10.1371/journal.pone.0071702] [PMID: 23951225]

[171]   Pantano D, Luccarini I, Nardiello P, Servili M, Stefani M, Casamenti F. Oleuropein aglycone and polyphenols from olive mill waste water ameliorate cognitive deficits and neuropathology. Br J Clin Pharmacol 2017; 83(1): 54-62.
[http://dx.doi.org/10.1111/bcp.12993] [PMID: 27131215]

[172]   Porquet D, Casadesús G, Bayod S, *et al.* Dietary resveratrol prevents Alzheimer's markers and increases life span in SAMP8. Age (Dordr) 2013; 35(5): 1851-65.
[http://dx.doi.org/10.1007/s11357-012-9489-4] [PMID: 23129026]

[173]   Porquet D, Griñán-Ferré C, Ferrer I, *et al.* Neuroprotective role of trans-resveratrol in a murine model of familial Alzheimer's disease. J Alzheimers Dis 2014; 42(4): 1209-20.
[http://dx.doi.org/10.3233/JAD-140444] [PMID: 25024312]

[174]   Mohan S, Gobinath T, Salomy A, *et al.* Biophysical interaction of resveratrol with sirtuin pathway: Significance in Alzheimer's disease. Front Biosci 2018; 23: 1380-90.
[http://dx.doi.org/10.2741/4650] [PMID: 29293440]

[175]   Jia Y, Wang N, Liu X. Resveratrol and Amyloid-Beta: Mechanistic Insights. Nutrients 2017; 9(10): E1122.
[http://dx.doi.org/10.3390/nu9101122] [PMID: 29036903]

[176]   Moussa C, Hebron M, Huang X, *et al.* Resveratrol regulates neuro-inflammation and induces adaptive immunity in Alzheimer's disease. J Neuroinflammation 2017; 14(1): 1.
[http://dx.doi.org/10.1186/s12974-016-0779-0] [PMID: 28086917]

[177]   Pacheco SM, Soares MSP, Gutierres JM, *et al.* Anthocyanins as a potential pharmacological agent to manage memory deficit, oxidative stress and alterations in ion pump activity induced by experimental sporadic dementia of Alzheimer's type. J Nutr Biochem 2018; 56: 193-204.
[http://dx.doi.org/10.1016/j.jnutbio.2018.02.014] [PMID: 29587242]

[178]   Reddy AC, Lokesh BR. Studies on spice principles as antioxidants in the inhibition of lipid peroxidation of rat liver microsomes. Mol Cell Biochem 1992; 111(1-2): 117-24.
[PMID: 1588934]

[179]   Ono K, Hasegawa K, Naiki H, Yamada M. Curcumin has potent anti-amyloidogenic effects for Alzheimer's beta-amyloid fibrils *in vitro*. J Neurosci Res 2004; 75(6): 742-50.
[http://dx.doi.org/10.1002/jnr.20025] [PMID: 14994335]

[180]   Kawamoto EM, Scavone C, Mattson MP, Camandola S. Curcumin requires tumor necrosis factor α signaling to alleviate cognitive impairment elicited by lipopolysaccharide. Neurosignals 2013; 21(1-2): 75-88.
[http://dx.doi.org/10.1159/000336074] [PMID: 22572473]

[181]   Begum AN, Jones MR, Lim GP, *et al.* Curcumin structure-function, bioavailability, and efficacy in models of neuroinflammation and Alzheimer's disease. J Pharmacol Exp Ther 2008; 326(1): 196-208.
[http://dx.doi.org/10.1124/jpet.108.137455] [PMID: 18417733]

[182]   Ma QL, Yang F, Rosario ER, *et al.* Beta-amyloid oligomers induce phosphorylation of tau and inactivation of insulin receptor substrate *via* c-Jun N-terminal kinase signaling: suppression by omega-3 fatty acids and curcumin. J Neurosci 2009; 29(28): 9078-89.
[http://dx.doi.org/10.1523/JNEUROSCI.1071-09.2009] [PMID: 19605645]

[183]   Baum L, Lam CW, Cheung SK, *et al.* Six-month randomized, placebo-controlled, double-blind, pilot clinical trial of curcumin in patients with Alzheimer disease. J Clin Psychopharmacol 2008; 28(1): 110-3.
[http://dx.doi.org/10.1097/jcp.0b013e318160862c] [PMID: 18204357]

[184]   Ringman JM, Frautschy SA, Teng E, *et al.* Oral curcumin for Alzheimer's disease: tolerability and efficacy in a 24-week randomized, double blind, placebo-controlled study. Alzheimers Res Ther 2012; 4(5): 43.

[http://dx.doi.org/10.1186/alzrt146] [PMID: 23107780]

[185] DiSilvestro RA, Joseph E, Zhao S, Bomser J. Diverse effects of a low dose supplement of lipidated curcumin in healthy middle aged people. Nutr J 2012; 11: 79.
[http://dx.doi.org/10.1186/1475-2891-11-79] [PMID: 23013352]

[186] Diamond BJ, Bailey MR. Ginkgo biloba: indications, mechanisms, and safety. Psychiatr Clin North Am 2013; 36(1): 73-83.
[http://dx.doi.org/10.1016/j.psc.2012.12.006] [PMID: 23538078]

[187] Liu X, Hao W, Qin Y, *et al.* Long-term treatment with Ginkgo biloba extract EGb 761 improves symptoms and pathology in a transgenic mouse model of Alzheimer's disease. Brain Behav Immun 2015; 46: 121-31.
[http://dx.doi.org/10.1016/j.bbi.2015.01.011] [PMID: 25637484]

[188] Wan W, Zhang C, Danielsen M, *et al.* EGb761 improves cognitive function and regulates inflammatory responses in the APP/PS1 mouse. Exp Gerontol 2016; 81: 92-100.
[http://dx.doi.org/10.1016/j.exger.2016.05.007] [PMID: 27220811]

[189] von Gunten A, Schlaefke S, Überla K. Efficacy of Ginkgo biloba extract EGb 761® in dementia with behavioural and psychological symptoms: A systematic review. World J Biol Psychiatry 2016; 17(8): 622-33.
[http://dx.doi.org/10.3109/15622975.2015.1066513] [PMID: 26223956]

[190] Yang G, Wang Y, Sun J, Zhang K, Liu J. Ginkgo biloba for mild cognitive impairment and alzheimer's disease: a systematic review and meta-analysis of randomized controlled trials. Curr Top Med Chem 2016; 16(5): 520-8.
[http://dx.doi.org/10.2174/1568026615666150813143520] [PMID: 26268332]

[191] DeKosky ST, Williamson JD, Fitzpatrick AL, *et al.* Ginkgo biloba for prevention of dementia: a randomized controlled trial. JAMA 2008; 300(19): 2253-62.
[http://dx.doi.org/10.1001/jama.2008.683] [PMID: 19017911]

CHAPTER 7

Calcium Deregulation in Alzheimer's Disease

Vitor S. Alves, Fernanda L. Ribeiro, Daniela R. de Oliveira and Fernando A. Oliveira[*]

Laboratory of Cellular and Molecular Neurobiology (LaNeC); Center for Mathematics, Computation and Cognition, Federal University of ABC (UFABC), São Bernardo do Campo, São Paulo, Brazil

Abstract: The first ideas proposed by Zaven Khachaturian about the calcium (Ca^{2+}) hypothesis of brain aging foster researchers into cellular and molecular mechanisms trying to explain Ca^{2+} alterations of brain function and cognitive deficits. Alzheimer's disease (AD) is dementia causally linked to aging, therefore Ca^{2+} cellular processes underlying aging-related impairments in the brain may share similarities to severe dementia, as in AD. The effective control of cytosolic Ca^{2+} is essential for the modulation of various processes and pathways of neuronal signaling, and its inefficiency or deregulation can lead to austere pathological conditions. This chapter shows pieces of evidence of Ca^{2+} deregulation in AD and its consequences, focusing on intrinsic properties of the neurons.

Keywords: Afterhyperpolarization, Aging, Alzheimer's Disease Diagnosis, Dementia, Learning and Memory, Neurodegeneration, Neuronal Susceptibility.

INTRODUCTION

Calcium (Ca^{2+}) is a ubiquitous intracellular signal which plays a fundamental role in neuronal physiology. Ca^{2+}-mediated signaling systems regulate several processes including exocytosis of neurotransmitters, protein expression and cell proliferation. At the presynaptic terminals, for example, Ca^{2+} influx triggers exocytosis of neurotransmitters through synaptic vesicles in microseconds [1 - 4]. Postsynaptically, a transient rise of the Ca^{2+} level in dendrites and dendritic spines regulates a variety of functions, including synaptic plasticity (*i.e.,* long-term potentiation - LTP, and long-term depression - LTD) [2, 5, 6] and gene transcription which lasts from minutes to hours [2, 7]. Ca^{2+} may impact many others processes that contribute to neuronal functions as well as membrane excitability [8], dendrite development [5] and synaptogenesis [9]. How is Ca^{2+}

[*] **Corresponding author Fernando A. Oliveira:** Center for Mathematics, Computation and Cognition, Federal University of ABC, Rua Arcturus, 03, Jardim Antares, CEP 09606-070, São Bernardo do Campo – SP, Brazil; Tel +55 11 2320 6274; E-mail: oliveira.fernando@ufabc.edu.br

able to regulate so many divergent cellular processes? The answer lies in the enormous versatility of the Ca^{2+} signaling mechanisms in terms of amplitude, speed, diffusion and local site of action in well-defined cellular domains.

Ca^{2+} concentration within the cytoplasm of neurons is tightly regulated through various mechanisms. In the mammalian brain, neurons have a low intracellular free Ca^{2+} concentration ($[Ca^{2+}]_i$; 50-100nM) and high extracellular Ca^{2+} levels (1.5-2 mM). However, during electrical activity, intracellular Ca^{2+} levels transiently can rise from tens to hundred times with different diffusion profiles. The level of intracellular Ca^{2+} is established by the balance between Ca^{2+} influx into the cytoplasm and efflux and/or sequestration driven by the combined actions of buffers, pumps and exchangers [10 - 13].

The complex Ca^{2+}-signaling pathways count with a broad toolkit of signaling components which are intricately arranged and can generate diverse Ca^{2+} signals with different spatial-temporal properties. In fact, the introduction of Ca^{2+} into the cytoplasm ('on' reactions) depends on an elaborate interplay between Ca^{2+} influx across plasma membrane through the opening of voltage-gated Ca^{2+} channels (VGCC), receptor-operated channels (ROCs), transient receptor potential (TRP) and store-operated channels (SOCs). Conversely, the removal (clearance and/or sequestration) of the exceeding intracellular Ca^{2+} ('off' reactions) is conducted by a variety of exchangers, pumps and buffers (Fig. **1**) [2, 13 - 22]. In this sense, neurons have developed extensive and complex Ca^{2+} signalling pathways to maintain Ca^{2+} homeostasis, therefore impairment of Ca^{2+} signaling results in cellular dysfunction. In fact, Ca^{2+} signaling disruption has been described during aging and neurodegenerative processes, as Alzheimer's disease (AD).

The Early Calcium Deregulation Theory

The assumption that Ca^{2+} homeostasis is essential for the normal function and survival of neurons date back from the early 1980s. Not surprisingly, Ca^{2+} deregulation might cause deleterious consequences in brain aging and potentially play a critical role in neurodegenerative disorders, such as AD. Since then, many hypotheses have been raised attempting to explain the two distinct versions of age-associated mental decline, the physiological aspects and the pathological process.

The "Ca^{2+} *hypothesis of brain aging*" was first proposed by Zaven Khachaturian (1984) in a meeting organized by the National Institute on Aging (NIA). The lack of hypotheses in the field of brain aging captured the attention of many investigators using descriptive studies; the pioneering ideas of Khachaturian led the field to a whole new era. In fact, he boosted the onset of the brain aging research concerning studies of molecular mechanisms in the cell, suggesting that alteration of intracellular Ca^{2+} concentration, $[Ca^{2+}]_i$, might account for a number of age-related neuronal changes. Based on this idea, cellular mechanisms engaged in maintaining the $[Ca^{2+}]_i$ homeostasis play a critical role during brain aging [23, 24]. The central idea of this hypothesis was determined by two factors: (1) the amount of the intracellular level of Ca^{2+} perturbation ($\Delta[Ca^{2+}]_i$) and (2) the time of the deregulation in Ca^{2+} homeostasis (ΔT), where the product is a constant (K), as the following equation shows:

$$K = \Delta[\,Ca^{2+}\,]_i \times \Delta T \qquad \textbf{(Equation 1)}$$

The relationship between $\Delta[Ca^{2+}]_i$ and ΔT are not linear, indicating that long-lasting period of a small change in $[Ca^{2+}]_i$ may cause the same cellular damage as large changes in $[Ca^{2+}]_i$ over a short period (Equation 2).

$$\text{Large } \Delta T \times \text{Small } \Delta[\,Ca^{2+}\,]_i = \text{Large } \Delta[\,Ca^{2+}\,]_i \times \text{Small } \Delta T = K \qquad \textbf{(Equation 2)}$$

Khachaturian's theory directed the scientific community towards the search for a unifying explanation of brain aging. Altered neuronal functions or cell death could be associated with age-related changes in the brain, thus Ca^{2+}-mediated signaling system and its regulation were expected to be the final common pathway for such cellular changes. In fact, a few years later, in 1987, the review article entitled "Ca^{2+} and the Aging Nervous System", by Gibson and Peterson, summarized a number of studies supporting the hypothesis that brain aging is directly associated with changes in Ca^{2+} homeostasis [25]. However, against the ideas proposed by Khachaturian, these studies showed a common feature observed during aging which was the decrease in Ca^{2+} permeation across membranes and its mobilization from organelles. The resulting reduction of Ca^{2+}-dependent functions including neurotransmitter release, axoplasmic transport and frequency potentiation was indicated to be crucial in age-related disorders, remarkably in AD.

In contrast, other research groups showed pieces of evidence for the 'increased Ca^{2+}-current' hypothesis of brain aging proposed by Khachaturian, which stated that the cause of altered Ca^{2+} homeostasis during brain aging is an enhanced neuronal Ca^{2+} concentration caused by the outsized Ca^{2+} influx. To support this idea, it was shown that the deleterious effects of aging in hippocampal neurons could be halted by Mg^{2+} which is a competitive inhibitor of Ca^{2+} [26, 27] and that Ca^{2+} could directly impact Ca^{2+}-dependent K^+-mediated afterhyperpolarization, one of the hallmarks of intrinsic cell property of learning and memory [28 - 32]. In addition, aged rats with elevated plasma levels of Mg^{2+}, which was provided by a special diet, showed stronger frequency potentiation and improved maze reversal learning [26]. Therefore, these pieces of evidence suggested that the deleterious effects of aging were straight associated with an increased Ca^{2+} and that they were arrested by Mg^{2+}.

Later, the intracellular Ca^{2+} deregulation was causally linked to some of the processes that underlie not only the neuronal deterioration occurring in normal aging but also in AD. Disterhoft *et al.* (1994) proposed based on several lines of evidence that aging and AD might have a causal connection. In fact, the incidence rates of AD increase with age, and pathological features of the AD have been observed in the normal aging brain, including changes in Ca^{2+} influx [34]. Multiple datasets indicated that the regulation of free intracellular Ca^{2+} in aging neurons might be disrupted, however further research was required at that time to determine if this disruption was qualitatively or quantitatively related with AD [33 - 36].

During the past 30 years, the Ca^{2+} hypothesis of brain aging and AD has been expanded. Several researchers conducted experiments to investigate the molecular mechanisms underlying the altered Ca^{2+} homeostasis and its neuronal damage during the aging brain and dementia. In fact, Ca^{2+}-dependent neuronal processes are disrupted during brain aging and AD, although the molecular bases accounted for these changes still remain unclear. In this chapter, before discussing the main findings of the altered Ca^{2+} homeostasis in AD and aging, the physiological function of the main players in Ca^{2+} signaling system will be briefly mentioned.

Calcium Signaling in Neuronal Physiology

The complex and diverse arrangements of the Ca^{2+} signaling pathways and components generate diverse Ca^{2+} signals with different spatial-temporal properties. The neuronal Ca^{2+} influx mechanisms, also known as the 'on' reactions, are traditionally regulated by four groups of the plasma membrane Ca^{2+} channel. These channels allow an intricate interplay between Ca^{2+} influx across plasma membrane through the opening of voltage-gated Ca^{2+} channels (VGCC), receptor-operated channels (ROCs) and transient receptor potential (TRP). Additionally, store-operated channels (SOCs) can increase $[Ca^{2+}]_i$ levels *via* coupling mechanisms with ryanodine receptors (RyRs) or inositol-1,4,5-triphosphate receptors ($InsP_3R$) in the endoplasmic reticulum membrane or with mitochondrial channels (*i.e.*, sodium-dependent Ca^{2+} [Na^+/Ca^{2+} exchanger]) (Fig. **1**).

On the other hand, in the course of Ca^{2+} transients, a second act takes place in the cell to maintain Ca^{2+}. $[Ca^{2+}]_i$ levels are sustained by processes that affect the diffusion or removal of Ca^{2+} from the cytosol, 'off' reactions, of which the main players are mobile or immobile Ca^{2+} buffers, plasma membrane Ca^{2+}-ATPase (PMCA), plasma membrane Na^+/Ca^{2+}-exchanger (NCX), Sarco(Endo)plasmic reticulum Ca^{2+}-ATPase (SERCA) and Ca^{2+} uniporters on the mitochondrial membrane (Fig. **1**).

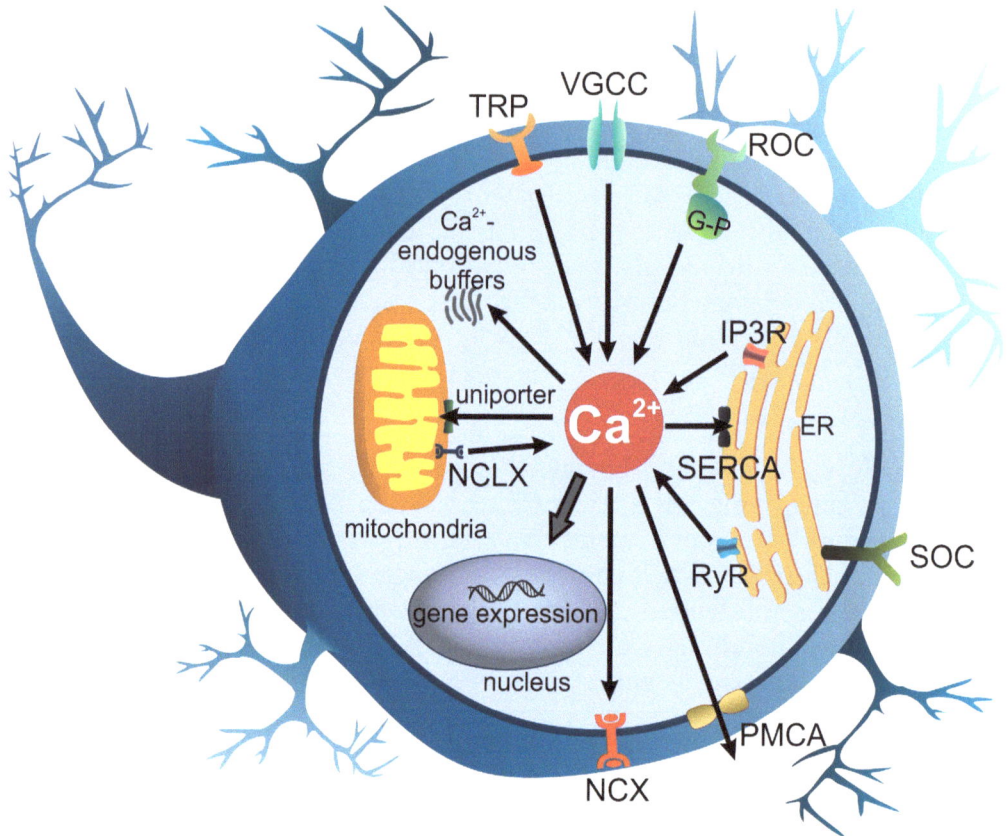

Fig. (1). Cellular components regulating Ca^{2+} signaling in the neuron. VGCC: voltage-gated Ca^{2+} channel; TRP: Transient receptor potential; IP3R: IP_3 receptor; RyR: ryanodine receptor; ER: endoplasmic reticulum; ROC: receptor-operated Ca^{2+} channels, activated by agonists acting on a range of G-protein-coupled receptors; SOC store-operated Ca^{2+} channels, activated following depletion of the Ca^{2+} stores within the sarcoplasmic reticulum; NCX: plasma membrane Na^+/Ca^{2+} exchanger; NCLX: Mitochondrial Na^+/Ca^{2+} exchanger; PMCA: Plasma membrane Ca^{2+}-ATPase; SERCA: Sarco(Endo)plasmic Reticulum Ca^{2+}-ATPase. The directions of the arrows represent what increases or decreases the intracellular Ca^{2+} concentration.

These diverse mechanisms show that neurons have developed extensive and intricate means to maintain Ca^{2+} homeostasis and its impairment might result in cellular dysfunction and neuronal loss. In the following sections, we will review some of the main contributors to the neuronal Ca^{2+} signaling and their functional changes in AD and aging.

Neuronal Calcium Deregulation in Alzheimer's Disease

Several Ca^{2+} mechanisms have been shown to be altered in the AD. It has been observed that the aging-related increase in Ca^{2+}-mediated responses depends on the increased activity of L-type VGCC (L-VGCC). The increased Ca^{2+} currents in aging neurons lead to larger post-burst afterhyperpolarization (AHP), resulting in neurons less excitable and, therefore, unable to properly intermediate the plastic changes that underlie learning and memory. The increased activity of L-VGCC appears to be crucial to these aging-associated changes [29, 37]. Additionally, a more recent study corroborates the potential role of L-VGCC in perturbed neuronal network activity in AD, suggesting that the selective hyper-phosphorylated tau pathology in hippocampal CA1 neurons in AD models correlates to an age-related elevation of L-VGCC density in these neurons, which might demonstrate a potential contribution of altered L-VGCC activity to the selective vulnerability of CA1 neurons to tau pathology in AD subjects [38].

Studies of the L-VGCC antagonist suggested that the age-related increase in Ca^{2+}-mediated responses might depend on greater activity through L-VGCC [39, 40]. Increased L-VGCC activity with aging was confirmed directly by single channel recording in partially dissociated hippocampal slices [41]. Moreover, changes in L-VGCCs appear to be functionally relevant, as L-VGCC antagonists improve learning and memory in aged animals [28, 29, 42] and some AD patients [43]. Furthermore, the increase in L-VGCC density is positively correlated with cognitive impairment in aged animals [41]. Corroborating these results AHP was shown to be increased in AD [44].

Besides that, Lopez et. al (2008) had been shown that resting Ca^{2+} concentration is enhanced in two different models of AD, 3xTg-AD and APP_{swe} [45]. These results corroborate with other studies found alteration on resting Ca^{2+} concentration in AD models [46, 47]. Resting $[Ca^{2+}]_i$ changes, based on the one compartment Ca^{2+} model, suggest neuronal alterations in membrane pumps [11]; these changes have been confirmed in several others studies [48 - 51]. Plasma membrane Ca^{2+}-ATPases, which has a high affinity but lower transport capacity, is capable of effectively binding to Ca^{2+} at very low concentrations, thus it is better suited to the task of maintaining cytoplasmic concentrations of Ca^{2+} that are within a cell in the resting state.

Studies have extensively linked aging and AD with Ca^{2+} deregulation on Ca^{2+} intracellular stores affecting Ca^{2+}-dependent mechanisms. Stutzmann *et al.* (2006, 2007) showed outsized amplitude hyperpolarization, AHP, due to enhanced Ca^{2+} released from the internal stores [52, 53]. In the AD, the perturbation of the endoplasmic reticulum Ca^{2+} homeostasis has been related to presenilin with several pieces of evidence towards to APP increasing ryanodine receptor expression and function, consequently enhancing Ca^{2+} release [54 - 56].

Ultimately alterations on Ca^{2+} buffer capacity have been reported on aging and AD. Endogenous buffer capacity is a very important Ca^{2+} mechanism to buffer Ca^{2+} and, in this sense, it can shape the $[Ca^{2+}]_i$ signal and might indicate a selective vulnerability of specific neurons in the pathophysiology of AD [15, 57 - 60]. Beyond all this, Ca^{2+} buffers can be mobile and/or immobile mediators within the cell with diverse Ca^{2+} dissociation constants; this configuration can lead to different Ca^{2+} diffusion profiles in the cytoplasm modifying intracellular microdomains and affecting distinct signaling pathways.

In addition to the changes described in this chapter AD could still cause changes in mechanisms associated to TRP, ROC or SOC [61 - 65], however, these changes were outside the scope of this chapter.

Clinical Studies Using Compounds

Since Ca^{2+} deregulation has been proposed in aging and AD [23, 24, 33] several compounds have been implied in Ca^{2+} signaling modulation to treat AD. As early as 1990, nimodipine, an L-type Ca^{2+} channel blocker (CCB), was tested in a multicenter clinical trial and was found to be an effective compound to treat old age dementias (primary degenerative and multi-infarct dementias) with practically no contralateral effects [66]. In the same time, Tollefson [67] reported nimodipine short-term effects to treat AD, but with a lot of debate on it [68].

The most likely Ca^{2+} compounds to AD treatment are still CCB, focusing mainly on L-VGCC [69, 70]. This can be attributed by the fact that L-VGCC is involved in the learning and memory mechanisms (*for more details see: Neuronal calcium deregulation in Alzheimer's disease section*) which is the first clinical aspect to be affected in AD patients.

Large population-based studies have suggested that dihydropyridines CCB, nilvadipine or amlodipine, can reduce the risk of developing AD [71, 72]. Nivaldipine was capable to slow the cognitive decline or stabilized it while amlodipine seems to have no protective effect [73, 74]. Interestingly, both drugs lowered blood pressure to the same level [74], suggesting a protective effect independent from the antihypertensive outcome. On the one hand, this difference might be explained by amlodipine retention on the blood-brain barrier [75]; on the other hand, it suggests a CCB direct effect on AD mechanisms which has already been shown previously [76]. Several ongoing studies are currently testing nivaldipine in mild-to-moderate AD [69, 77, 78].

Still, it's interesting to note that CCBs are drugs initially used to treat hypertension. Hypertension is a condition considered a risk factor for AD [79 - 81], therefore many clinical trial testing CCBs are involved with hypertensive patients

[43, 70, 71, 82]. This fact causes a confusion in the data interpretation since one can claim that the results obtained are because of the control of the high blood pressure instead of a direct effect on the AD mechanisms. Always considering this aspect in mind, some reports have been shown that the data are still inconclusive about antihypertensive drugs improving cognition [80]; however, others have been showing cognitive improvements with CCB drugs [73, 74, 78, 83]. Besides that, both agree that a good vascular condition leads to a healthy brain, but more studies are needed about the CCBs action, cognition and AD mechanisms.

Summary

- There is a Ca^{2+} deregulation on aging and Alzheimer's disease.
- Intracellular Ca^{2+} concentration affects learning and memory mechanisms.
- Resting Ca^{2+} concentration is increased in Alzheimer's disease.
- Ca^{2+} signaling is altered in Alzheimer's disease.
- The L-type Ca^{2+} channel is one of the main player in Alzheimer's disease.
- L-type Ca^{2+} channel blocker is effective in stabilized the AD cognitive decline.

CONSENT FOR PUBLICATION

Not applicable.

CONFLICT OF INTERESTS

The authors declare no conflict of interests.

ACKNOWLEDGEMENT

This work was supported by FAPESP – São Paulo Research Foundation grants: 2012/50336-2 and 2016/50484-2 to FAO.

REFERENCES

[1]   Südhof TC. Calcium control of neurotransmitter release. Cold Spring Harb Perspect Biol 2012; 4(1): a011353-3.
[http://dx.doi.org/10.1101/cshperspect.a011353] [PMID: 22068972]

[2]   Berridge MJ, Bootman MD, Roderick HL. Calcium signalling: dynamics, homeostasis and remodelling. Nat Rev Mol Cell Biol 2003; 4(7): 517-29.
[http://dx.doi.org/10.1038/nrm1155] [PMID: 12838335]

[3]   Neher E, Sakaba T. Multiple roles of calcium ions in the regulation of neurotransmitter release. Neuron 2008; 59(6): 861-72.
[http://dx.doi.org/10.1016/j.neuron.2008.08.019] [PMID: 18817727]

[4]   Augusto Oliveira F, Silveira PE, Lopes MJ, Kushmerick C, Naves LA. Angiotensin II increases evoked release at the frog neuromuscular junction through a receptor sensitive to A779. Brain Res 2007; 1175: 48-53.

[http://dx.doi.org/10.1016/j.brainres.2007.06.013] [PMID: 17888412]

[5]   Lohmann C, Wong ROL. Regulation of dendritic growth and plasticity by local and global calcium dynamics. Cell Calcium 2005; 37(5): 403-9.
        [http://dx.doi.org/10.1016/j.ceca.2005.01.008] [PMID: 15820387]

[6]   Higley MJ, Sabatini BL. Calcium signaling in dendrites and spines: practical and functional considerations. Neuron 2008; 59(6): 902-13.
        [http://dx.doi.org/10.1016/j.neuron.2008.08.020] [PMID: 18817730]

[7]   Lyons MR, West AE. Mechanisms of specificity in neuronal activity-regulated gene transcription. Prog Neurobiol 2011; 94(3): 259-95.
        [http://dx.doi.org/10.1016/j.pneurobio.2011.05.003] [PMID: 21620929]

[8]   Südhof TC. The synaptic vesicle cycle. Annu Rev Neurosci 2004; 27: 509-47.
        [http://dx.doi.org/10.1146/annurev.neuro.26.041002.131412] [PMID: 15217342]

[9]   Michaelsen K, Lohmann C. Calcium dynamics at developing synapses: mechanisms and functions. Eur J Neurosci 2010; 32(2): 218-23.
        [http://dx.doi.org/10.1111/j.1460-9568.2010.07341.x] [PMID: 20646046]

[10]   Egelman DM, Montague PR. Calcium dynamics in the extracellular space of mammalian neural tissue. Biophys J 1999; 76(4): 1856-67.
        [http://dx.doi.org/10.1016/S0006-3495(99)77345-5] [PMID: 10096884]

[11]   Helmchen F, Tank DW. A single-compartment model of calcium dynamics in nerve terminals and dendrites. Cold Spring Harb Protoc 2015; 2015
        [http://dx.doi.org/10.1101/pdb.top085910]

[12]   Maravall M, Mainen ZF, Sabatini BL, Svoboda K. Estimating intracellular calcium concentrations and buffering without wavelength ratioing. Biophys J 2000; 78(5): 2655-67.
        [http://dx.doi.org/10.1016/S0006-3495(00)76809-3] [PMID: 10777761]

[13]   Berridge MJ, Lipp P, Bootman MD. The versatility and universality of calcium signalling. Nat Rev Mol Cell Biol 2000; 1(1): 11-21.
        [http://dx.doi.org/10.1038/35036035] [PMID: 11413485]

[14]   Matthews EA, Dietrich D. Buffer mobility and the regulation of neuronal calcium domains. Front Cell Neurosci 2015; 9: 48.
        [http://dx.doi.org/10.3389/fncel.2015.00048] [PMID: 25750615]

[15]   Oh MM, Oliveira FA, Waters J, Disterhoft JF. Altered calcium metabolism in aging CA1 hippocampal pyramidal neurons. J Neurosci 2013; 33(18): 7905-11.
        [http://dx.doi.org/10.1523/JNEUROSCI.5457-12.2013] [PMID: 23637181]

[16]   Anwar H, Hong S, De Schutter E. Controlling Ca^{2+}-activated K+ channels with models of Ca^{2+} buffering in Purkinje cells. Cerebellum 2012; 11(3): 681-93.
        [http://dx.doi.org/10.1007/s12311-010-0224-3] [PMID: 20981513]

[17]   Petersen OH. The effects of Ca^{2+} buffers on cytosolic Ca^{2+} signalling. J Physiol 2017; 595(10): 3107-8.
        [http://dx.doi.org/10.1113/JP273852] [PMID: 28058721]

[18]   Schwaller B. The use of transgenic mouse models to reveal the functions of Ca^{2+} buffer proteins in excitable cells. Biochim Biophys Acta 2012; 1820(8): 1294-303.
        [http://dx.doi.org/10.1016/j.bbagen.2011.11.008] [PMID: 22138448]

[19]   Saftenku EÈ. Models of calcium dynamics in cerebellar granule cells. Cerebellum 2012; 11(1): 85--.
        [http://dx.doi.org/10.1007/s12311-010-0216-3] [PMID: 20922512]

[20]   Augustine GJ, Neher E. Neuronal Ca^{2+} signalling takes the local route. Curr Opin Neurobiol 1992; 2(3): 302-7.
        [http://dx.doi.org/10.1016/0959-4388(92)90119-6] [PMID: 1643411]

[21]   Neher E. Usefulness and limitations of linear approximations to the understanding of Ca++ signals.

Cell Calcium 1998; 24(5-6): 345-57.
[http://dx.doi.org/10.1016/S0143-4160(98)90058-6] [PMID: 10091004]

[22]   Faas GC, Raghavachari S, Lisman JE, Mody I. Calmodulin as a direct detector of Ca²⁺ signals. Nat Neurosci 2011; 14(3): 301-4.
[http://dx.doi.org/10.1038/nn.2746] [PMID: 21258328]

[23]   Khachaturian ZS. Scientific challenges and opportunities related to Alzheimer's disease. Clin Pharm 1984; 3(5): 522-3.
[PMID: 6149032]

[24]   Khachaturian ZS. Hypothesis on the regulation of cytosol calcium concentration and the aging brain. Neurobiol Aging 1987; 8(4): 345-6.
[http://dx.doi.org/10.1016/0197-4580(87)90073-X] [PMID: 3627349]

[25]   Gibson GE, Peterson C. Calcium and the aging nervous system. Neurobiol Aging 1987; 8(4): 329-43.
[http://dx.doi.org/10.1016/0197-4580(87)90072-8] [PMID: 3306433]

[26]   Landfield PW, Morgan GA. Chronically elevating plasma Mg2+ improves hippocampal frequency potentiation and reversal learning in aged and young rats. Brain Res 1984; 322(1): 167-71.
[http://dx.doi.org/10.1016/0006-8993(84)91199-5] [PMID: 6097334]

[27]   Landfield PW. 'Increased calcium-current' hypothesis of brain aging. Neurobiol Aging 1987; 8(4): 346-7.
[http://dx.doi.org/10.1016/0197-4580(87)90074-1] [PMID: 3627350]

[28]   McKay BM, Matthews EA, Oliveira FA, Disterhoft JF. Intrinsic neuronal excitability is reversibly altered by a single experience in fear conditioning. J Neurophysiol 2009; 102(5): 2763-70.
[http://dx.doi.org/10.1152/jn.00347.2009] [PMID: 19726729]

[29]   Disterhoft JF, Wu WW, Ohno M. Biophysical alterations of hippocampal pyramidal neurons in learning, ageing and Alzheimer's disease. Ageing Res Rev 2004; 3(4): 383-406.
[http://dx.doi.org/10.1016/j.arr.2004.07.001] [PMID: 15541708]

[30]   Oh MM, Oliveira FA, Disterhoft JF. Learning and aging related changes in intrinsic neuronal excitability. Front Aging Neurosci 2010; 2: 2.
[http://dx.doi.org/10.3389/neuro.24.002.2010] [PMID: 20552042]

[31]   Landfield P, Pitler T. Prolonged Ca²⁺-dependent afterhyperpolarizations in hippocampal neurons of aged rats. Science (80-) 1984; 226: 1089-92.

[32]   Cruz JS, Kushmerick C, Moreira-Lobo DC, Oliveira FA. Thiamine deficiency *in vitro* accelerates A-type potassium current inactivation in cerebellar granule neurons. Neuroscience 2012; 221: 108-14.
[http://dx.doi.org/10.1016/j.neuroscience.2012.06.053] [PMID: 22771620]

[33]   Disterhoft JF, Moyer JR Jr, Thompson LT. The calcium rationale in aging and Alzheimer's disease. Evidence from an animal model of normal aging. Ann N Y Acad Sci 1994; 747: 382-406.
[http://dx.doi.org/10.1111/j.1749-6632.1994.tb44424.x] [PMID: 7847686]

[34]   Landfield PW, Thibault O, Mazzanti ML, Porter NM, Kerr DS. Mechanisms of neuronal death in brain aging and Alzheimer's disease: role of endocrine-mediated calcium dyshomeostasis. J Neurobiol 1992; 23(9): 1247-60.
[http://dx.doi.org/10.1002/neu.480230914] [PMID: 1469387]

[35]   Mattson MP, Chan SL. Neuronal and glial calcium signaling in Alzheimer's disease. Cell Calcium 2003; 34(4-5): 385-97.
[http://dx.doi.org/10.1016/S0143-4160(03)00128-3] [PMID: 12909083]

[36]   Bezprozvanny I, Mattson MP. Neuronal calcium mishandling and the pathogenesis of Alzheimer's disease. Trends Neurosci 2008; 31(9): 454-63.
[http://dx.doi.org/10.1016/j.tins.2008.06.005] [PMID: 18675468]

[37]   Thibault O, Gant JC, Landfield PW. Expansion of the calcium hypothesis of brain aging and

Alzheimer's disease: minding the store. Aging Cell 2007; 6(3): 307-17.
[http://dx.doi.org/10.1111/j.1474-9726.2007.00295.x] [PMID: 17465978]

[38]   Wang Y, Mattson MP. L-type Ca^{2+} currents at CA1 synapses, but not CA3 or dentate granule neuron
        synapses, are increased in 3xTgAD mice in an age-dependent manner. Neurobiol Aging 2014; 35(1):
        88-95.
        [http://dx.doi.org/10.1016/j.neurobiolaging.2013.07.007] [PMID: 23932880]

[39]   Campbell LW, Hao S-YY, Thibault O, Blalock EM, Landfield PW. Aging changes in voltage-gated
        calcium currents in hippocampal CA1 neurons. J Neurosci 1996; 16(19): 6286-95.
        [http://dx.doi.org/10.1523/JNEUROSCI.16-19-06286.1996] [PMID: 8815908]

[40]   Moyer JR Jr, Thompson LT, Black JP, Disterhoft JF. Nimodipine increases excitability of rabbit CA1
        pyramidal neurons in an age- and concentration-dependent manner. J Neurophysiol 1992; 68(6): 2100-
        9.
        [http://dx.doi.org/10.1152/jn.1992.68.6.2100] [PMID: 1491260]

[41]   Thibault O, Landfield PW. Increase in single L-Type calcium channels in hippocampal neurons during
        aging. Science (80-) 1996; 272: 1017-20.

[42]   Deyo RA, Straube KT, Moyer JR Jr, Disterhoft JF. Nimodipine ameliorates aging-related changes in
        open-field behaviors of the rabbit. Exp Aging Res 1989; 15(3-4): 169-75.
        [http://dx.doi.org/10.1080/03610738908259771] [PMID: 2638635]

[43]   Forette F, Seux ML, Staessen JA, *et al.* The prevention of dementia with antihypertensive treatment:
        new evidence from the Systolic Hypertension in Europe (Syst-Eur) study. Arch Intern Med 2002; 162
        (18): 2046-52.
        [http://dx.doi.org/10.1001/archinte.162.18.2046] [PMID: 12374512]

[44]   Kaczorowski CC, Sametsky E, Shah S, Vassar R, Disterhoft JF. Mechanisms underlying basal and
        learning-related intrinsic excitability in a mouse model of Alzheimer's disease. Neurobiol Aging 2011;
        32(8): 1452-65.
        [http://dx.doi.org/10.1016/j.neurobiolaging.2009.09.003] [PMID: 19833411]

[45]   Lopez JR, Lyckman A, Oddo S, Laferla FM, Querfurth HW, Shtifman A. Increased intraneuronal
        resting [Ca^{2+}] in adult Alzheimer's disease mice. J Neurochem 2008; 105(1): 262-71.
        [http://dx.doi.org/10.1111/j.1471-4159.2007.05135.x] [PMID: 18021291]

[46]   Arbel-Ornath M, Hudry E, Boivin JR, *et al.* Soluble oligomeric amyloid-β induces calcium
        dyshomeostasis that precedes synapse loss in the living mouse brain. Mol Neurodegener 2017; 12(1):
        27.
        [http://dx.doi.org/10.1186/s13024-017-0169-9] [PMID: 28327181]

[47]   Ferreiro E, Oliveira CR, Pereira C. Involvement of endoplasmic reticulum Ca^{2+} release through
        ryanodine and inositol 1,4,5-triphosphate receptors in the neurotoxic effects induced by the amyloid-
        beta peptide. J Neurosci Res 2004; 76(6): 872-80.
        [http://dx.doi.org/10.1002/jnr.20135] [PMID: 15160398]

[48]   Berrocal M, Corbacho I, Vázquez-Hernández M, Ávila J, Sepúlveda MR, Mata AM. Inhibition of
        PMCA activity by tau as a function of aging and Alzheimer's neuropathology. Biochim Biophys Acta
        - Mol Basis Dis 2015; 1852: 1465-76.

[49]   Berrocal M, Sepulveda MR, Vazquez-Hernandez M, Mata AM. Calmodulin antagonizes amyloid-β
        peptides-mediated inhibition of brain plasma membrane Ca^{2+}-ATPase. Biochim Biophys Acta - Mol
        Basis Dis 2012; 1822: 961-.

[50]   Green KN, Demuro A, Akbari Y, *et al.* SERCA pump activity is physiologically regulated by
        presenilin and regulates amyloid β production. J Cell Biol 2008; 181(7): 1107-16.
        [http://dx.doi.org/10.1083/jcb.200706171] [PMID: 18591429]

[51]   Berrocal M, Marcos D, Sepúlveda MR, Pérez M, Avila J, Mata AM. Altered Ca^{2+} dependence of
        synaptosomal plasma membrane Ca^{2+}-ATPase in human brain affected by Alzheimer's disease.

FASEB J 2009; 23(6): 1826-34.
[http://dx.doi.org/10.1096/fj.08-121459] [PMID: 19144698]

[52]   Stutzmann GE, Smith I, Caccamo A, Oddo S, Laferla FM, Parker I. Enhanced ryanodine receptor recruitment contributes to Ca²⁺ disruptions in young, adult, and aged Alzheimer's disease mice. J Neurosci 2006; 26(19): 5180-9.
[http://dx.doi.org/10.1523/JNEUROSCI.0739-06.2006] [PMID: 16687509]

[53]   Stutzmann GE, Smith I, Caccamo A, Oddo S, Parker I, Laferla F. Enhanced ryanodine-mediated calcium release in mutant PS1-expressing Alzheimer's mouse models. Ann N Y Acad Sci 2007; 1097: 265-77.
[http://dx.doi.org/10.1196/annals.1379.025] [PMID: 17413028]

[54]   Oulès B, Del Prete D, Greco B, *et al*. Ryanodine receptor blockade reduces amyloid-β load and memory impairments in Tg2576 mouse model of Alzheimer disease. J Neurosci 2012; 32(34): 11820-34.
[http://dx.doi.org/10.1523/JNEUROSCI.0875-12.2012] [PMID: 22915123]

[55]   Chakroborty S, Briggs C, Miller MB, *et al*. Stabilizing ER Ca²⁺ channel function as an early preventative strategy for Alzheimer's disease. PLoS One 2012; 7(12): e52056.
[http://dx.doi.org/10.1371/journal.pone.0052056] [PMID: 23284867]

[56]   Del Prete D, Checler F, Chami M. Ryanodine receptors: physiological function and deregulation in Alzheimer disease. Mol Neurodegener 2014; 9: 21.
[http://dx.doi.org/10.1186/1750-1326-9-21] [PMID: 24902695]

[57]   Riascos D, de Leon D, Baker-Nigh A, *et al*. Age-related loss of calcium buffering and selective neuronal vulnerability in Alzheimer's disease. Acta Neuropathol 2011; 122(5): 565-76.
[http://dx.doi.org/10.1007/s00401-011-0865-4] [PMID: 21874328]

[58]   Schnurra I, Bernstein H-G, Riederer P, Braunewell K-H. The neuronal calcium sensor protein VILIP-1 is associated with amyloid plaques and extracellular tangles in Alzheimer's disease and promotes cell death and tau phosphorylation *in vitro*: a link between calcium sensors and Alzheimer's disease? Neurobiol Dis 2001; 8(5): 900-9.
[http://dx.doi.org/10.1006/nbdi.2001.0432] [PMID: 11592857]

[59]   Begley JG, Duan W, Chan S, Duff K, Mattson MP. Altered calcium homeostasis and mitochondrial dysfunction in cortical synaptic compartments of presenilin-1 mutant mice. J Neurochem 1999; 72(3): 1030-9.
[http://dx.doi.org/10.1046/j.1471-4159.1999.0721030.x] [PMID: 10037474]

[60]   Lally G, Faull RLM, Waldvogel HJ, Ferrari S, Emson PC. Calcium homeostasis in ageing: studies on the calcium binding protein calbindin D28K. J Neural Transm (Vienna) 1997; 104(10): 1107-12.
[http://dx.doi.org/10.1007/BF01273323] [PMID: 9503262]

[61]   Yamamoto S, Wajima T, Hara Y, Nishida M, Mori Y. Transient receptor potential channels in Alzheimer's disease. Biochim Biophys Acta - Mol Basis Dis 2007; 1772: 958-67.

[62]   Whitehead G, Regan P, Whitcomb DJ, Cho K. Ca²⁺-permeable AMPA receptor: A new perspective on amyloid-beta mediated pathophysiology of Alzheimer's disease. Neuropharmacology 2017; 112(Pt A): 221-7.
[http://dx.doi.org/10.1016/j.neuropharm.2016.08.022] [PMID: 27561971]

[63]   Zhang Y, Li P, Feng J, Wu M. Dysfunction of NMDA receptors in Alzheimer's disease. Neurol Sci 2016; 37(7): 1039-47.
[http://dx.doi.org/10.1007/s10072-016-2546-5] [PMID: 26971324]

[64]   Pchitskaya E, Popugaeva E, Bezprozvanny I. Calcium signaling and molecular mechanisms underlying neurodegenerative diseases. Cell Calcium 2017; 4-11.
[http://dx.doi.org/10.1016/j.ceca.2017.06.008] [PMID: 28728834]

[65]   Popugaeva E, Pchitskaya E, Bezprozvanny I. Dysregulation of neuronal calcium homeostasis in

Alzheimer's disease - A therapeutic opportunity? Biochem Biophys Res Commun 2017; 483(4): 998-1004.
[http://dx.doi.org/10.1016/j.bbrc.2016.09.053] [PMID: 27641664]

[66]   Ban TA, Morey L, Aguglia E, *et al.* Nimodipine in the treatment of old age dementias. Prog Neuropsychopharmacol Biol Psychiatry 1990; 14(4): 525-51.
[http://dx.doi.org/10.1016/0278-5846(90)90005-2] [PMID: 2236581]

[67]   Tollefson GD. Short-term effects of the calcium channel blocker nimodipine (Bay-e-9736) in the management of primary degenerative dementia. Biol Psychiatry 1990; 27(10): 1133-42.
[http://dx.doi.org/10.1016/0006-3223(90)90050-C] [PMID: 2187540]

[68]   Jarvik LF. Calcium channel blocker nimodipine for primary degenerative dementia. Biol Psychiatry 1991; 30(11): 1171-2.
[http://dx.doi.org/10.1016/0006-3223(91)90186-P] [PMID: 1777531]

[69]   Meulenbroek O, O'Dwyer S, de Jong D, *et al.* European multicentre double-blind placebo-controlled trial of Nilvadipine in mild-to-moderate Alzheimer's disease-the substudy protocols: NILVAD frailty; NILVAD blood and genetic biomarkers; NILVAD cerebrospinal fluid biomarkers; NILVAD cerebral blood flow. BMJ Open 2016; 6(7): e011584.
[http://dx.doi.org/10.1136/bmjopen-2016-011584] [PMID: 27436668]

[70]   Hwang D, Kim S, Choi H, *et al.* Calcium-Channel Blockers and Dementia Risk in Older Adults - National Health Insurance Service - Senior Cohort (2002-2013). Circ J 2016; 80(11): 2336-42.
[http://dx.doi.org/10.1253/circj.CJ-16-0692] [PMID: 27666598]

[71]   Forette F, Seux M-L, Staessen JA, *et al.* Prevention of dementia in randomised double-blind placebo-controlled Systolic Hypertension in Europe (Syst-Eur) trial. Lancet 1998; 352(9137): 1347-51.
[http://dx.doi.org/10.1016/S0140-6736(98)03086-4] [PMID: 9802273]

[72]   Hanon O, Forette F. Prevention of dementia: lessons from SYST-EUR and PROGRESS. J Neurol Sci 2004; 226: 71-4.
[http://dx.doi.org/10.1016/j.jns.2004.09.015] [PMID: 15537524]

[73]   Hanyu H, Hirao K, Shimizu S, Sato T, Kiuchi A, Iwamoto T. Nilvadipine prevents cognitive decline of patients with mild cognitive impairment. Int J Geriatr Psychiatry 2007; 22: 1264-6.
[http://dx.doi.org/10.1002/gps.1851] [PMID: 18033677]

[74]   Hanyu H. Favourable effects of nilvadipine on cognitive function and regional cerebral blood flow on SPECT in hypertensive patients with mild cognitive impairment. Nucl Med Commun 2007; 28: 281-7.
[http://dx.doi.org/10.1097/MNM.0b013e32804c58aa] [PMID: 17325591]

[75]   Uchida S, Yamada S, Nagai K, Deguchi Y, Kimura R.. Brain pharmacokinetics and *in vivo* receptor binding of 1,4-dihydropyridine calcium channel antagonists. Life Sci 1997; 61: 2083-90.
[http://dx.doi.org/10.1016/S0024-3205(97)00881-3] [PMID: 9395249]

[76]   Paris D, Bachmeier C, Patel N, *et al.* Selective antihypertensive dihydropyridines lower Aβ accumulation by targeting both the production and the clearance of Aβ across the blood-brain barrier. Mol Med 2011; 17: 149-62.
[http://dx.doi.org/10.2119/molmed.2010.00180] [PMID: 21170472]

[77]   Lawlor B, Kennelly S, O'Dwyer S, *et al.* NILVAD protocol: a European multicentre double-blind placebo-controlled trial of nilvadipine in mild-to-moderate Alzheimer's disease. BMJ Open 2014; 4(10): e006364.
[http://dx.doi.org/10.1136/bmjopen-2014-006364] [PMID: 25300460]

[78]   Kennelly S, Abdullah L, Kenny RA, Mathura V, Luis CA, Mouzon B, *et al.* Apolipoprotein E genotype-specific short-term cognitive benefits of treatment with the antihypertensive nilvadipine in Alzheimer's patients-an open-label trial. Int J Geriatr Psychiatry 2011; 27

[79]   van der Flier WM, Skoog I, Schneider JA, *et al.* Vascular cognitive impairment. Nat Rev Dis Primers 2018; 4: 18003.

[http://dx.doi.org/10.1038/nrdp.2018.3] [PMID: 29446769]

[80]   Iadecola C, Yaffe K, Biller J, *et al.* American Heart Association Council on Hypertension; Council on Clinical Cardiology; Council on Cardiovascular Disease in the Young; Council on Cardiovascular and Stroke Nursing; Council on Quality of Care and Outcomes Research; and Stroke Council. Impact of Hypertension on Cognitive Function: A Scientific Statement From the American Heart Association. Hypertension 2016; 68(6): e67-94.
[http://dx.doi.org/10.1161/HYP.0000000000000053] [PMID: 27977393]

[81]   Nagai M, Dote K, Kato M, *et al.* Visit-to-Visit Blood Pressure Variability and Alzheimer's Disease: Links and Risks. J Alzheimers Dis 2017; 59(2): 515-26.
[http://dx.doi.org/10.3233/JAD-161172] [PMID: 28598842]

[82]   Murray MD, Lane KA, Gao S, *et al.* Preservation of cognitive function with antihypertensive medications: a longitudinal analysis of a community-based sample of African Americans. Arch Intern Med 2002; 162(18): 2090-6.
[http://dx.doi.org/10.1001/archinte.162.18.2090] [PMID: 12374517]

[83]   Nimmrich V, Eckert A.. Calcium channel blockers and dementia. Br J Pharmacol 2013; 169: 1203-10.
[http://dx.doi.org/10.1111/bph.12240]

SUBJECT INDEX

www.ingramcontent.com/pod-product-compliance
Lightning Source LLC
Chambersburg PA
CBHW050832220326
41598CB00006B/356